Imaging in Tuberculosis
Clinicopathological Correlation

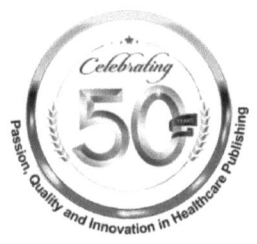

Imaging in Tuberculosis
Clinicopathological Correlation

Editors

Rakesh K Gupta MD
Director and Head
Department of Radiology
Fortis Memorial Research Institute
Gurugram, Haryana, India

Raju Sharma MD MAMS FICR
Professor
Department of Radiology
All India Institute of Medical Sciences
New Delhi, India

Foreword

Vishwa M Katoch

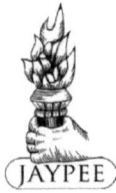

JAYPEE BROTHERS MEDICAL PUBLISHERS
The Health Sciences Publisher
New Delhi | London | Panama

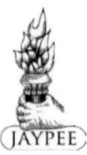
Jaypee Brothers Medical Publishers (P) Ltd

Headquarters
Jaypee Brothers Medical Publishers (P) Ltd
4838/24, Ansari Road, Daryaganj
New Delhi 110 002, India
Phone: +91-11-43574357
Fax: +91-11-43574314
Email: jaypee@jaypeebrothers.com

Overseas Offices

J.P. Medical Ltd	Jaypee-Highlights Medical Publishers Inc	Jaypee Brothers Medical Publishers (P) Ltd
83 Victoria Street, London	City of Knowledge, Bld. 235, 2nd Floor, Clayton	Bhotahity, Kathmandu, Nepal
SW1H 0HW (UK)	Panama City, Panama	Phone: +977-9741283608
Phone: +44 20 3170 8910	Phone: +1 507-301-0496	Email: kathmandu@jaypeebrothers.com
Fax: +44 (0)20 3008 6180	Fax: +1 507-301-0499	
Email: info@jpmedpub.com	Email: cservice@jphmedical.com	

Website: www.jaypeebrothers.com
Website: www.jaypeedigital.com

© 2019, Jaypee Brothers Medical Publishers

The views and opinions expressed in this book are solely those of the original contributor(s)/author(s) and do not necessarily represent those of editor(s) of the book.

All rights reserved. No part of this publication may be reproduced, stored or transmitted in any form or by any means, electronic, mechanical, photocopying, recording or otherwise, without the prior permission in writing of the publishers.

All brand names and product names used in this book are trade names, service marks, trademarks or registered trademarks of their respective owners. The publisher is not associated with any product or vendor mentioned in this book.

Medical knowledge and practice change constantly. This book is designed to provide accurate, authoritative information about the subject matter in question. However, readers are advised to check the most current information available on procedures included and check information from the manufacturer of each product to be administered, to verify the recommended dose, formula, method and duration of administration, adverse effects and contraindications. It is the responsibility of the practitioner to take all appropriate safety precautions. Neither the publisher nor the author(s)/editor(s) assume any liability for any injury and/or damage to persons or property arising from or related to use of material in this book.

This book is sold on the understanding that the publisher is not engaged in providing professional medical services. If such advice or services are required, the services of a competent medical professional should be sought.

Every effort has been made where necessary to contact holders of copyright to obtain permission to reproduce copyright material. If any have been inadvertently overlooked, the publisher will be pleased to make the necessary arrangements at the first opportunity. The **CD/DVD-ROM** (if any) provided in the sealed envelope with this book is complimentary and free of cost. **Not meant for sale.**

Inquiries for bulk sales may be solicited at: jaypee@jaypeebrothers.com

Imaging in Tuberculosis: Clinicopathological Correlation / Rakesh K Gupta, Raju Sharma

> Cover images: (*Top left*) Axial contrast enhanced CT of the abdomen showing ascites and a 'sliced bread' appearance of the mesentery. Aspirated fluid showed low serum ascites albumin gradient with lymphocytosis and elevated levels of adenosine deaminase. Diagnosis: Peritoneal tuberculosis; (*Top right*) T2 weighted sagittal image of the cervical spine showing collapse of C4 vertebra with a prevertebral and extradural intraspinal collection suggestive of abscess. Diagnosis: Tubercular spondylodiscitis; (*Bottom left*) STIR coronal (fat suppressed) MR image of the wrist showing hyperintensity in the carpals, and lower end of radius and ulna, erosions in the scaphoid, synovial thickening and joint effusion. Diagnosis: Osteoarticular tuberculosis; (*Bottom right*) Ziehl-Neelsen staining: Multiple acid-fast bacilli identified singly and in clusters within the necrotic debris (1,000x).

First Edition: **2019**

ISBN: 978-93-88958-97-4

Printed at

CONTRIBUTORS

EDITORS

Rakesh K Gupta MD
Director and Head
Department of Radiology
Fortis Memorial Research Institute
Gurugram, Haryana, India

Raju Sharma MD MAMS FICR
Professor
Department of Radiology
All India Institute of Medical Sciences
New Delhi, India

CONTRIBUTING AUTHORS

Abhishek Behera MD
Senior Resident
Department of Nuclear Medicine
All India Institute of Medical Sciences
New Delhi, India

Ajoy K Verma MD
Specialist, Department of Microbiology
National Institute of Tuberculosis and
Respiratory Diseases
New Delhi, India

Ankur Goyal MD DNB MNAMS FICR
Assistant Professor
Department of Radiodiagnosis
All India Institute of Medical Sciences
New Delhi, India

Arun K Gupta MD FAMS
Professor and Head
Department of Radiodiagnosis
All India Institute of Medical Sciences
New Delhi, India

Ashok Srinivasan MD DABR
Associate Professor and Director Neuroradiology
University of Michigan Health System
Ann Arbor, USA

Ashesh Dhungana MD DM
Ex-Senior Resident
Department of Pulmonology and
Sleep Disorders
All India Institute of Medical Sciences
New Delhi, India

Ashu S Bhalla MD MAMS FICR
Professor
Department of Radiodiagnosis
All India Institute of Medical Sciences
New Delhi, India

Chandan J Das MD DNB FICR FRCP (Edin)
Associate Professor
Department of Radiodiagnosis
All India Institute of Medical Sciences
New Delhi, India

Chandra M Pandey PhD
Professor and Head
Department of Biostatistics
SGPGI MS
Lucknow, Uttar Pradesh, India

Chirag K Ahuja MD DM
Assistant Professor
Department of Radiodiagnosis
PGIMER
Chandigarh, India

Devasenathipathy Kandasamy MD DNB FRCR
Associate Professor
Department of Radiodiagnosis
All India Institute of Medical Sciences
New Delhi, India

GC Khilnani MD FCCP FICCM FICP MAMS
Ex-Professor and Head
Department of Pulmonology and
Sleep Disorders
All India Institute of Medical Sciences
New Delhi, India

Gurpreet S Gulati MD
Professor
Department of Cardiac Radiology
All India Institute of Medical Sciences
New Delhi, India

Jeffrey Hawk MD DABR
Ex-Fellow
Department of Radiology
University of Michigan Health System
Ann Arbor, USA

Jitender Saini MD DM
Additional Professor
Department of Neuroimaging and
Interventional Radiology
National Institute of Mental Health and
Neuroscience
Bengaluru, Karnataka, India

Karthik Rayasam MD
Ex-Senior Resident
Department of Radiology
PGIMER
Chandigarh, India

Krishan Chugh MD
Director and Head
Department of Pediatrics
Fortis Memorial Research Institute
Gurugram, Haryana, India

Krishan K Agarwal MD
Ex-Senior Resident
Department of Nuclear Medicine
All India Institute of Medical Sciences
New Delhi, India

Madhusudhan KS MD MAMS FICR
Associate Professor
Department of Radiodiagnosis
All India Institute of Medical Sciences
New Delhi, India

Mahesh Prakash MD
Professor
Department of Radiodiagnosis
PGIMER
Chandigarh, India

Manisha Jana MD DNB FRCR
Associate Professor
Department of Radiodiagnosis
All India Institute of Medical Sciences
New Delhi, India

Mudit Gupta MD
Radiologist
Saral Diagnostic Center
New Delhi, India

Munish Guleria MD
Assistant Professor
Department of Radiology
PGIMER and Dr RML Hospital
New Delhi, India

Naveen Kalra MD MAMS FICR
Professor
Department of Radiodiagnosis, PGIMER
Chandigarh, India

Neetu Talwar MD
Senior Consultant
Department of Pediatrics
Fortis Memorial Research Institute
Gurugram, Haryana, India

Contributors

Niranjan Khandelwal MD FAMS FICR
Ex-Professor and Head
Department of Radiodiagnosis
PGIMER
Chandigarh, India

Nuzhat Husain MD FICP IFCAP
Professor and Head
Department of Pathology
RML Institute of Medical Sciences
Lucknow, Uttar Pradesh, India

Raju P Dungeni MD DM
Ex-Senior Resident
Department of Pulmonology and
Sleep Disorders
All India Institute of Medical Sciences
New Delhi, India

Rakesh Kumar MD PhD FAMS
Professor
Department of Nuclear Medicine
All India Institute of Medical Sciences
New Delhi, India

Randeep Guleria MD DM FAMS
Director
Department of Pulmonology and
Sleep Disorders
All India Institute of Medical Sciences
New Delhi, India

Sanjeev Kumar MD
Assistant Professor
Department of Cardiac Radiology
All India Institute of Medical Sciences
New Delhi, India

Saumya Shukla MD
Assistant Professor
Department of Pathology
RML Institute of Medical Sciences
Lucknow, Uttar Pradesh, India

Shivanand Gamanagatti MD MAMS FICR
Professor
Department of Radiodiagnosis
All India Institute of Medical Sciences
New Delhi, India

FOREWORD

It is my privilege to write this foreword for the book titled *"Imaging in Tuberculosis: Clinicopathological Correlation"* edited by Professor Rakesh K Gupta and Professor Raju Sharma. This book has important contributions by several eminent experts from India and abroad on key issues relevant for diagnosis and treatment of tuberculosis in children as well as adults. Tuberculosis in humans involve almost all organs, has varying and many a times confusing presentations. Advances in pathology, microbiology, and molecular biology techniques, optics and robotics, as well as imaging technologies offer the opportunity to arrive at diagnosis of tuberculosis with high sensitivity and specificity. This book has chapters not only on important forms of tuberculosis (central nervous system, spine, head and neck, pulmonary, lymph node, abdominal, urogenital tract, bone and joints, and cardiovascular), but also addressed epidemiology/public health issues. There are other well-written chapters on clinical perspective, laboratory and molecular diagnosis, pathology relevant to radiologist, basics of antitubercular therapy, and multidrug-resistant tuberculosis. Lastly, chapters on whole body imaging in tuberculosis and positron emission tomography/computed tomography will be of immense interest to radiologists as well as clinicians interested in applying these advanced techniques to solve diagnostic dilemma in those forms of tuberculosis where the lesions may not be easy to access and differential diagnosis may be challenging to solve.

Considering the importance of the topics covered in a comprehensive manner, I am highly optimistic that this book will be of interest to a wide spectrum of users—medical students at undergraduate and postgraduate level, doctors ranging from general physicians, medical specialists, other specialists, surgeons, and super-specialists. On the whole, this will be useful to both medical professionals as well as technologists interested in using modern methods, especially imaging techniques, to reach at the diagnosis of tuberculosis with fair amount of certainty. I compliment the contributors as well as Professor Rakesh K Gupta and Professor Raju Sharma in bringing out this book. I expect that this book will be a popular resource on this subject in the coming years.

Vishwa M Katoch MD FNASc FASc FAMS FNA
NASI-ICMR Chair on Public Health Research
Rajasthan University of Health Sciences
Jaipur, Rajasthan, India

PREFACE

Tuberculosis is a common and challenging clinical problem with protean manifestations and can affect any organ system. The disease is endemic in India and can masquerade as a plethora of disease entities. Imaging plays a vital role in detection of the disease, in narrowing the differential diagnosis and provides subtle differentiating features because of the non-specific clinical presentation, radiologist may be the first to raise a suspicion of this disease.

This book focuses on the imaging manifestations of tuberculosis and leading experts from across the country have contributed to this effort. Pulmonary tuberculosis is well recognized, but its important to take cognizance of the fact that extrapulmonary tuberculosis accounts for one-fifth of all the cases and keeping that in mind the book includes chapters on all organ systems. The initial chapters also cover epidemiology, clinical features, pathology of this condition and the treatment and issues related to drug resistance. Recent advances in imaging with specific application in imaging a multisystem disease like whole body MR and PET-CT are also covered. An emerging application of imaging in this context is treatment response assessment as increasingly clinical improvement is not accepted as an end-point of therapy. This is also covered in the relevant sections of the book.

We hope this book will be useful to the students and practicing radiologists and internists. We will be happy to receive constructive criticism of this work from the readers to enhance its quality in the future!

Rakesh K Gupta
Raju Sharma

CONTENTS

1. **Epidemiology of Tuberculosis** — 1
   Chandra M Pandey

2. **Tuberculosis: Clinical Features** — 7
   Krishan Chugh, Neetu Talwar

3. **Laboratory and Molecular Diagnosis of Tuberculosis** — 17
   Ajoy K Verma

4. **Pathology Relevant to Radiologist** — 25
   Saumya Shukla, Nuzhat Husain

5. **Basics of Antitubercular Therapy** — 40
   Randeep Guleria, Ashesh Dhungana

6. **Multidrug-resistant Tuberculosis** — 46
   GC Khilnani, Raju P Dungeni

7. **Central Nervous System Tuberculosis** — 51
   Rakesh K Gupta, Mudit Gupta

8. **Spinal Tuberculosis** — 73
   Shivanand Gamanagatti, Jitender Saini

9. **Head and Neck Tuberculosis** — 86
   Jeffrey Hawk, Ashu S Bhalla, Ashok Srinivasan

10. **Imaging in Chest Tuberculosis** — 98
    Ashu S Bhalla, Ankur Goyal

11. **Lymph Node Tuberculosis** — 111
    Naveen Kalra, Chirag K Ahuja, Niranjan Khandelwal

12. **Imaging in Abdominal Tuberculosis** — 121
    Raju Sharma, Madhusudhan KS, Devasenathipathy Kandasamy

13. **Imaging in Urogenital Tuberculosis** — 145
    Chandan J Das, Ankur Goyal

14. **Tuberculosis of Bones and Joints** — 159
    Mahesh Prakash, Karthik Rayasam

15.	Cardiovascular Tuberculosis	176
	Munish Guleria, Sanjeev Kumar, Gurpreet S Gulati	
16.	Whole Body Imaging in Tuberculosis	197
	Mudit Gupta, Rakesh K Gupta	
17.	Tuberculosis in the Pediatric Patient	207
	Manisha Jana, Arun K Gupta	
18.	Positron Emission Tomography-Computed Tomography: Does It Have a Role in Tuberculosis?	226
	Rakesh Kumar, Krishan K Agarwal, Abhishek Behera	

Index — 239

PLATE 1

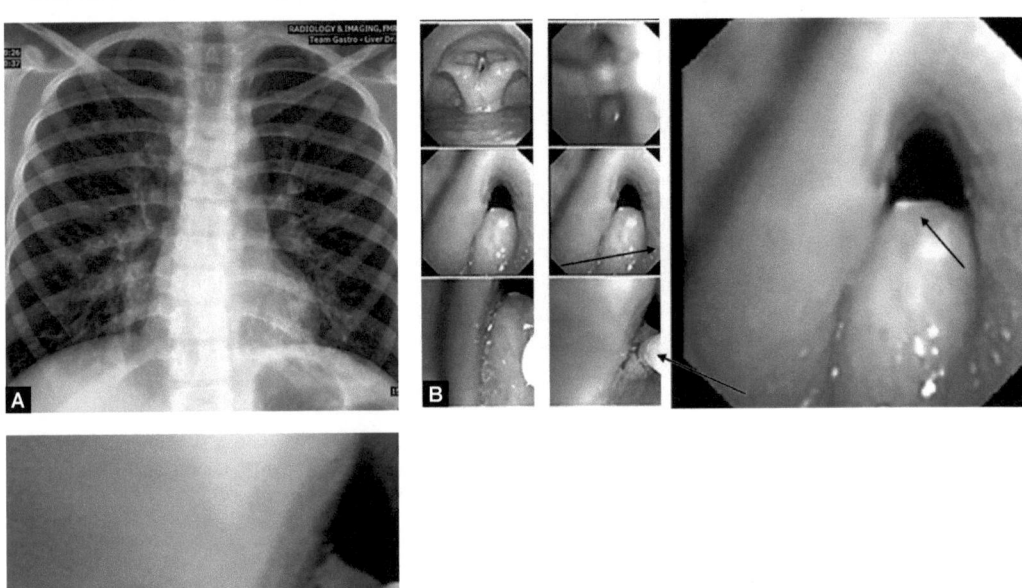

FIG. 1: A, A 10-year-old child diagnosed with human immunodeficiency virus with Kaposi's sarcoma with persistent fever, lethargy, and poor oral intake of 2 weeks duration; **B,** Flexible bronchoscopy revealed a mass at the entry of the left main bronchus with a yellow colored tip (caseating mass of lymph nodes); and **C,** Transbronchial needle aspiration of the mass was done *(Chapter 2)*

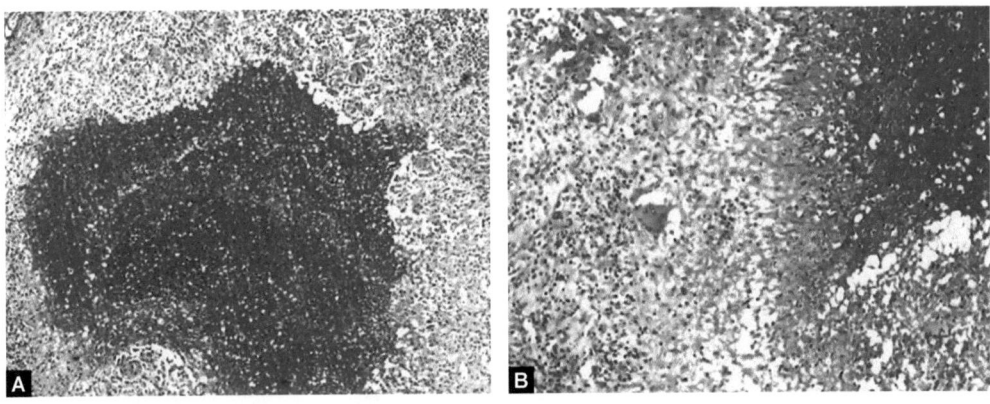

FIG. 1: Photomicrograph depicting the classical "soft granuloma" with central area of caseous necrosis surrounded by loose aggregates of epithelioid cells with Langhans type of giant cell and minimal lymphocytic cuffing (A = H&E 50x, B = H&E 100x) *(Chapter 4)*

PLATE 2

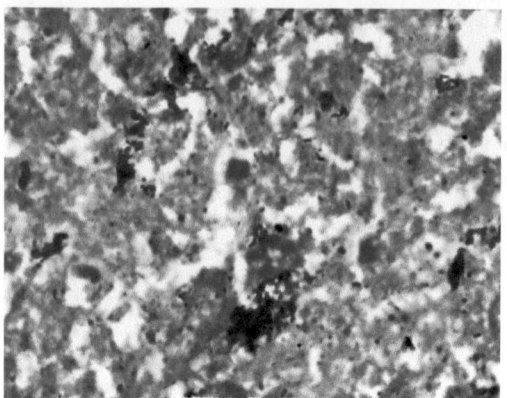

FIG. 2: Ziehl-Neelsen staining: Multiple acid-fast bacilli identified singly and in clusters within the necrotic debris (1,000x) *(Chapter 4)*

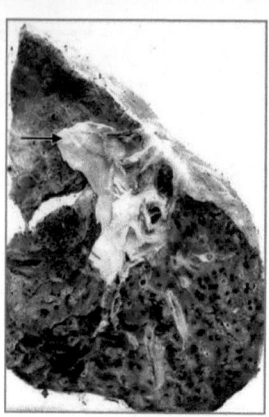

FIG. 4: Ghon's complex: Gross specimen of the lung with a minute parenchymal lesion and hilar lymphadenopathy (arrow) *(Chapter 4)*

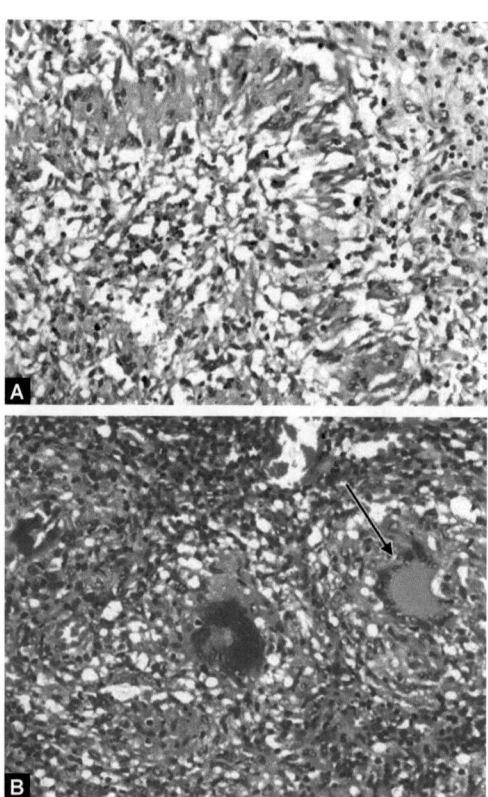

FIG. 3: A, The granuloma of tuberculosis with slipper-shaped epithelioid histiocytes; **B,** Multinucleated Langhans giant cell (arrow) having peripherally arranged nuclei with central clear cytoplasmic area (A = H&E 200x, B = H&E 200x) *(Chapter 4)*

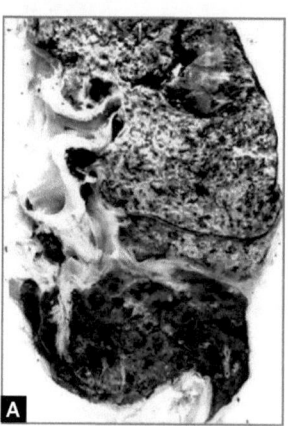

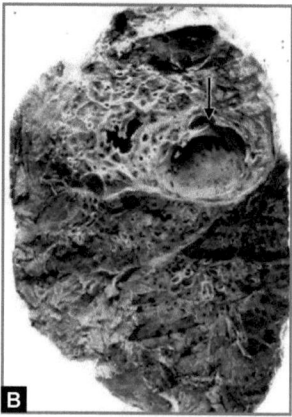

FIG. 5: Fibrocaseous tuberculosis: Gross specimen of the lung showing numerous yellow gray caseating nodules with a cavity (arrow) with an irregular wall and pleural thickening *(Chapter 4)*

PLATE 3

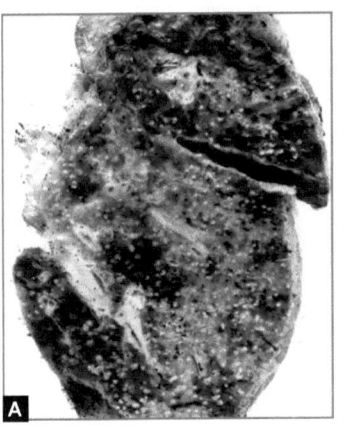 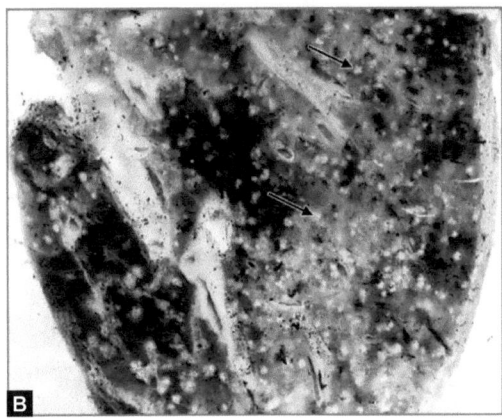

FIG. 6: Miliary tuberculosis: Gross specimen of the lung with numerous small, discrete yellow gray nodules involving the entire lung *(Chapter 4)*

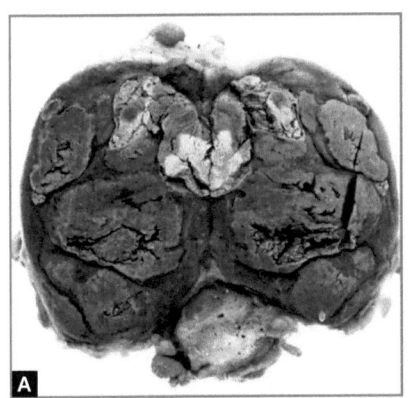 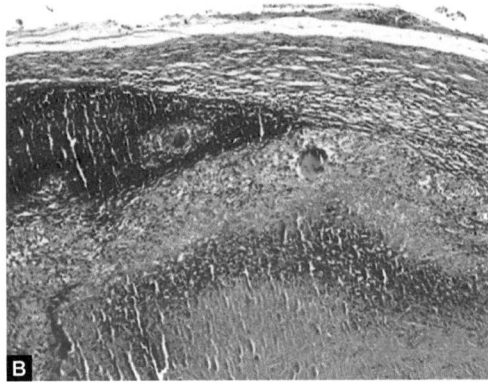

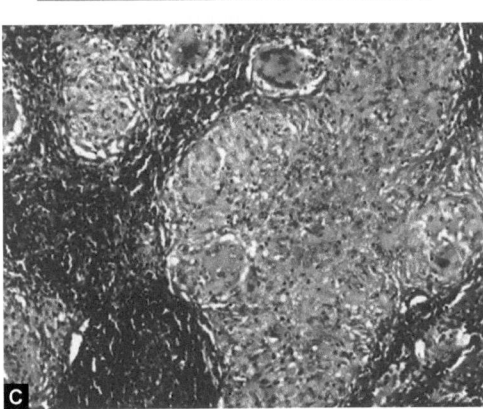

FIG. 7: Tubercular lymphadenitis. **A,** Gross specimen of a matted group of lymph nodes with caseation; **B and C,** Photomicrograph with partial effacement of nodal architecture by numerous epithelioid granulomas with central caseous necrosis and Langhans giant cell (B = H&E 50x, C = H&E 100x) *(Chapter 4)*

PLATE 4

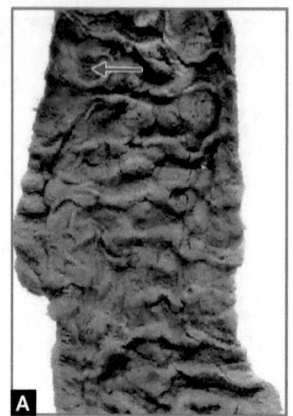
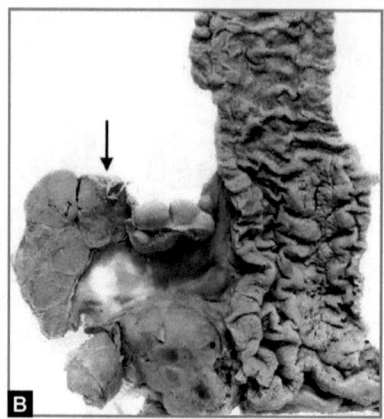

FIG. 8: Ileal tuberculosis with mesenteric lymphadenopathy: **A,** The cut open specimen of the ileum with numerous small ulcers with necrotic base (red arrow); **B,** matted group of enlarged mesenteric lymph nodes (black arrow) *(Chapter 4)*

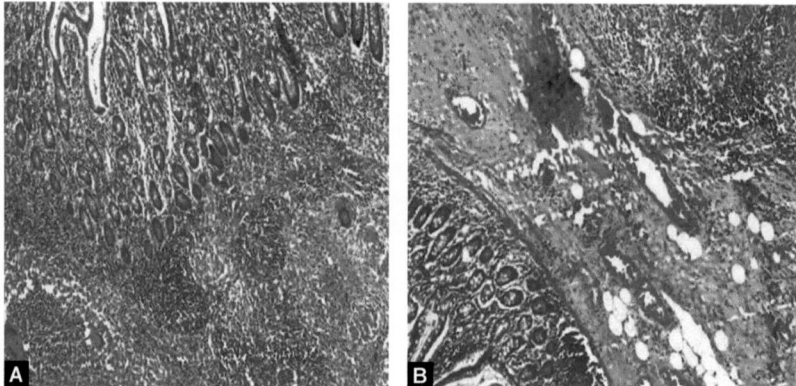

FIG. 9: Intestinal tuberculosis. Necrotizing granulomas in the mucosa and submucosa (A, B = H&E 50x) *(Chapter 4)*

PLATE 5

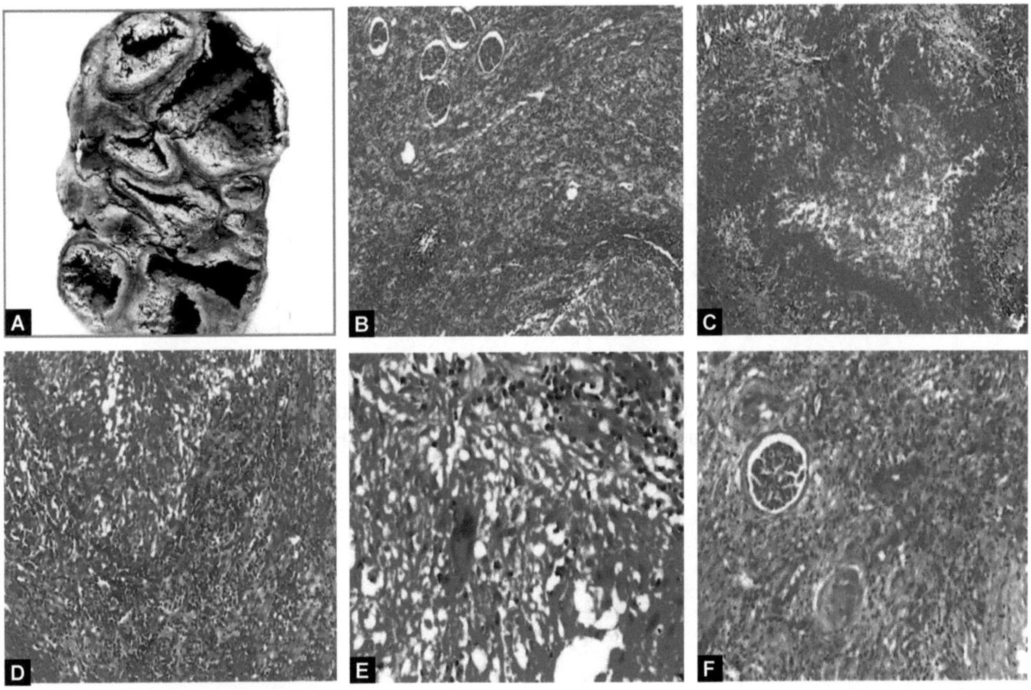

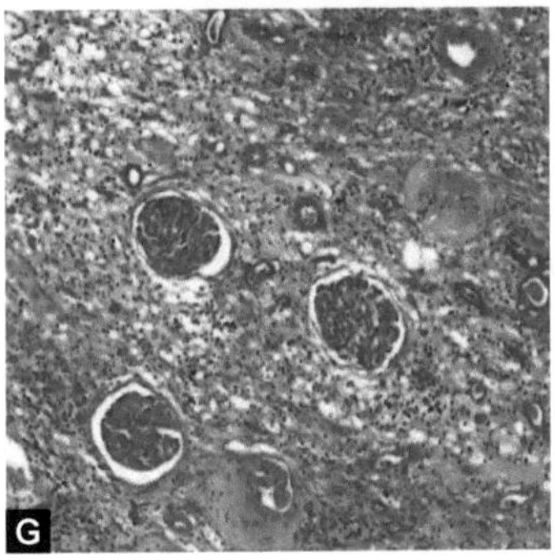

FIG. 10: **A,** Gross specimen of the kidney with hydronephrosis, cystic dilatation, atrophy and thinning of the renal cortex; **B to E**, Renal tuberculosis: Granulomatous inflammation with central caseous necrosis, interspersed Langhans giant cell, neutrophilic and lymphocytic infiltrate (B = H&E 50x; C, D = H&E 100x; E = H&E 200x). **F and G,** Photomicrograph showing secondary changes in renal parenchyma characterized by glomerular sclerosis and thyroidization of tubules (F,G = H&E 100x) *(Chapter 4)*

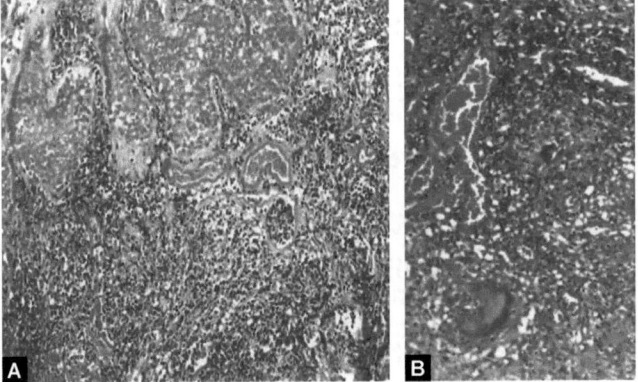

FIG. 11: Tuberculous orchitis: Tuberculous granulomatous inflammation involving the testis (A = H&E 100x, B = H&E 200x) *(Chapter 4)*

PLATE 6

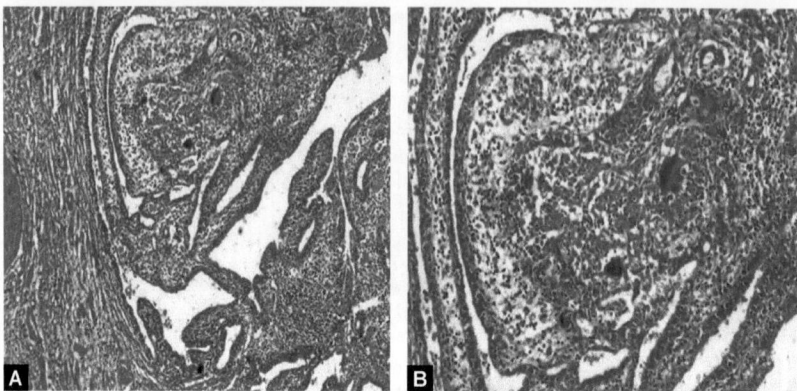

FIG. 12: Tuberculous salpingitis. Granulomatous inflammation with epithelioid granulomas, Langhans type giant cells along with lymphoplasmacytic and neutrophilic infiltrate (A = H&E 50x, B = H&E 100x) *(Chapter 4)*

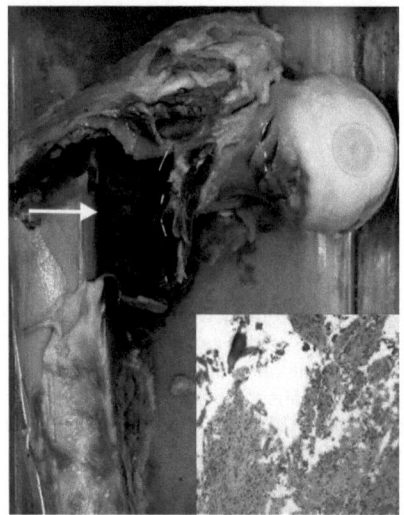

FIG. 13: Gross specimen of the femur with a cavity (arrow) near the head indicative of osteomyelitis. Inset: The microscopic evaluation revealed necrotizing granulomatous inflammation composed of epithelioid granulomas, Langhans giant cell, and caseous necrosis along with destruction of the bone (H&E 100x) *(Chapter 4)*

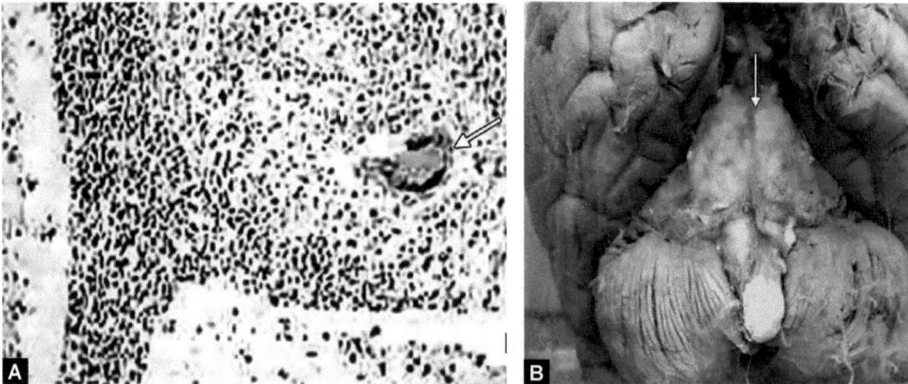

FIG. 14: Tubercular meningitis. **A,** The histology revealed inflammation of the meninges along with lymphocytic infiltration and scattered Langhans giant cell (arrow) (H&E 100x); **B,** Gross specimen of the brain with exudates at the basal meninges (arrow) *(Chapter 4)*

PLATE 7

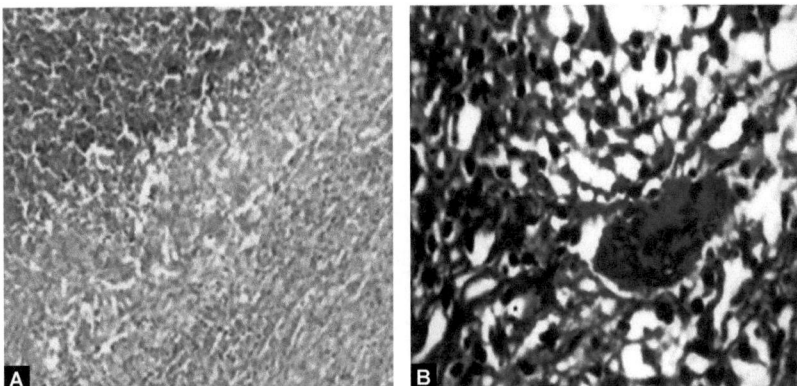

FIG. 15: Tuberculoma. **A,** Photomicrograph showing necrosis surrounded by a thin layer of granulomatous infiltrate, fibrosis, and gliosis; **B,** A cellular region of the same lesion with Langhans giant cell (A = H&E 50x, B = H&E 200x) *(Chapter 4)*

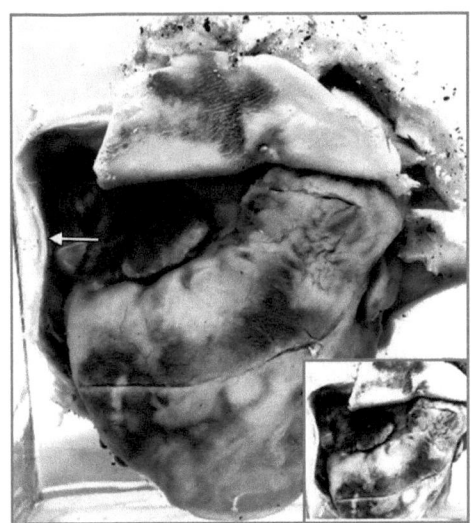

FIG. 16: Tuberculous pericarditis: The gross specimen of the heart with thickening of the pericardium (arrow) along with fibrinous exudates. Inset: Closer view of the thickened wall with the classical bread and butter appearance *(Chapter 4)*

PLATE 8

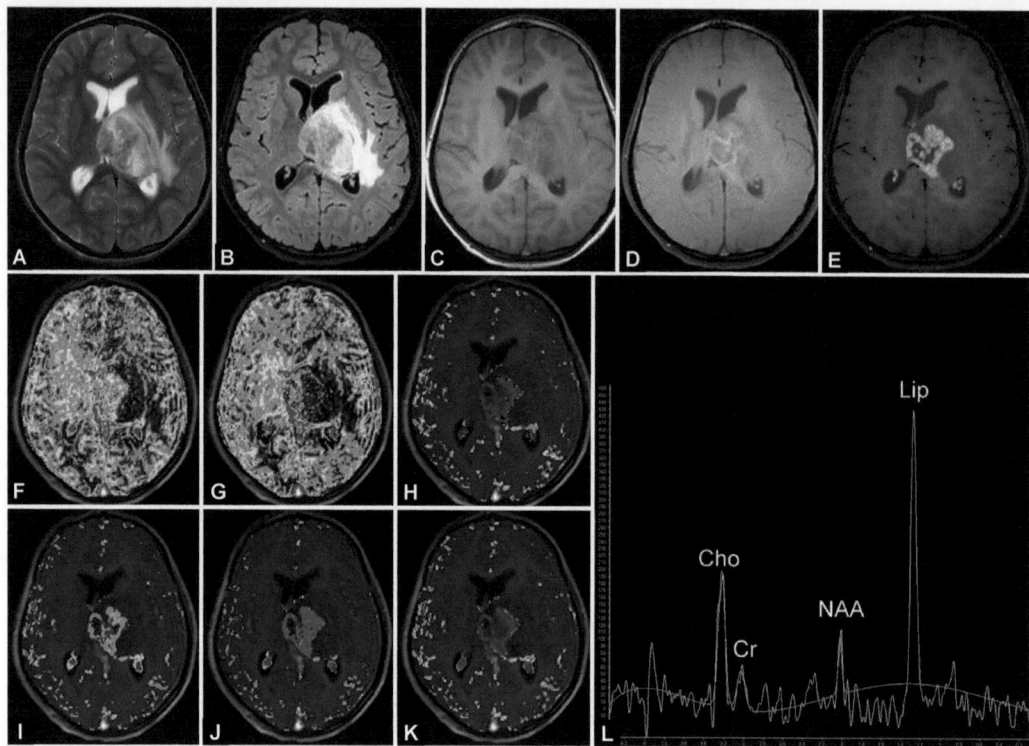

FIG. 14: Heterogeneous tuberculoma. A 13-year-old boy presented with right sided weakness. **A** and **B**, Axial T2 weighted and FLAIR images show a central hypointense lesion with surrounding peripheral hyperintensity which appears **C**, heterogeneous on T1 weighed image. **D** and **E**, MTT1 image shows a bright rim around T2 hypointense lesion that shows enhancement on post contrast T1 weighted image. **F** to **K**, T1-DCE images of rCBF, rCBV, Vp, Ve, leakage, and Kep demonstrate poor perfusion in the capsule with contrast pooling in the extra-vascular extra-cellular space. **L**, SVS at 135 ms demonstrates dominant lipid peak at 1.3 ppm. Note marginal increase in Cho at 3.2ppm to indicate cellularity of tuberculoma; and contamination of NAA at 2.0 ppm and Cr at 3.0 ppm from surrounding tissue *(Chapter 7)*

PLATE 9

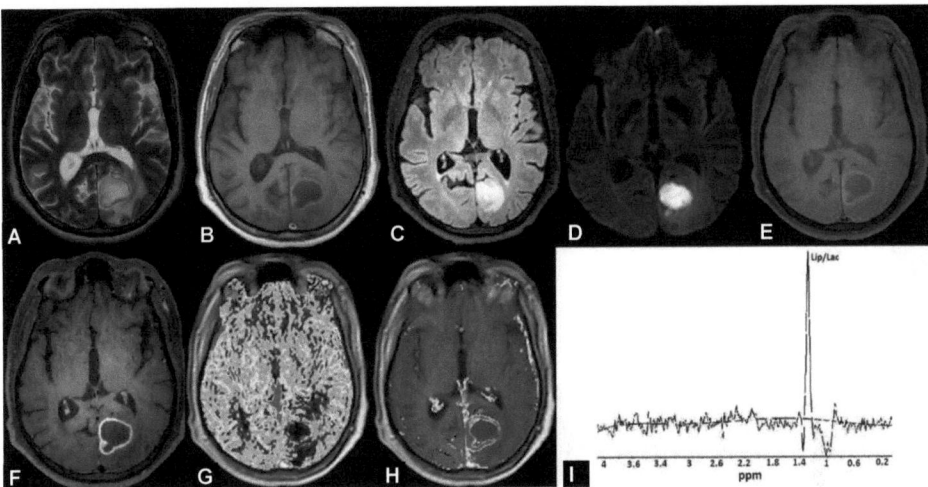

FIG. 15: Tubercular abscess in the left occipital region of a 65-year-old man. **A,** A well-defined hyperintense lesion is seen with a hypointense wall on T2-weighted image. **B,** T1-weighted image shows hypointense lesion with minimally hyperintense wall. **C,** On FLAIR images it appears hyperintense. **D,** Diffusion-weighted image shows homogeneous hyperintensity in the cavity. **E,** On MT T1-weighted image shows increased brightness of the T2 hypointense wall compared to image **B**. **F,** Postcontrast T1-weighted image shows rim enhancement. **G,** On DCE perfusion magnetic resonance imaging there is decreased CBV on corrected CBV map. **H,** Note the leakage of contrast suggesting break in blood brain barrier on leakage map. **I,** Proton magnetic resonance spectroscopy from the center of the lesion with a voxel size of 1.2 mL shows predominant lipid/lactate peak (Lip/Lac, 1.3 ppm) *(Chapter 7)*

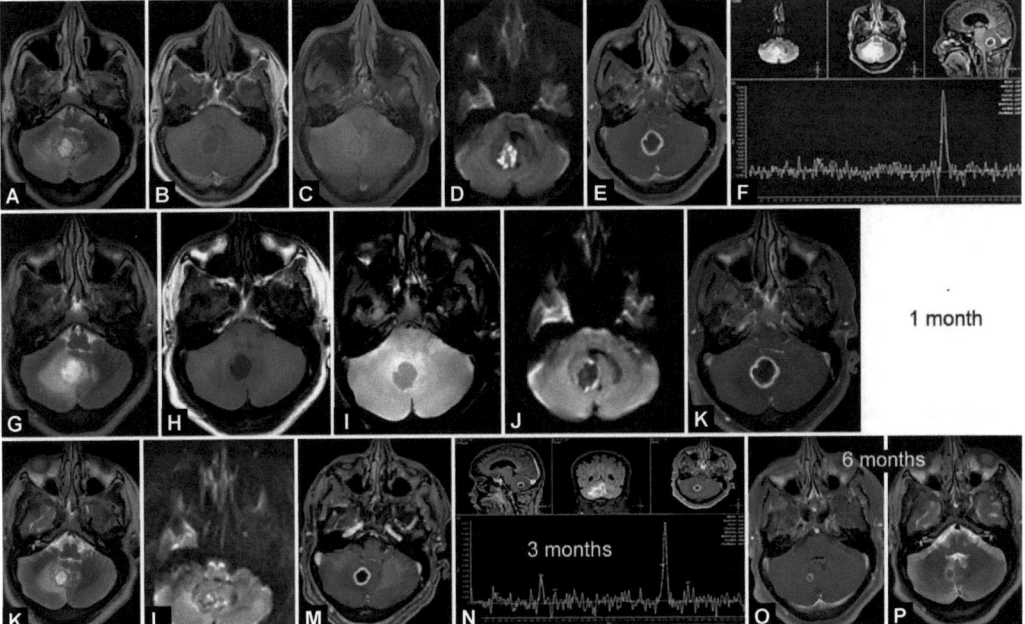

FIG. 23: Tubercular abscess on treatment. **A,** Well-defined paramedian cerebellar abscess with hyperintense contents and hypointense rim on T2WI, **B,** hypointense contents on T1WI, **C,** hyperintense rim on MT, **D,** restricting contents on DWI, **E,** rim-enhancement on post-contrast T1WI, **F,** lipid/lactate peak resonating at 1.3 ppm with single voxel spectroscopy with RoI in the contents. Lesion showed gradual resolution on ATT **G-K,** at month, **K–N,** three months and **O, P,** at 6 months *(Chapter 7)*

PLATE 10

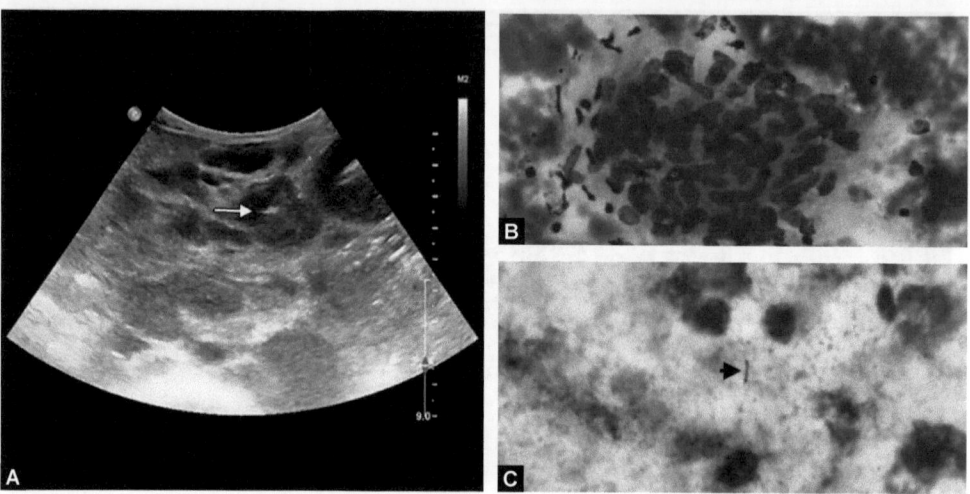

FIG. 1: Axial transabdominal ultrasound **A,** shows presence of multiple large mesenteric and retroperitoneal lymph nodes showing hypoechoic centres suggestive of necrosis. Needle-in-situ noted in one of the mesenteric lymph node (arrow). **B,** cytopathology smear shows an epitheloid cell granuloma (May Grünwald-Giemsa x 40X); and **B,** presence of an acid-fast bacillus (Ziehl–Neelsen stain x 100X) *(Chapter 11)*

Courtesy: Images B and C: Dr Nalini Gupta, Professor, Department of Cytology, PGIMER, Chandigarh, India.

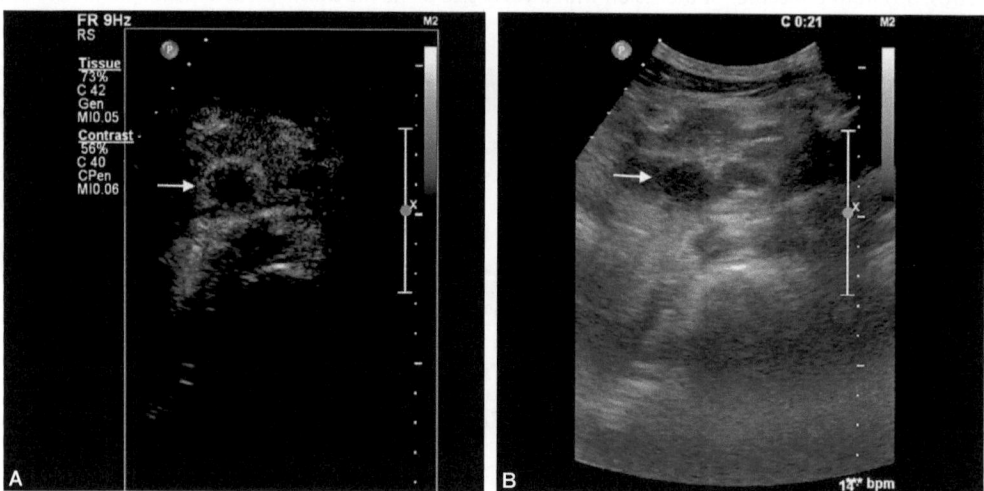

FIG. 2: Contrast enhanced **A,** and corresponding gray scale **B,** ultrasound images demonstrate presence of central necrosis and peripheral enhancement (arrow) in a patient of tubercular lymphadenitis at the porta hepatis *(Chapter 11)*

PLATE 11

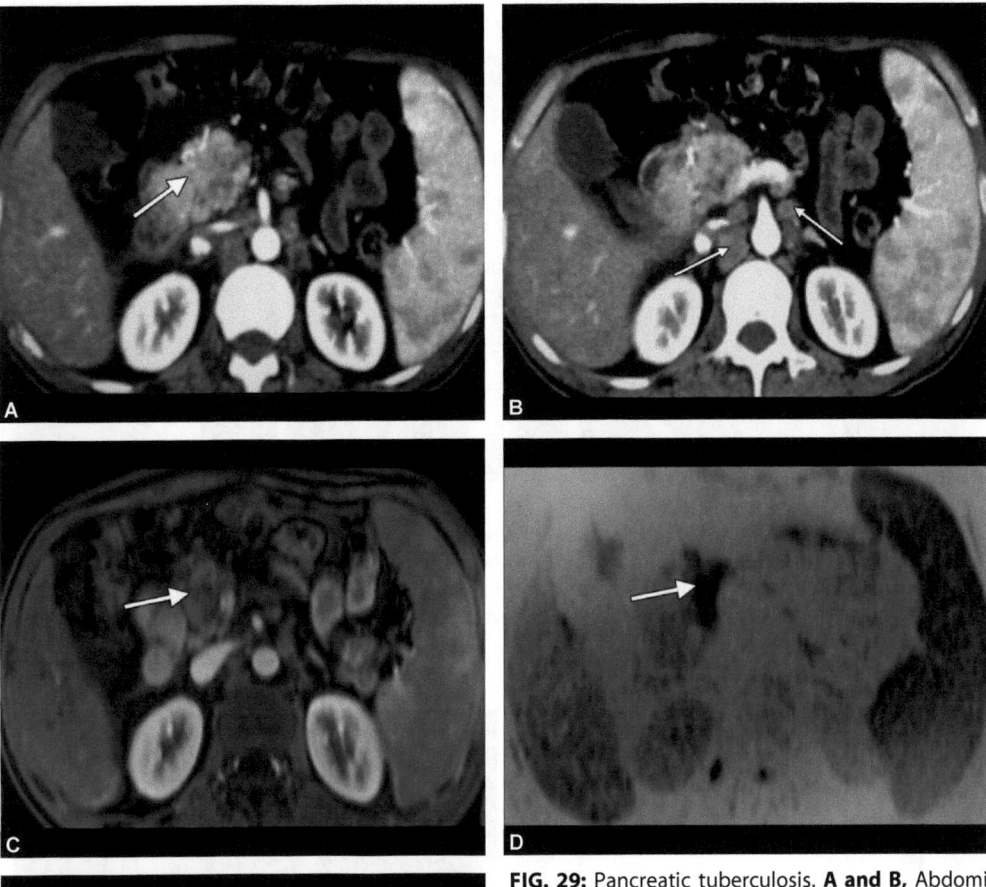

FIG. 29: Pancreatic tuberculosis. **A and B,** Abdominal contrast-enhanced computed tomography images show hypodense mass lesion (thick arrow) in the head of pancreas with multiple necrotic lymph nodes in retroperitoneum (thin arrow) and there is associated splenomegaly; **C and D,** postcontrast T1-weighted fat suppressed image also shows pancreatic focal lesion which is showing diffusion restriction on inverted grey scale image of diffusion-weighted sequence (B 1000); and **E,** tracer uptake on fluorodeoxyglucose positron emission tomography-CT scan. Based on the earlier imaging features this patient was diagnosed to have pancreatic carcinoma. However, endoscopic ultra-sonography-guided fine-needle aspiration cytology revealed tuberculosis which is a rare entity and a close mimicker of pancreatic carcinoma *(Chapter 12)*

PLATE 12

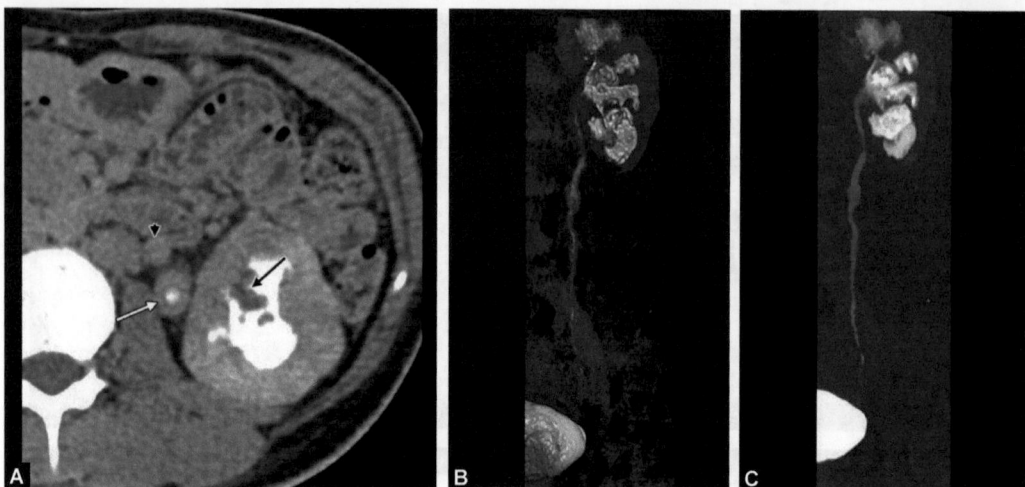

FIG. 7: Computed tomography (CT) urography. **A,** Axial urogram phase CT image demonstrates left hydronephrosis with irregular margins, hypodense filling defects (due to papillary sloughing) (black arrow), ureteric wall thickening (white arrow) and left paraaortic lymph node (black arrow head); **B,** coronal volume rendered image; and **C,** thick maximum intensity projection image better demonstrate irregular caliectasis with debris and multiple ureteric strictures resulting in beaded appearance *(Chapter 13)*

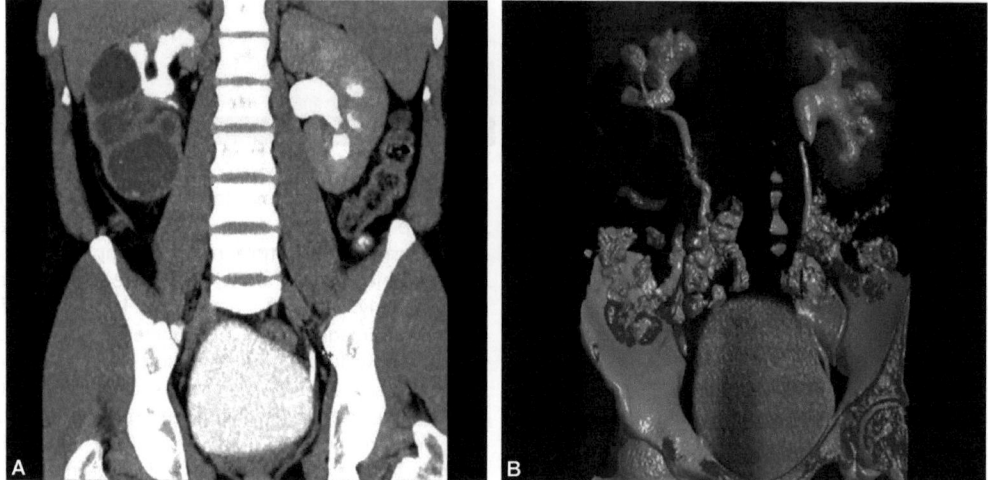

FIG. 19: Genitourinary tuberculosis in an adolescent male. **A,** Coronal maximum intensity projection; **B,** volume rendering technique image reveal focal caliectasis of the mid and lower pole of right kidney, with lack of contrast accumulation (phantom calyces) *(Chapter 17)*

PLATE 13

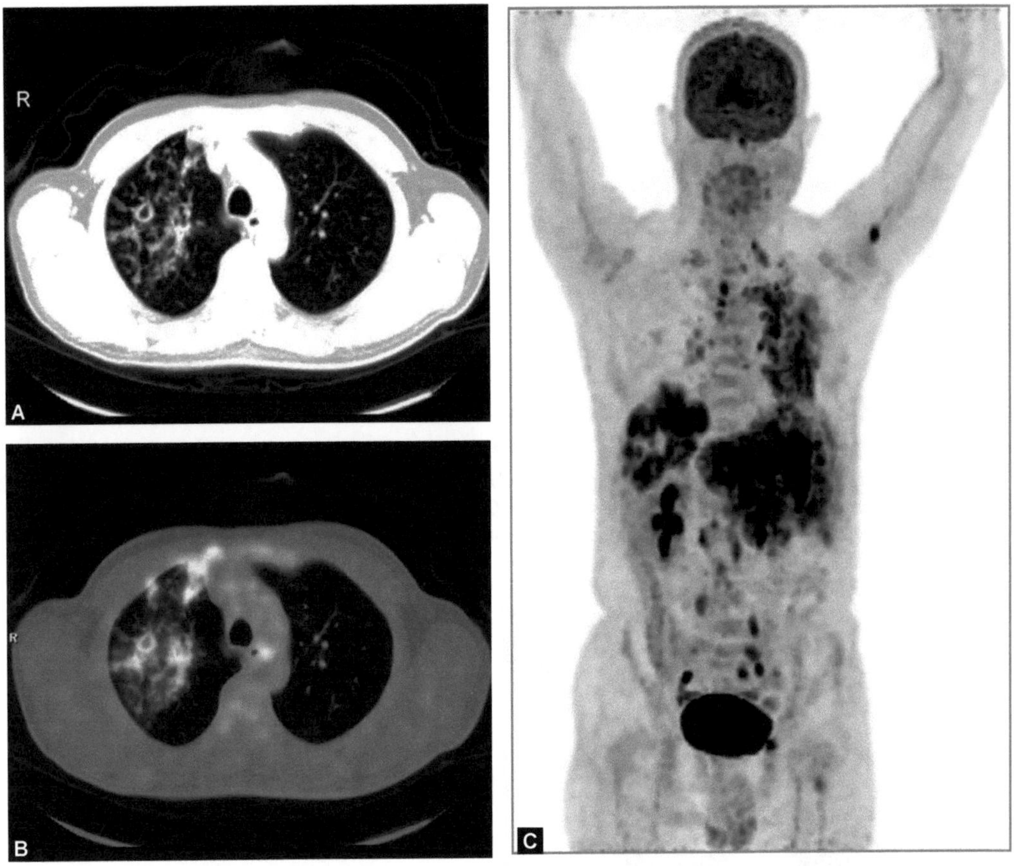

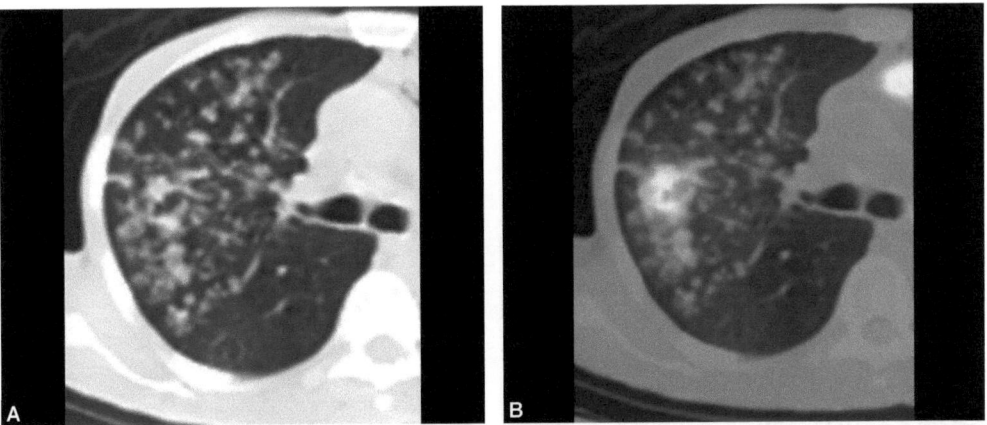

FIG. 1: A 45-year-old male, known case of Type 2 diabetes presented with hemoptysis, positron emission tomography/computed tomography (PET/CT) scan showing lung parenchymal changes, micro and macronodules with cavitations surrounded suggestive of active pulmonary tuberculosis *(Chapter 18)*

CT, computed tomography; PET, positron emission tomography; TB, tuberculosis.

FIG. 2: A 63-year-old male, known case of pulmonary tuberculosis underwent PET/CT which demonstrated the "tree-in-bud sign" which is reliable marker of active TB *(Chapter 18)*

PLATE 14

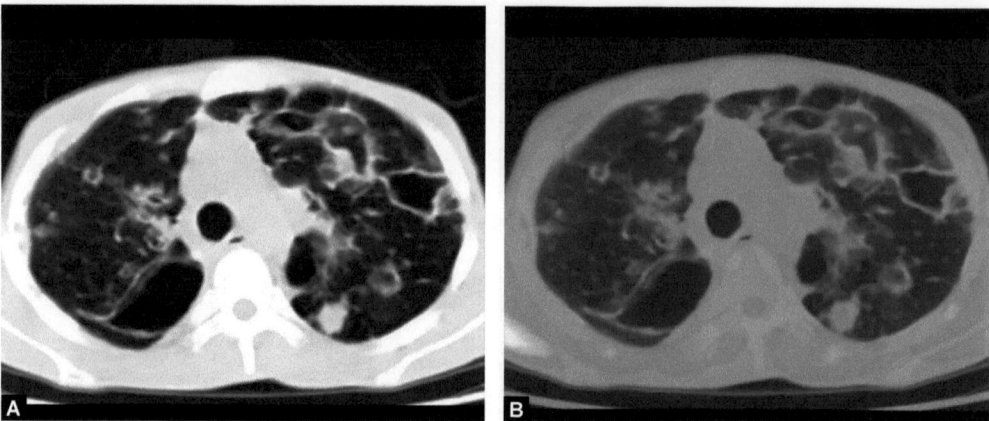

CT, computed tomography; FDG, fluorodeoxyglucose; PET, positron emission tomography.

FIG. 3: A 54-year-old male, known case of pulmonary tuberculosis, treated with antitubercular treatment in 2008. Now presented with chest pain and breathlessness, PET/CT scan was done to see activity of disease which showed multiple fibrocavitary lesions with no significant FDG uptake suggestive of no disease activity *(Chapter 18)*

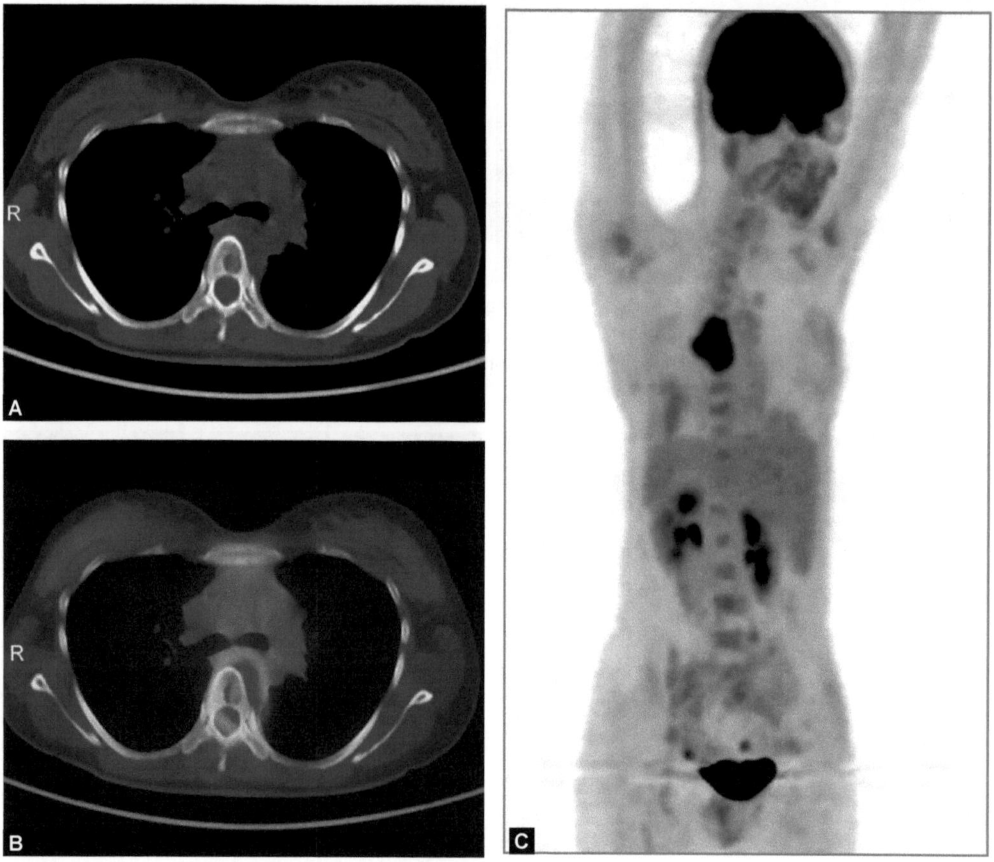

CT, computed tomography; FDG, fluorodeoxyglucose; PET, positron emission tomography.

FIG. 4: A patient with a vertebral lesion consistent with Pott's spine showing FDG uptake indicative of active disease *(Chapter 18)*

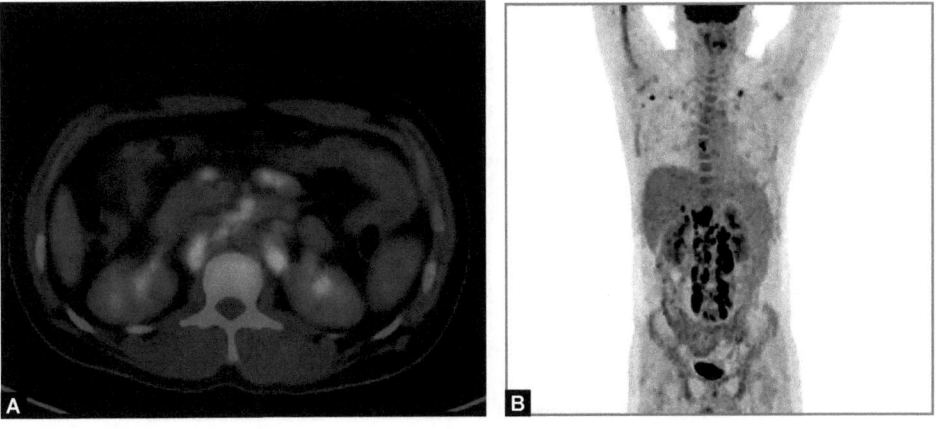

CT, computed tomography; FDG, fluorodeoxyglucose; PET, positron emission tomography.

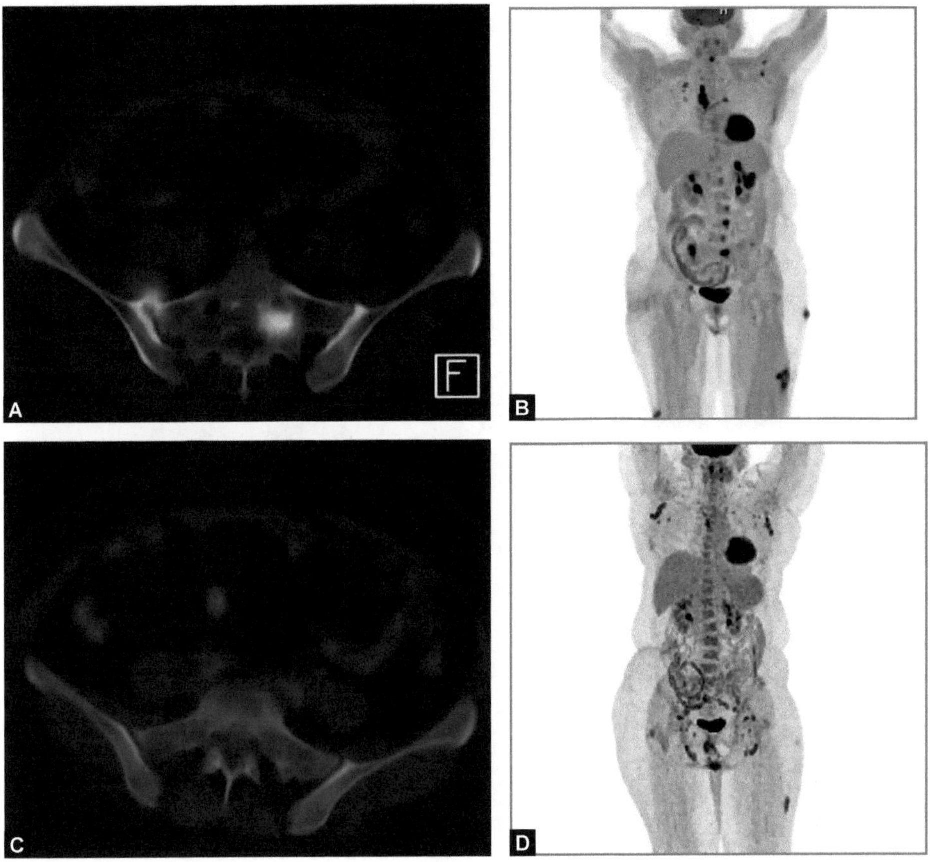

FIG. 5: A 23-year-old female presented with miliary disseminated tuberculosis. PET/CT was advised to see the extent of disease which showed lytic lesion with prevertebral soft tissue component and increased FDG uptake, these consistent Pott's spine *(Chapter 18)*

CT, computed tomography; FDG, fluorodeoxyglucose; PET, positron emission tomography.

FIG. 6: A 30-year-old male, presented with abdominal lymphadenopathy, PET/CT scan showing multiple retroperitoneal lymph nodes with increased FDG uptake suggestive of active disease *(Chapter 18)*

PLATE 16

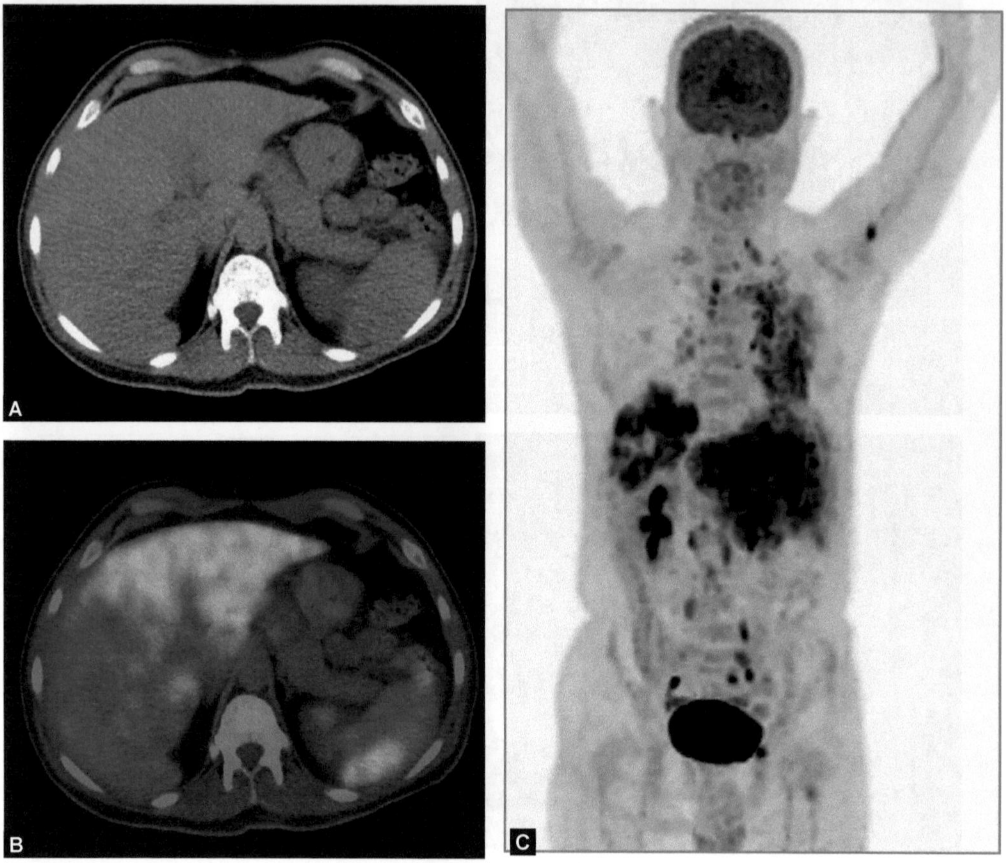

CT, computed tomography; FDG, fluorodeoxyglucose; PET, positron emission tomography.

FIG. 7: A 45-year-old male, known case of Type 2 diabetes, diagnosed as pulmonary tuberculosis, PET/CT scan showing areas of increased FDG uptake in liver and spleen. Projection image show abnormal uptake in lungs and multiple lymph nodes, in addition to liver and spleen *(Chapter 18)*

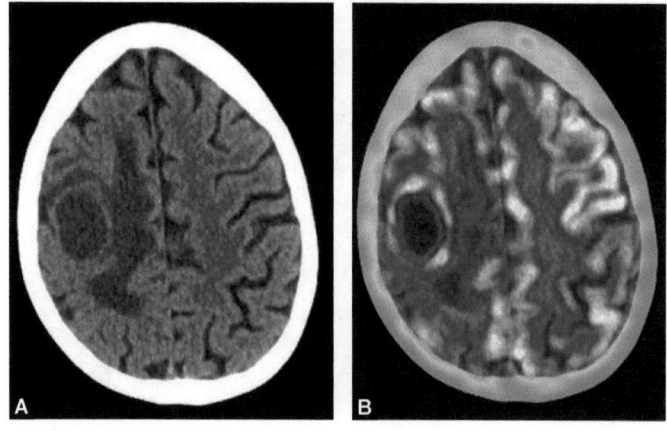

CT, computed tomography; FDG, fluorodeoxyglucose; PET, positron emission tomography.

FIG. 8: A 19-year-old male known case of disseminated multidrug-resistant tuberculosis presented with seizures. PET/CT shows right frontal lesion with perilesional edema and FDG uptake in margins suggestive of active disease *(Chapter 18)*

PLATE 17

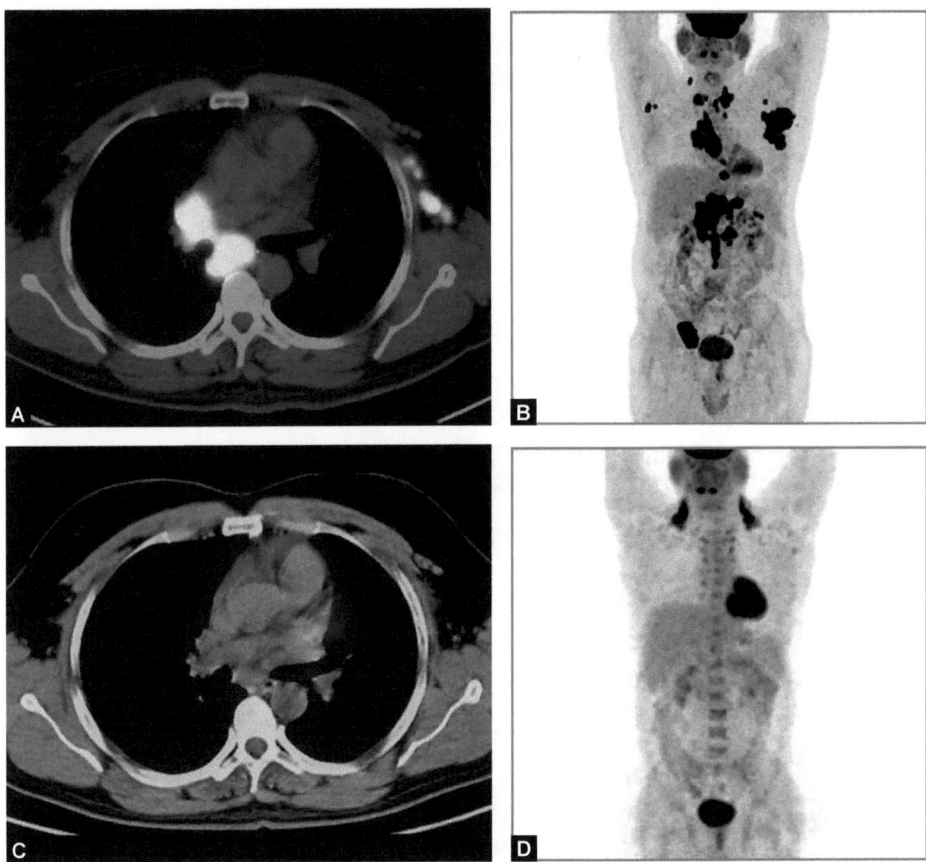

CT, computed tomography; FDG, fluorodeoxyglucose; PET, positron emission tomography.

FIG. 9: A 32-year-old male, disseminated tuberculosis, underwent baseline and 6-months post-treatment PET/CT scan to see therapy response. Baseline PET/CT showed multiple focal areas of increased FDG uptake in multiple lymph nodes (upper row). Post-treatment PET/CT scan showed complete resolution of FDG uptake suggestive of complete response (lower row) *(Chapter 18)*

PLATE 18

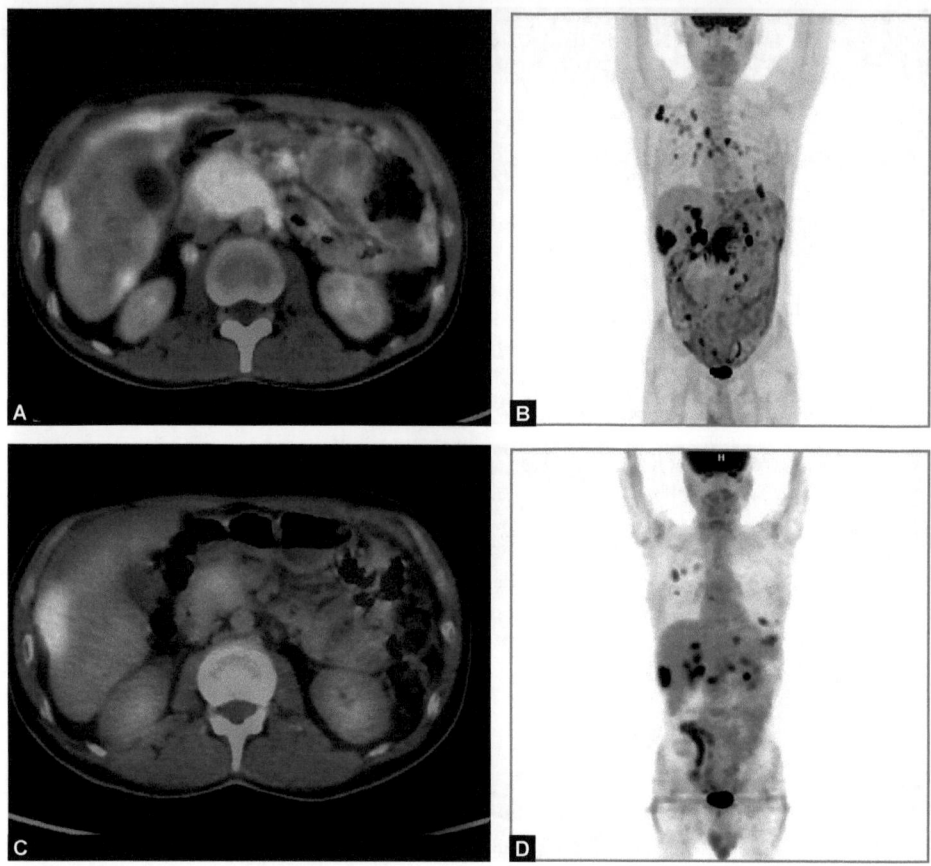

CT, computed tomography; FDG, fluorodeoxyglucose; PET, positron emission tomography.

FIG. 10: A 38-year-old male, disseminated tuberculosis, underwent baseline and 9-month post-treatment PET/CT scan to see therapy response. Baseline PET/CT showed multiple focal areas of increased FDG uptake in multiple lymph nodes and liver (upper row). Post-treatment PET/CT scan showed decrease in FDG uptake suggestive of partial response (lower row) *(Chapter 18)*

CHAPTER 1

Epidemiology of Tuberculosis

Chandra M Pandey

INTRODUCTION

Relics found in ancient Egypt, India, and China mention the presence of *Mycobacterium tuberculosis*. Tuberculosis (TB) had numerous names in ancient times including consumption (because of the severe weight loss and infection seemed to consume the patient), phthisis pulmonalis and the white plague. The term "white plague" for TB was coined in 18th century when it reached the peak in Western Europe. Scrofula, the TB of cervical lymph nodes was termed as the king's evil and was believed that the kings of England and France could cure scrofula simply by touching those affected. Poet John Keats and Percy Bysshe Shelley, the authors Robert Louis Stevenson, Emily Bronte and Edgar Allan Poe, the musicians Niccolo Paganini and Frederic Chopin were some famous people who suffered from this disease.[1] In 1937, the lady Governor General of India, issued a public appeal, for antituberculosis fund, and nearly ten million rupees were collected. A small portion of this money was retained and rest was distributed to various States. Subsequently, establishment of the TB clinic in New Delhi, creation of the Lady Linlithgow Sanatorium at Kasauli and a scheme for organizing home treatment as an essential part of India's anti-TB campaign was started using this fund. The Tuberculosis Association of India was formed in February 1939 with the retained funds.

Tuberculosis is a contagious and often severe airborne disease caused by a bacterial (*Mycobacterium tuberculosis*) infection. Tuberculosis typically affects the lungs, but it also may affect any other organ of the body.[2] It is transmitted from person to person via droplets from the throat and lungs of people with the active respiratory disease.[3]

A bacteriologically confirmed TB is one where specimen is positive by smear microscopy or culture. A clinically diagnosed TB is one that does not fulfill the criteria of bacteriological confirmation but has been diagnosed with active TB by a medical practitioner and the patient is prescribed a full course of TB treatment.[4,5]

About 9.6 million people were estimated to have TB in 2014. Out of which 5.4 million were men, 3.2 million women and 1.0 million children. According to World Health Organization (WHO) global TB report 2015, the incidence of TB has been declining globally for several years and has reached at an average rate of 1.5% per year between 2000 and 2014. The case fatality rate has also declined by 47% between 1990 and 2015. A decline of about 40% has been projected during 1990–2015. All six WHO regions have achieved Millennium Development Goal set for halting and reversing the burden of TB by the year 2015.[6] Despite these achievements, TB remains one of the biggest threats to mankind. In 2014, TB killed 1.5 million people [1.1 million human immunodeficiency virus (HIV) –ve and 0.4 million HIV +ve]. The death toll comprised of 0.89 million men, 0.48 women and 0.14 children respectively. Tuberculosis with HIV has been ranked as a leading cause of death worldwide. The African region accounted for 74% of these cases. Globally, 51% of notified TB patients were HIV +ve in 2014, with a slight increase from 49% in 2013. About 0.9 million people living with HIV were treated with isoniazid preventive therapy in 2014. Majority of these were from South African region. The foundation of the current global strategy for TB began in early 1990s, when the rising trends of TB led to the provision of directly observed treatment short-course (DOTS) strategy. The DOTS was implemented in 184 countries and provided treatment to more than 32 million patients out of whom more than 25 million achieved cure. Despite this achievement TB has been a major concern for WHO due to continuously increasing drug resistant trait.[7] In some countries with alarmingly high incidence the Bacillus Calmette-Guérin (BCG) is used as preventive vaccination. Although BCG is helpful in preventing people from TB, it is not considered effective enough to justify for wide use.

CLASSIFICATION OF TUBERCULOSIS

The TB has been classified based on anatomical site, primarily as pulmonary and extrapulmonary tuberculosis (EPTB). It has also been classified according to drug resistance, treatment history, presence of HIV, and active or latent TB.[8-10] The details of these subgroups are given as under.

Pulmonary Tuberculosis

Pulmonary TB is more common than EPTB and the diagnosed case must have TB involving lung parenchyma or tracheobronchial tree.[11-14] The pulmonary TB is a contagious infection involving lungs and it can spread to other organs. Most people recover from primary TB infection without further evidence of the disease. The infection may stay dormant for years. In some cases it becomes reactivate. Generally people showing TB symptoms became infected with the bacteria in the past. In some cases the disease becomes symptomatic within few weeks of primary infection showing breathing difficulty, chest pain, cough (usually with mucus), coughing up blood, excessive sweating (especially at night), fatigue, fever, weight loss, wheezing as symptoms of pulmonary TB.[15,16] Once the bacteria reaches the lungs of an individual:

- The bacteria may be killed by strong immune system
- It may become latent and stops growing inside the body and does not cause disease. About one-third of global population has latent TB
- It may cause active TB in people with weak immune system and may develop full blown case of TB.

People with latent TB may develop active TB if immunity is compromised. Symptoms often improve in 2–3 weeks of treatment. A chest X-ray may not indicate this improvement till several weeks or months. Outcome is excellent if pulmonary TB is diagnosed early and effective treatment is started quickly.[15,16] The pulmonary TB has following subtypes:

- Primary tuberculosis pneumonia: Tuberculosis presents as pneumonia. Patients suffer from high fever and productive cough. Occurs most often in extremely young children, elderly and in patients with immunosuppression, such as people with HIV/acquired immunodeficiency syndrome (AIDS), and in patients on long-term corticosteroid therapy
- Tuberculosis pleurisy: It usually appears soon after initial infection due to rupture of granuloma at edge of lung into the pleural space. Bacteria grow in this pleural space and the increased amount of fluid exerts pressure on walls of lungs causing dyspnea and sharp chest pain that worsens with a deep breath. Mild fever is common in these cases. Generally the infection resolves without any treatment, but about two-third of cases with TB pleurisy develop active pulmonary TB within 5 years
- Cavitary tuberculosis: It involves the upper lobes of the lung. The bacteria cause progressive lung destruction by forming cavities, or enlarged air spaces. This type of TB occurs in reactivation disease. The upper lobes of the lung are affected because they are highly oxygenated, a favorable environment for *Mycobacterium tuberculosis* to grow. This commonly does not occur soon after primary infection. The patients may suffer with coughing of blood, night sweats,

fever, weight loss and weakness. The disease can further cause TB empyema, a chronic, active infection containing a large number of tubercle bacilli in the pleural space
- Miliary tuberculosis: "Miliary" describes the appearance of millet seeds like nodules on chest X-ray throughout the lungs. It can occur soon after primary infection. The patient becomes acutely ill and suffers high fever and risk of death. Other symptoms may include night sweat and weight loss. The condition may get difficult to diagnose as initial chest X-ray may appear normal. Immune-compromised and children exposed to bacteria are at high-risk for this condition.

Extrapulmonary Tuberculosis

Extrapulmonary tuberculosis occurs in any other part of the body outside the lungs. It can infect almost any part of the body including the inner organs, like liver, kidney, spleen, brain, spine and bones, etc. In fact, the body parts which are not susceptible to TB are only our nails and hair. About 20% TB patients are infected with EPTB and these strains are often difficult to diagnose. Extrapulmonary tuberculosis is especially common in regions where prevalence of TB is low. Factors associated with the development of EPTB are poorly understood, however, the patients can have the same symptoms as reported with pulmonary TB. Following are the common forms of EPTB:
- Tubercular lymphadenitis/Scrofula: Lymph nodes have uncontrolled replication of TB bacteria, causing the lymph node to become enlarged. The infected lymph nodes swell and present like a cold abscess breaking the outer skin forming a draining sinus. The infection is most common in posterior cervical and supraclavicular chains
- Tuberculous peritonitis: *M. tuberculosis* can involve the outer linings of the intestines and the linings inside the abdominal wall producing increased fluid, as in TB pleuritis. Increased fluid leads to abdominal distension and pain. Patients are moderately ill and have fever. The infection is most common in alcoholic patients with cirrhosis
- Tuberculous pericarditis: The pericardium is affected in this condition. This causes the space between the pericardium and the heart to fill with fluid, impeding the heart's ability to fill with blood and beat efficiently. Patient may suffer positional chest pain, fever, dyspnea and hypotension
- Osteal tuberculosis: Infection of any bone can occur, but one of the most common sites is the spine. Spinal infection can lead to compression fractures and deformity of the back and compression of spinal cord with severe consequences. Infected joints swell and are painful
- Laryngeal tuberculosis: The TB of larynx, or the vocal cord area. The condition is extremely infectious[15-19]
- Renal tuberculosis: Kidney disease caused by *Mycobacterium tuberculosis*. Symptoms are often delayed after the initial infection. Patients present urinary symptoms like conventional bacterial cystitis, suprapubic pain, flank frequency and nocturia. Symptoms like fever, weight loss and night sweats are uncommon. The infection my affect adjoining reproductive organs
- Tuberculous meningitis: Meningitis is the most serious form of TB and has high morbidity and mortality. Headache, sleepiness and coma are typical symptoms. The patient may also develop a stroke. This is believed to be prevented by BCG immunization in childhood
- Hepatic tuberculosis: The *Mycobacterium tuberculosis* infection of the liver is known as hepatic TB. The most common signs and symptoms are fever, hepatomegaly, abdominal pain and weight loss. It is common in patients with advanced pulmonary TB or HIV. Sometimes the infection spreads to gall bladder causing obstructive jaundice. However in most cases the liver heals well if the principal infection is treated adequately
- Other sites: Though quite uncommon but bacteria can infect adrenal glands, skin, ruptured aorta and wall of blood vessels, etc.[20-22]

Drug-resistant Tuberculosis

Though TB involves complex drug treatment, the basic drugs for TB are isoniazid, rifampicin, pyrazinamide, ethambutol and streptomycin. These drugs have generally the strongest activity against the TB causing bacteria. Drug-resistant TB was recognized during late 1940s when streptomycin, the first drug to treat TB initially showed rapid improvement but reported treatment failure after 3 months of drug usage. *Mycobacterium tuberculosis* obtained from patients with treatment failure was found streptomycin resistant. This resistance to single antibiotic therapy led to multidrug chemotherapy for TB. Among globally known cases of TB about 3.6% of new and 20.2% of earlier treated cases had multidrug-resistant TB (MDR-TB). The Eastern Europe and Central Asia had highest prevalence of MDR-TB. However, adequate data for certain African regions is not available. According to National TB programs, in 2012 about 3,00,000 new cases were reported out of which 94,000 were drug-resistant and more than half of TB cases were from India, China and the Russian Federation. The success rate of treatment was 40% against the target of 75% (WHO 2011a). The estimated deaths from MDR-TB in 2012 were 1,70,000 (1,00,000–2,40,000). Extensively drug-resistant TB (XDR-TB) has been so far reported from 92 countries and is about approximately 10% of the MDR-TB cases. The earlier estimates for MDR-TB were found rising with 480,000 new cases in 2014. New traits of totally drug-resistant TB and rifampicin-resistant TB (RR-TB) were notified but statistical estimate of its burden is not available. Globally 27 countries have been declared as high burden MDR (>10% of new cases or 4,000 MDRs) these are: Armenia, Azerbaijan, Bangladesh, Belarus, Bulgaria, China, Democratic Republic of the Congo, Estonia, Ethiopia, Georgia, India, Indonesia, Kazakhstan, Kyrgyzstan, Latvia, Lithuania, Myanmar, Nigeria, Pakistan, Philippines, Republic of Moldova, Russian Federation, South Africa, Tajikistan, Ukraine, Uzbekistan and Vietnam. The diagnosing of MDR-TB is another challenge. Although, new tests like GeneXpert are available, but not affordable in underdeveloped and high burden areas. Progressively increasing trait of MDR-TB and XDR-TB, fuelled by poverty and limited access to effective treatment has compelled WHO, Global Drug Facility (GDF) and their international partners to develop newer generation of antitubercular drugs.[23-27]

Tuberculosis with Human Immunodeficiency Virus

The risk of TB is estimated to be 26–31 times higher in people living with HIV than those without HIV. In 2014 about 1.2 million people living with HIV reported TB. If people have HIV and active or latent TB together, the condition is termed as HIV-TB coinfection. A rapid progress of both diseases is observed under the HIV-TB coinfection. With HIV infection the progression of latent to active TB is also accelerated. This coinfection is reported to have higher mortality. The risk of death in coinfected cases is twice that of HIV infected individuals without TB. Tuberculosis also occurs earlier in case of HIV infection than many other opportunistic infections. World health organization recommends that all HIV-infected TB patients should be put on antiretroviral therapy (ART). This may have potential to reduce mortality. However, tuberculous meningitis with HIV is associated with more severe adverse events if immediate ART is given. It is recommended to postpone ART until the onset of anti-TB treatment.[28,29]

FACT SHEET

The epidemiological study of TB indicates that the Millennium Development Goal of TB elimination by 2050 will not be achieved. The majority of TB cases are occurring as endemic in population dense regions of Africa and Asia. Poor healthcare system has led to an increase in drug-resistant TB, which becomes more complicated with the HIV coinfection. The increasing drug resistance trait may reverse the achievements in controlling the TB. A well-coordinated global effort should be made to fight the TB.

The current global TB strategy began in the 1990s, when the increasing trends of TB led to the creation of DOTS strategy. The DOTS framework was implemented in 184 countries and covered more than 32 million patients receiving treatment and more than 25 million achieving cure. However, these achievements had insignificant impact on rising epidemic of TB. The global program to stop TB by 2015 was initiated in 2006. This was in line with the goals set by the WHO (70% detection and 85% cure rates by 2005) and ultimately to achieve Millennium Development Goal (<1 case per million population) by 2050. The total estimated cost of program was $56 billion including $9 billion for research and development but the program could not arrange the total funds and was started with financial deficit. Due to nexus between known risk factors like poverty, poor nutrition, and population crowding, combined with rising trend in drug resistance, the problem has become more complex. It is high time to address the issue by various governments and nongovernment organizations based on most recent epidemiological data and available resources. The WHO believes that, the cases of TB are decreasing slowly since 2000.

ERADICATION OF TUBERCULOSIS

In recent years United States (US) has recorded lowest TB rates. The achievement was brought through following a strategy of focusing and treating the latent TB infection. The following points came in view:

- It was estimated that about 11 million people in US were having latent TB infection
- If not treated 5–10% of this population will develop TB disease (i.e., about 550,000 to 1.1 million people in US)
- Diagnostic and treatment of latent TB can be difficult.[29]

CONCLUSION

Several gaps are found in proper and effective efforts for controlling TB worldwide. As a result the global reduction in the burden of TB is much below the targeted Millennium Development Goal of TB elimination by 2050. Additionally these gaps have favored the spread and rise of drug-resistant TB in most populous countries like India and China. The lethal combination of TB with HIV is acting as a power source for epidemic in many countries. Although the higher burden of disease has largely affected the resource-limited nations. The increasingly globalized environment calls for responsibility and urgent action in all international arenas. Several solutions are available, but the funding gaps are the major obstacle to realize these initiatives. Strategies that should be considered include policies that enhance DOTS by improving diagnostics to increase case detection and closing the funding gap in DOTS-based programs. Risk factors for continued TB transmission could be addressed by reducing socioeconomic health disparities and improving financial support to national TB control programs. Better management of HIV and TB coinfection may occur by enhancing diagnostic applications of both disease processes and using prophylactic therapy. Underlying any effort in TB elimination, however, will be increased funding and political will from both the international community and national health sectors. Progressively increasing trait of MDR-TB and XDR-TB, fuelled by limited access to effective treatment and poverty, needs proper attention of WHO, GDF and Global Lighting Forum and their international partners to develop newer generation of antitubercular drugs.

REFERENCES

1. Mandal A. (2014). History of Tuberculosis. [online] Available from www.news-medical.net/health/History-of-Tuberculosis.aspx. [Accessed March, 2017].
2. National Institute of Allergy and Infectious Diseases (NIH). (2017). Tuberculosis (TB). [online] Available from www.niaid.nih.gov/diseases-conditions/tuberculosis-tb. [Accessed March, 2017].
3. World Health Organization (WHO). (2017). Tuberculosis (TB). [online] Available from www.who.int/tb/en/.[Accessed March, 2017].
4. World Health Organization (WHO). (2014). Definitions and reporting framework for tuberculosis – 2013 revision (updated December 2014). [online] Available from apps.who.int/iris/bitstream/10665/79199/1/9789241505345_eng.pdf. [Accessed March, 2017].
5. World Health Organization (WHO). (2016). Global Health Observatory data repository. [online] Available from apps.who.int/gho/data/node.home. [Accessed March, 2017].
6. National Institute of Allergy and Infectious Diseases (NIH). (2017). Tuberculosis-Disease and Conditions. [online] Available from: https://www.niaid.nih.gov/diseases-conditions/tuberculosis-tb [Accessed March, 2017].
7. World Health Organization (WHO). (2015). Global Tuberculosis Report 2015. [online] Available from apps.who.int/

8. Newfoundland and Labrador Heritage Web Site. (2012). Labrador Boundary Dispute Documentation. [online] Available from www.heritage.nf.ca/articles/politics/pdf/labrador-boundary-dispute-documents.pdf [Accessed March, 2017].
9. Newfoundland and Labrador Heritage Web Site. (2013). The Amulree Commission Report, 1933. [online] Available from www.heritage.nf.ca/articles/politics/pdf/amulee-report-1933.pdf [Accessed March, 2017].
10. Newfoundland and Labrador Heritage Web Site. (2017). Dictionary of Newfoundland English. [online] Available from www.heritage.nf.ca/dictionary/ [Accessed March, 2017].
11. Centers for Disease Control and Prevention (CDC). (2011). Tuberculosis: General Information. [online] Available from www.cdc.gov/tb/publications/factsheets/general/tb.htm [Accessed March, 2017].
12. Centers for Disease Control and Prevention (CDC). (2012). Trends in Tuberculosis – United States, 2011. [online] Available from www.cdc.gov/mmwr/preview/mmwrhtml/mm6111a2.htm. [Accessed March, 2017].
13. American Lung Association. (2017). Tuberculosis (TB). [online] Available from www.lung.org/lung-health-and-diseases/lung-disease-lookup/tuberculosis/. [Accessed March, 2017].
14. Ellner JJ. Tuberculosis. In: Goldman L, Schafer AI (Eds). Goldman's Cecil Medicine, 24th edition. Philadelphia: Elsevier Saunders; 2012. p. 24.
15. Fitzgerald DW, Sterling TR, Haas DW. Mycobacterium tuberculosis. In: Bennett JE, Dolin R, Blaser MJ (Eds). Mandell, Douglas, and Bennett's Principles and Practice of Infectious Diseases, 8th edition. Philadelphia: Elsevier Churchill Livingstone; 2014.
16. Centers for Disease Control and Prevention (CDC). (2004). Trends in Tuberculosis—United States, 1998–2003. [online] Available from www.cdc.gov/mmwr/preview/mmwrhtml/mm5310a2.htm. [Accessed March, 2017].
17. Fanning A. Tuberculosis: 6. Extrapulmonary disease. CMAJ. 1999;160(11):1597-603.
18. Weir MR, Thornton GF. Extrapulmonary tuberculosis. Experience of a community hospital and review of the literature. Am J Med. 1985;79(4):467-78.
19. World Health Organization (WHO). (2006). Report of the meeting of the WHO Global Task Force on XDR-TB. [online] Available from www.who.int/tb/xdr/globaltaskforcereport_oct06.pdf. [Accessed March, 2017].
20. World Health Organization (WHO). (2009). Global Tuberculosis Control: Epidemiology, Strategy, Financing. [online] Available from www.reliefweb.int/sites/reliefweb.int/files/resources/878BDA5E2504C9F449257584001B5E60-who_mar2009.pdf. [Accessed March, 2017].
21. World Health Organization (WHO). (2011). Global Tuberculosis Control. [online] Available from www.apps.who.int/iris/bitstream/10665/44728/1/9789241564380_eng.pdf. [Accessed March, 2017].
22. Centers for Disease Control and Prevention (CDC). (1996). Tuberculosis Morbidity—United States, 1995. [online] Available from www.cdc.gov/mmwr/preview/mmwrhtml/00041404.htm. [Accessed March, 2017].
23. Centers for Disease Control and Prevention (CDC). (2013). Reported Tuberculosis in the United States. [online] Available from www.cdc.gov/tb/statistics/reports/2013/pdf/report2013.pdf. [Accessed March, 2017].
24. World Health Organization (WHO). (2008). Implementing the WHO Stop TB Strategy: a handbook for national tuberculosis control programmes. [online] Available from whqlibdoc.who.int/publications/2008/9789241546676_eng.pdf. [Accessed March, 2017].
25. World Health Organization (WHO). (2014). Global Tuberculosis Report. [online] Available from apps.who.int/iris/bitstream/10665/137094/1/9789241564809_eng.pdf. [Accessed March, 2017].
26. World Health Organization (WHO). (2015). The Global Plan to Stop TB 2011-2015. [online] Available from www.stoptb.org/assets/documents/global/plan/tb_globalplantostoptb2011-2015.pdf. [Accessed March, 2017].
27. Ambe G, Lönnroth K, Dholakia Y, Copreaux J, Zignol M, Borremans N, et al. Every provider counts: effect of a comprehensive public-private mix approach for TB control in a large metropolitan area in India. Int J Tuberc Lung Dis. 2005;9(5):562-8.
28. Bierrenbach AL, Stevens AP, Gomes AB, Noronha EF, Glatt R, Carvalho CN, et al. Impact on tuberculosis incidence rates of removal of repeat notification records. Rev Saude Publica. 2007;41 Suppl 1:67-76.
29. World Health Organization (WHO). (1991). The Forty-fourth World Health Assembly. [online] Available from www.who.int/tobacco/framework/wha_eb/wha44_26/en/. [Accessed March, 2017].

CHAPTER 2

Tuberculosis: Clinical Features

Krishan Chugh, Neetu Talwar

INTRODUCTION

Tuberculosis (TB) is one of the most common infectious diseases worldwide, affecting almost a third of the global population. It is caused by *Mycobacterium tuberculosis*. Although any organ in the body can get affected, pulmonary infections are the most common.

KEY FACTS ON CLINICAL FEATURES IN TUBERCULOSIS

- Tuberculosis may remain completely asymptomatic till the disease is quite advanced
- The usual symptoms of TB, like low-grade fever, loss of weight, poor appetite, and productive cough can either go undetected both by the patient as well as the physician or wrongly attributed to some other disease
- Delay in diagnosis leads to silent transmission of the disease
- The estimated lifetime risk of a young child developing TB infection as diagnosed by positive Mantoux test is about 10%[1]
- Of these infected children, approximately 5% are likely to develop the disease in the first year after infection and the remaining 5% during their lifetime.[1] Thus, in TB, infection and disease are two different entities—an infected child may never develop symptoms (i.e., disease) in his lifetime
- About 40% of the untreated children infected below 1 year of age, develop radiologically significant lymphadenopathy or parenchymal lesions in contrast to 24% of children between 1 and 10 years and 16% of children with 11–15 years of age[2]
- Older children and adults who develop the disease, often have reactivation of the infection acquired earlier.

WHO IS AT HIGH RISK?

The risk factors for developing TB are young age (<3 years), malnutrition, unvaccinated [Bacillus Calmette-Guerin (BCG)] population, rural area, exposure to biomass cooking fuel, smoking, and a history of contact with a known TB case. Immunocompromised patients such as those with human immunodeficiency virus (HIV), malnutrition, or diabetes are not only at risk of developing the infection but are also more likely to develop a severe and disseminated infection.[3]

DISEASE PROGRESS

The clinical presentations of childhood TB have undergone significant variations due to widespread BCG vaccination. There is a decreased incidence of disseminated and severe disease, but a higher rate of localized illness like localized central nervous system (CNS) infection. The progress of the disease has been described in table 1.

CLINICAL FEATURES

Primary Infection

Usually this phase passes off unrecognized with no specific clinical or radiological manifestations. The only way to diagnose is by a positive Mantoux test.

Table 1: Tuberculosis march (of clinical features)

Phase	Mantoux test	Chest X-ray	Time after primary infection	Point to note
Phase I	Positive	Primary complex seen	After 3–8 weeks	–
Phase II	Positive	–	After 1–3 months	Highest risk of developing tuberculous meningitis and miliary tuberculosis
Phase III	Positive	Present	After 3–7 months	Period of pleural effusion over 5 years, period of bronchial disease below 5 years
Phase IV	Positive	Present	Lasts 1–3 years after primary infection and continues till the primary complex is calcified	Phase of development of osteoarticular tuberculosis in children below 5 years
Phase V	–	Present	Occurs more than 3 years after primary infection	Late manifestations of tuberculosis including pulmonary reactivation disease occur

PULMONARY TUBERCULOSIS

This is the most common manifestation of TB. Symptoms vary according to the site of involvement, whether it is the parenchyma, endobronchial tree or the pleura. Accordingly clinical features have been described.

Clinical Presentations of Pulmonary Tuberculosis

Pulmonary Primary Complex

Pulmonary primary complex (PPC) is the most common presentation of TB. Symptoms are vague-like cough, low-grade fever with an evening rise of temperature, lethargy, poor appetite and even these symptoms may not always be present. Radiological features may also be absent or may be nonspecific like a doubtful shadow persisting despite a course of antibiotics. In such a clinical setting, history of a contact especially a sputum positive contact should be actively elicited.

Progressive Primary Disease

Progressive primary disease is because of the progression of the PPC. Now the symptoms may be the presence of moderate to high-grade fever and cough. Productive cough and hemoptysis would be the signs of advanced disease and are indicative of formation of cavity or ulceration of bronchus.[4] These symptoms are usually present in adolescents and adults. If they are seen in the younger age group, HIV and other immunodeficiencies must be ruled out.

Endobronchial Tuberculosis

When the spread is to the endobronchial tree, the child will develop persistent fever and cough, expectoration may be present and breathlessness. Respiratory distress, wheezing, and cyanosis could be present. Radiological presentation is usually in the form of broncho-pneumonia. However, X-ray may not show any significant abnormality (Fig. 1). Airway compression would be indicated by emphysema (if partial compression) and collapse (with complete compression).

Miliary Tuberculosis

Miliary TB results from hematogenous spread of the disease leading to seeding throughout the body with progressive, innumerable small foci. The age groups most affected are infants and small children. Onset is usually sudden with the symptoms of high-grade fever, cyanosis, and breathlessness. Respiratory system examination reveals bilateral, fine crepitations. In addition, significant systemic findings are the presence of hepatosplenomegaly.

On the contrary, the other presentation of this alarming condition may be a slow, insidious onset with a lethargic child, low-grade persistent fever, and sick looking with a loss of weight and appetite.

Miliary TB may spread to the brain and meninges resulting in TB meningitis.

Tuberculosis: Clinical Features

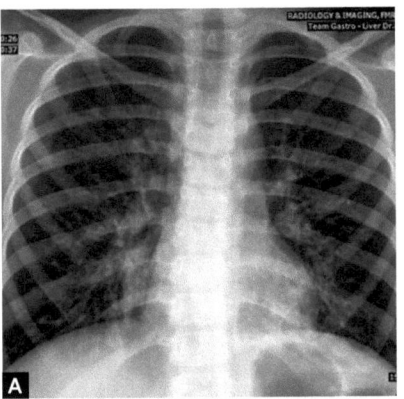
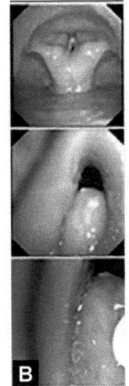
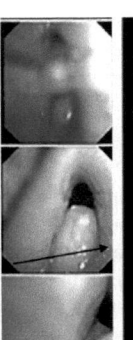
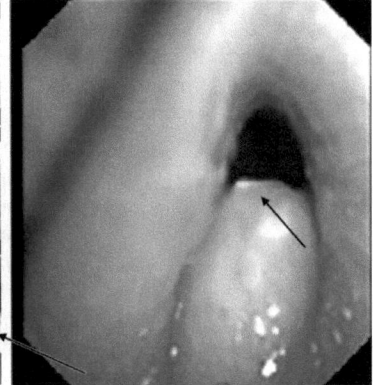
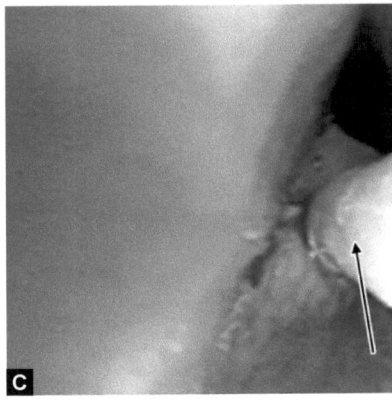

FIG. 1: A, A 10-year-old child diagnosed with human immunodeficiency virus with Kaposi's sarcoma with persistent fever, lethargy, and poor oral intake of 2 weeks duration; **B,** Flexible bronchoscopy revealed a mass at the entry of the left main bronchus with a yellow colored tip (caseating mass of lymph nodes); and **C,** Transbronchial needle aspiration of the mass was done *(For color version, see Plate 1)*

Pleural Effusion

Pleural effusion may result from primary complex in young persons. The patient may have respiratory distress and breathlessness. Fever is commonly present.[4] On the contrary, the patient may appear to be quite comfortable despite a massive pleural effusion.

Diagnosis

Following important points help in the diagnosis of pulmonary TB:
- Clinical features
- Presence of TB contact in family or neighborhood
- Positive tuberculin skin test (TST)
- Radiological features
- Demonstration of possible acid-fast bacilli (AFB) remains the gold standard for diagnosis, but may not always be present.

Specimen Collection

Specimens to be collected for the diagnosis of pulmonary TB are sputum, gastric lavage, bronchoalveolar lavage collected by flexible bronchoscopy, and pleural fluid.

Laboratory Tests

Tables 2 and 3 list the site-specific investigations to be done in a case of pulmonary TB.

LATENT TUBERCULOSIS

Latent tuberculosis infection (LTBI) occurs when there is a persistent immune response to stimulation by *Mycobacterium tuberculosis* antigens without any evidence of clinically manifested active TB. Almost a third of the world's population has LTBI, and have a risk of developing TB later, a process called as "TB reactivation".[5]

Table 2: Diagnostic investigations for pulmonary tuberculosis

Suspected site of disease	Possible imaging techniques	Specimen	Routine test	Additional tests
Pulmonary (adult)	• X-ray • Lung ultrasound	• Three respiratory samples—preferably spontaneously produced, deep cough sputum samples, otherwise induced sputum or bronchoscopy and lavage • Preferably one early morning sample	• Microscopy • Culture • Histology	• Cartridge-based nucleic acid amplification test (CBNAAT)
Pulmonary (young people aged 16–17 years)	• X-ray • Computed tomography thorax	• Three respiratory samples—preferably spontaneously produced, deep cough sputum samples, otherwise induced sputum or gastric lavage • Preferably one early morning sample	• Microscopy • Culture • Histology	• CBNAAT
Pulmonary (children aged 15 years or younger)	• X-ray • Computed tomography thorax	• Three respiratory samples: preferably spontaneously produced, deep cough sputum samples, otherwise induced sputum or gastric lavage • Preferably one early morning sample	• Microscopy • Culture • Histology • CBNAAT (one per specimen type)	• Interferon-γ release assay and/or tuberculin skin test (with expert input)

Table 3: Site-specific investigations for pleural tuberculosis

Suspected site of disease	Possible imaging techniques	Specimen	Routine test	Additional tests on primary specimen
Pleural	• X-ray • Bronchoscopy	• Three respiratory samples: preferably spontaneously produced, deep cough sputum samples, otherwise induced sputum or gastric lavage • Preferably one early morning sample • Pleural biopsy	• Microscopy • Culture • Histology • Cartridge-based nucleic acid amplification test	–
		• Pleural fluid	–	Adenosine deaminase assay

Diagnosis of Latent Tuberculosis Infection

The traditional method of diagnosing LTBI is the TST. However, newer diagnostic tests are now available commercially, e.g., QuantiFeron®-TB Gold In-Tube (QFT-IT) and the T-Spot, TB.

TUBERCULOUS LYMPHADENITIS

Tuberculous lymphadenitis is the most common form of extrapulmonary TB in children and is usually due to *M. tuberculosis*. One or more lymph nodes may be affected. The affected lymph nodes may be a localized group (regional adenopathy) or at multiple sites. These may be unilateral or bilateral.

Clinical Features

Tuberculous lymphadenitis most frequently involves the cervical lymph nodes followed by mediastinal, axillary, mesenteric, porta hepatis, perihepatic, and inguinal lymph nodes (Table 4). Symptoms usually develop gradually and insidiously.[6-8] The three characteristic features of tuberculous lymphadenitis are:
1. Affection of multiple nodes
2. Matting
3. Caseation.

Lymph nodes affected by TB are usually nontender, hence the terminology—"cold abscess".

NEUROTUBERCULOSIS

Tuberculous involvement of the brain and spinal cord is more common in children below 5 years of age.

Clinical Picture of Central Nervous System Tuberculosis

Tuberculous meningitis (TBM) is the most common type of neurotuberculosis in our country.[9] Different stages of CNS tuberculosis can be differentiated on the basis of clinical features as follows:[10]
- Stage I (early): Conscious, nonspecific symptoms without any neurological symptoms
- Stage II (intermediate): Signs of meningeal irritation are present, with or without affection of the sensorium, with or without minor neurological deficits like cranial nerve palsy or limb paresis
- Stage III (advanced): Severe clouding of the sensorium, convulsions and focal neurological deficits, involuntary movements.

Laboratory Diagnosis

This is based on the findings in the cerebrospinal fluid (CSF). But, these tests are neither sensitive nor specific (Table 5).

Table 4: Site-specific investigations for lymph node tuberculosis				
Suspected site of disease	Possible imaging techniques	Specimen	Routine test	Additional tests on primary specimen
Lymph node (including intrathoracic mediastinal adenopathy)	• Ultrasound • Computed tomography • Magnetic resonance imaging	Biopsy	• Microscopy • Culture • Histology	Cartridge-based nucleic acid amplification test
		Aspirate	• Microscopy • Culture • Cytology	

Table 5: Site-specific investigations for central nervous system tuberculosis				
Suspected site of disease	Possible imaging techniques	Specimen	Routine test	Additional tests on primary specimen
Central nervous system	• CT • MRI	Biopsy of suspected tuberculoma	• Microscopy • Culture • Histology	• CBNAAT
		Cerebrospinal fluid	• Microscopy • Culture • Cytology • CBNAAT	• Adenosine deaminase assay
Meningeal	• CT • MRI	Cerebrospinal fluid	• Microscopy • Culture • Cytology • CBNAAT	• Nucleic acid amplification test • Adenosine deaminase assay

CT, computed tomography; MRI, magnetic resonance imaging; CBNAAT, cartridge-based nucleic acid amplification test.

Molecular Diagnostic Tests

Detection of *M. tuberculosis* antigens and antibodies in the CSF has no value.[11]

Recent data shows that commercial nucleic acid amplification tests for the diagnosis of TBM show a combined average sensitivity of 56% and specificity of 98%. Hence, due to the high specificity, a positive commercial nucleic acid amplification tests is regarded as a definite test in cases of suspected TBM. It is of particular value in those patients who have already received TB treatment.[12]

Radiological Evidence

Radiology has an established role in the diagnosis of CNS tuberculosis. Hydrocephalus and basal meningeal enhancement are the most common findings.

Computed Tomography Findings in Tuberculous Meningitis

Combination of infarcts, hydrocephalus, and basal meningeal enhancement has a 100% specificity in the diagnosis of TBM. Basal meningeal enhancement is the most sensitive finding.[13]

Magnetic Resonance Imaging in Tuberculous Meningitis

Magnetic resonance imaging (MRI) is very useful in the detection of abnormalities like meningeal enhancement, infarcts and tuberculomas especially in the area of the brain stem. In patients with coinfection of HIV and TBM, hydrocephalus and basal meningeal enhancement are not very frequently seen. The positive findings in such cases are infarcts, gyral enhancement, and mass lesions. Cerebral atrophy is also commonly present.[14]

Spinal TB is diagnosed by CSF examination and MRI of the spine.[15] One should actively rule out TB elsewhere in the body, especially in all cases of TBM.

Parenchymal Neurotuberculosis

Parenchymal tuberculous affection results in the formation of a tuberculoma or tuberculous granuloma. Tuberculoma usually occurs in solid organs.

Clinical Features

The clinical presentation is determined by the size and location of the tuberculoma as well as the concurrent absence or presence of meningitis. The child usually presents with seizures without any meningeal signs and without any evidence of TB elsewhere in the body. If the location of the neurotuberculoma is infratentorial then the child will present with features of raised intracranial tension.

ABDOMINAL TUBERCULOSIS[16]

Clinical Features

Usually the symptoms are vague and non-specific. In children peritoneum and abdominal lymph nodes are more commonly involved as compared to the intestine per se. Contiguous extension is common, especially tuberculous salpingitis and TB of the spine.

Peritoneal Tuberculosis

The presenting features of this type of TB are abdominal distension and ascites. Constitutional symptoms like fever and night sweats may be present. Abdominal examination reveals a diffuse tenderness with a doughy feeling. Enlarged mesenteric lymph nodes may be the other presentation.

Small Intestinal and Ileocecal Tuberculosis

Older children and adults are more commonly affected. The various types are:
- Ulcerative: Presenting with chronic diarrhea and features of malabsorption
- Stricturous: May present with subacute intestinal obstruction
- Hypertrophic: May also present with the earlier feature as well as a vague lump in the abdomen. Involvement of other sites like colorectal and anal areas is rare. In disseminated disease, spleen, pancreas, and the hepatobiliary region can be involved.[17]

Diagnosis of Abdominal Tuberculosis

Diagnosis is achieved by demonstration of the AFB.

The following samples can be tested (Table 6):
- Ascitic fluid: The yield is usually low for smear[18,19] as well as for culture.[20] However, if the sample is concentrated, the yield of culture can be increased by approximately 80%
- Fine-needle aspiration cytology: Fine-needle aspiration cytology from an intra-abdominal mass can give a quick diagnosis. Mass could either be a lymph node mass, rolled up omentum or intestines. Ultrasound and computed tomography (CT)-guided aspiration can be done if the mass is deep-seated. This sample can further be tested for smear, culture or histopathology[20]
- Biopsy: Biopsy material can be obtained by upper or lower gastrointestinal endoscopy, peritoneal biopsy, laparoscopy, peritoneoscopy, laparotomy, liver biopsy, and splenic aspirate.
- Gastric aspirate
- Stool
- Sputum
- Urine.

Other Investigations

Other tests to prove the diagnosis of TB are Mantoux test, chest X-ray, family screening, plain X-ray abdomen, abdominal ultrasound, percutaneous fistulogram, barium meal and follow through, and a barium enema.

Enzyme-linked immunosorbent assay tests for antigens and antibodies are not recommended for the diagnosis. Polymerase chain reaction (PCR) and certain newer seromarkers such as C-X-C motif chemokine IP-10 (CXCL-10) are being investigated for the diagnosis.[21,22]

GENITOURINARY TUBERCULOSIS

Genitourinary tuberculosis (GUTB) often presents insidiously and with nonspecific complaints. This very often leads to the diagnosis being missed or delayed. The risk is of a rapid progression to a nonfunctioning kidney. Investigations which are helpful in the diagnosis of GUTB are given in table 7.[23]

SKELETAL TUBERCULOSIS

Tuberculous arthritis usually involves only one joint. Although any joint may be involved, the hips and knees are affected most commonly, followed by the ankle, elbow, wrist, and shoulder.[24] Pain may precede radiographic changes by weeks to months. Tubercular osteomyelitis is often diagnosed late, as the onset is insidious and the acute symptoms of pyogenic osteomyelitis are generally not present (Table 8).

Table 6: Site-specific investigations for gastrointestinal tuberculosis				
Suspected site of disease	Possible imaging techniques	Specimen	Routine test	Additional tests on primary specimen
Gastrointestinal	• Ultrasound • Computed tomography • Laparoscopy	• Biopsy of omentum • Biopsy of bowel • Biopsy of liver	• Microscopy • Culture • Histology	–
		• Ascitic fluid	• Microscopy • Culture • Cytology	• Cartridge-based nucleic acid amplification test • Adenosine deaminase assay

Table 7: Site-specific investigations for genitourinary tuberculosis				
Suspected site of disease	Possible imaging techniques	Specimen	Routine test	Additional tests on primary specimen
Genitourinary	• Ultrasound • Intravenous urography • Laparoscopy	• Early morning urine	• Culture	–
		• Biopsy from site of disease, such as endometrial curettings or renal biopsy	• Microscopy • Culture • Histology	–

Table 8: Site-specific investigations for bone and joint tuberculosis

Suspected site of disease	Possible imaging techniques	Specimen	Routine test	Additional test on primary specimen
Bone or joint tuberculosis	• X-ray • Computed tomography • Magnetic resonance imaging	• Biopsy or aspirate of paraspinal abscess • Biopsy of joint • Aspiration of joint fluid	• Culture • Cartridge-based nucleic acid amplification test	–

DISSEMINATED TUBERCULOSIS

Disseminated TB or miliary TB is a potentially lethal condition and often goes undetected due to the nonspecific symptoms. An underlying immune deficiency or HIV status should always be investigated. Table 9 lists the investigations, which help in the diagnosis of this condition.[25] In addition, evaluation of the fundus should be done.

LOCALIZED TUBERCULOSIS

Localized tuberculous abscess can be evaluated in table 10.

HUMAN IMMUNODEFICIENCY VIRUS AND TUBERCULOSIS

Recent data suggests that HIV infection is probably one of the most important factors leading to increased incidence of TB in adults as well as in the children.[26]

Two mechanisms serve to lead to an increased incidence of TB in patients infected with HIV:

1. Individuals coinfected with HIV-TB can transmit the *Mycobacterium tuberculosis* infection to others, thus putting them at high risk for developing significant disease including drug-resistant TB

Table 9: Site-specific investigations for disseminated tuberculosis

Suspected site of disease	Possible imaging techniques	Specimen	Routine test	Additional tests on primary specimen
Disseminated	• Computed tomography of the thorax and head • Magnetic resonance imaging • Ultrasound of the abdomen	• Biopsy of site of disease, including lung, liver, and bone marrow	• Microscopy • Culture • Histology	• Additional tests appropriate to site • Cartridge-based nucleic acid amplification test
		• Aspirate bone marrow • Bronchial wash • Cerebrospinal fluid	• Microscopy (if sample available) • Culture • Cytology	
		• Blood	• Culture	

Table 10: Site-specific investigations for localized tuberculous abscess

Suspected site of disease	Possible imaging techniques	Specimen	Routine test	Additional tests on primary specimen
Abscess outside of the lymph nodes	Ultrasound or other appropriate imaging	Aspirate	• Microscopy • Culture • Cytology	Cartridge-based nucleic acid amplification test
		Biopsy	• Microscopy • Culture • Histology	

2. Individuals of populations with a high incidence of HIV infection are at higher risk of developing HIV and subsequently more prone to developing TB.

There is no difference in the clinical features of TB in HIV-infected children, however, as mentioned before they are at a higher risk of developing more severe and disseminated disease.[27]

CONCLUSION

Diagnosis of childhood tuberculosis continues to remain a challenge, especially in immunocompromised and those with HIV co-infection. The spectrum of the disease may range from a latent or an asymptomatic presentation to a rapidly progressive disseminated or miliary TB.

This review sums up the clinical, radiological, and bacteriological approaches to diagnose the diverse presentations of TB infection and disease in children.

Fever which is low grade and intermittent, weight loss or failure to thrive, and cough persisting for more than 2 weeks remain the most useful symptoms for diagnosing pulmonary tuberculosis. Extrapulmonary TB, which is not so uncommon, would present with additional specific symptoms or signs. Index of suspicion should be high in the evaluation of certain groups of patients, since they may not have a typical presentation. These patients are children below 5 years, unvaccinated children, poor nutritional status, contact history of pulmonary TB, and those on immunosuppressive drugs. Evidence of an adult TB index case is clue for diagnosis of childhood TB in low-endemic countries.

Although Mantoux test remains in the forefront of laboratory tests, other investigations, relevant to system affected should be performed. Bacteriological confirmation should be aggressively sought and fluids and tissues obtained whenever possible and sent for CBNAAT, culture for mycobacteria, and drug sensitivity. Chest radiographs provide important information in many patients and advanced imaging can be applied in case of (and should be restricted to) inconclusive diagnosis.

Continuous assessment and evaluation of the patient, along with appropriate investigations in suspected cases would definitely march us towards a TB free India.

REFERENCES

1. Comstock GW, Livesay VT, Woolpert SF. The prognosis of a positive tuberculin reaction in childhood and adolescence. Am J Epidemiol. 1974;99(2):131-8.
2. Miller FJ, Seale RM, Taylor MD. Tuberculosis in children. Boston: Little Brown & Co; 1963.
3. Mukherjee A, Lodha R, Kabra SK. Changing trends in childhood tuberculosis. Indian J Pediatr. 2011;78(3):328-33.
4. Seth V, Kabra SK. Pulmonary tuberculosis. In: Seth V, Kabra SK (Eds). Essentials of Tuberculosis in Children, 4th edition. New Delhi: Jaypee Brothers Medical Publishers (P) Ltd; 2011. pp.101-21.
5. World Health Organization (WHO). (2015). Guidelines on the management of latent tuberculosis infection. [online] Available from www.who.int/tb/publications/latent-tuberculosis-infection/en/. [Accessed March, 2017].
6. Mohapatra PR, Janmeja AK. Tuberculous lymphadenitis. J Assoc Physicians India. 2009;57:585-90.
7. Jones PG, Campbell PE. Tuberculous lymphadenitis in childhood: the significance of anonymous mycobacteria. Br J Surg. 1962;50:302-14.
8. Marais BJ, Donald PR. Tuberculous lymphadenitis. In: Seth V, Kabra SK (Eds). Essentials of Tuberculosis in Children, 4th edition. New Delhi: Jaypee Brothers Medical Publishers (P) Ltd; 2011. pp.122-7.
9. Udani PM. Pathology and pathogenesis. In: Seth V, Kabra SK (Eds). Essentials of Tuberculosis in Children, 4th edition. New Delhi: Jaypee Brothers Medical Publishers (P) Ltd; 2011. pp.150-60.
10. Seth V. Neurotuberculosis. In: Parthasarathy A, Menon PSN, Nair MKC, Kundu R (Eds). IAP Textbook of Pediatrics, 6th edition. New Delhi: Jaypee Brothers Medical Publishers (P) Ltd; 2016. pp.327-32.
11. Gupta BK, Bharat V, Bandyopadhyay D. Sensitivity, specificity, negative and positive predictive values of adenosine deaminase in patients of tubercular and nontubercular serosal effusion in India. J Clin Med Res. 2010;2(3):121-6.
12. Dayal R, Senthilkumar P, Katoch VM, Chauhan DS, Yadav NK. Diagnostic value of real time PCR for neurotuberculosis. Indian Pediatr. 2010;47(7):631-2.
13. Alva R, Alva P. A study of CT findings in children with neurotuberculosis. Int J Biomed Res. 2014;5(11):685-7.
14. Ahluwalia VV, Sagar GD, Singh TP, et al. MRI spectrum of CNS tuberculosis. JIACM. 2013;14(2):83-90.
15. Rasouli MR, Mirkoohi M, Vaccaro AR, et al. Spinal Tuberculosis: Diagnosis and Management. Asian Spine J. 2012;6(4):294-308.
16. Debi U, Ravisankar V, Prasad KK, et al. Abdominal tuberculosis of the gastrointestinal tract: Revisited. World J Gastroenterol. 2014;20(40):14831-40.
17. Rasheed S, Zinicola R, Watson D, et al. Intra-abdominal and gastrointestinal tuberculosis. Colorectal Dis. 2007;9(9):773-83.

18. Steingart KR, Henry M, Ng V, et al. Fluorescence versus conventional sputum smear microscopy for tuberculosis: a systematic review. Lancet Infect Dis. 2006;6(9):570-81.
19. Marais BJ, Brittle W, Painczyk K, et al. Use of light-emitting diode fluorescence microscopy to detect acid-fast bacilli in sputum. Clin Infect Dis. 2008;47(2):203-7.
20. Bemer P, Palicova F, Rüsch-Gerdes S, et al. Multicenter evaluation of fully automated BACTEC Mycobacteria Growth Indicator Tube 960 system for susceptibility testing of Mycobacterium tuberculosis. J Clin Microbiol. 2002;40(1):150-4.
21. Steingart KR, Henry M, Laal S, et al. A systematic review of commercial serological antibody detection tests for the diagnosis of extrapulmonary tuberculosis. Postgrad Med J. 2007;83(985):705-12.
22. Imazio M, Adler Y. Management of pericardial effusion. Eur Heart J. 2013;34:1186-97.
23. Merchant S, Bharati A, Merchant N. Tuberculosis of the genitourinary system-Urinary tract tuberculosis: Renal tuberculosis-Part I. Indian J Radiol Imaging. 2013;23(1):46-63.
24. Choi JA, Koh SH, Hong SH, et al. Rheumatoid arthritis and tuberculous arthritis: differentiating MRI features. AJR Am J Roentgenol. 2009;193(5):1347-53.
25. Sharma SK, Mohan A, Sharma A. Challenges in the diagnosis & treatment of miliary tuberculosis. Indian J Med Res. 2012;135(5):703-30.
26. World Health Organization (WHO). (2016). Tuberculosis and HIV. [online] Available from www.who.int/hiv/topics/tb/en/. [Accessed March, 2017].
27. Padmapriyadarsini C, Narendran G, Swaminathan S. Diagnosis and treatment of tuberculosis in HIV co-infected patients. Indian J Med Res. 2011;134(6):850-65.

CHAPTER 3

Laboratory and Molecular Diagnosis of Tuberculosis

Ajoy K Verma

INTRODUCTION

Tuberculosis (TB) is a comprehensive term that describes various clinical illnesses caused by *Mycobacterium tuberculosis*. In 1993, World Health Organization (WHO) had declared TB a major threat to public health worldwide, still its management continues to be a challenge for public health administrators in developing countries. Tuberculosis has been present in humans since Neolithic as well as pre-Columbian ages, mentioned in their literature and spotted even in the spines of Egyptian mummies from 3000–2400 BC. Tuberculosis spread fast during industrial revolution in the 17th and 18th centuries when people started living in crowded areas around the industrial hubs in developed countries. Similarly, in latter part of 19th and 20th century it has shifted from developed economies to developing world.[1]

Tuberculosis is an infectious disease caused by the bacillus *Mycobacterium tuberculosis*. It is chiefly known for its predilection for the lungs but can affect any part of the human body and is called as extrapulmonary TB. The disease mainly spreads through air when infected person releases the tubercle bacilli droplet in air while coughing and sneezing. It involves all groups of people like men and women, young children and old persons but more commonly observed in young adults of reproductive age group with more number of cases in men than women.[2]

SPECIMEN COLLECTION, STORAGE AND TRANSPORT FOR TUBERCULOSIS DIAGNOSIS

Samples are collected in a clean, sterile, clear, leak proof and watertight 50 mL plastic cups, McCartney bottle, or 50 mL falcon tubes.

Specimens

- Pulmonary specimens: Sputum, broncho-alveolar lavage (BAL), transbronchial biopsy, transtracheal biopsy, laryngeal swab and gastric aspirate
- Extrapulmonary specimens: Urine, pus, pus swab, bone marrow, blood, pleural fluid, cerebrospinal fluid, body fluids, biopsy materials, menstrual blood, fecal sample, or any other suspected materials.

Sputum Collection

The current national and international policy is collection and examination of two sputum smears for the diagnosis of pulmonary TB. In the two sputum examination, 1st sputum is collected in morning and 2nd on the spot. Morning specimen is considered as superior, since the mucociliary clearance of the lungs is lower during the night and the caliber of the bronchial tree is narrower.[3]

Gastric lavage samples are processed as soon as possible. If processing is to be done after a gap of more than 4 hours, it should be collected in a container having 100 mg sodium carbonate, so as to neutralize the acid.

Storage of Sputum Specimens

Check that the tube is tightly capped, properly labeled, and that the screening and/or subject ID on the tube and the requisition forms should match. Refrigerate specimens at 2–8°C until ready for transport to the laboratory. Refrigeration reduces the growth of contaminants in the specimen. If a refrigerator is not available, specimens should be placed in coolers with ice packs.

PROCESSING OF SAMPLES

Petroff's Method

In petroff's method, 4–5 mL of sputum mixes with equal the volume of 4% sodium hydroxide (NaOH) solution in a sterile McCartney bottle. The bottles are kept in shaking incubator at 37°C incubator for 20 minutes. Then centrifuge at 3,000 × g for 15 minutes. After centrifugation, supernatant fluid is discarded and pellet is mix well with residual 2–3 mL fluids for smear examination and culture.

N-acetyl-L-cysteine/ Sodium Hydroxide Method

Sputum samples are digested and decontaminated by N-acetyl-L-cysteine/NaOH (NALC-NaOH). Add equal volume of the NALC-NaOH in the specimen in a sterile 50 mL conical tube. Mix each specimen on the vortex until liquefied for 5–20 seconds. Let the specimen stand for 15 minutes, at room temperature. Fill each tube to the 50 mL mark with a 6.8 pH phosphate buffer after the 15 minute period of decontamination has finished. In a centrifuge, using safety cups, centrifuge each sample at 3,000 x g for 15 minutes. Decant supernatant into a splash-proof can containing concentrated disinfectant (Vesphene), leaving as little of the supernatant as possible without disturbing the sediment. Resuspend the sediment with phosphate buffer 1.5–2 mL and use this to inoculate media and prepare smear.

MICROSCOPY

Sputum microscopy is the most efficient, rapid, inexpensive and less labor intensive way of identifying sources of TB infection.

Ziehl-Neelsen Staining

Ziehl-Neelsen (ZN) staining is a method for detection acid-fast bacilli (AFB) through microscopic examination. If smear is properly prepared the number of bacilli seen in the smear is directly related to the number of bacilli present in per milliliter of sputum. The property of acid-fastness of mycobacteria is based on the presence of mycolic acid in their cell walls. Primary stain, i.e., carbol fuchsin binds cell wall mycolic acids. Intense decolorization does not release primary stain from the cell wall easily so AFBs keep the red color of fuchsin following acid treatment. Counterstain (methylene blue) provides contrasting background to improve visualization. Smear prepared by spreading the material carefully over an area equal to about 1–2 cm. The thickness of smear should be such that a newspaper held under the slide can be read through the smear. The smeared slide should be left to air dry at room temperature. After the air dry, fix the slide by passing them through a Bunsen burner or spirit flame three times in quick succession.[4]

Fluorescent Staining (Auramine O Stain)

In fluorescent stain, auramine binds cell wall mycolic acids which resist decolorization with strong acid and give AFB a fluorescent bright golden yellow color of auramine. Fluorescent stains are usually organic substances which absorb ultraviolet (UV) light and remit part of the energy as light of longer wavelength which can be observed through the eyepiece as fluorescence. When exposed to UV light, the fluorescent bacilli are perceived as brightly colored organisms against a dark background. The most important advantage of the fluorescence technique is that slides can be examined at a lower magnification, thus allowing the examination of a much larger area per unit of time. Fluorescence microscopy for sputum smear examination is recommended by the WHO for detection of AFB in high TB burden countries and has sensitivity 8–10% more in comparison to ZN staining.[5]

Light-emitting Diode Fluorescent Microscopy

Light-emitting diode (LED) technology allows the use of fluorescent microscopy with a much less expensive light source. It is recommended that conventional fluorescence microscopy be replaced by LED microscopy. Light-emitting diode fluorescent microscopy (LED-FM) has higher sensitivity 8–10% more and similar specificity as compared with ZN staining sputum smear microscopy in detecting sputum smear positive TB cases and is more efficient.[6]

CULTURE

Culture is more sensitive than smear microscopy for the detection of *M. tuberculosis* and can detect as low as 100 viable mycobacteria/mL in sample. Culture is used for diagnosis, surveillance, treatment failure, detection of drug resistance and species identification. It is an important diagnostic tool in detecting TB in human immunodeficiency virus (HIV)-positive patients where the bacillary load in sputum is less. In spite of many drawbacks, it is a gold standard method for detection of *Mycobacterium tuberculosis* complexes (MTBCs). In general, the sensitivity of culture is 80–85% with a specificity of approximately 98%.[7,8]

Culture in Solid Media

The media that allow abundant growth of *M. tuberculosis* are egg-enriched media with glycerol and asparagine [viz. Lowenstein-Jensen (LJ)] or agar-based media supplemented with bovine albumin (viz. Middlebrook 7H10 or 7H11). Culture increases the number of TB cases found, often by 30–50% and detects cases which are smear-negative. Since culture techniques detect fewer bacilli, the efficiency of diagnosing cases of failure at the end of treatment may improve considerably. Culture results interpreted as negative when no growth seen after 8 weeks of incubation or positive with actual number of colonies (1–100 colonies), positive (2+) when more than 100 discrete colonies and positive (3+) while there is confluent growth.

Culture in Liquid Media

The most commonly used liquid medium known to result in the better recovery and faster growth of mycobacteria is modified Middlebrook 7H9 broth. The common liquid media are Dubos medium, Middlebrook 7H9 broth, Proskauer and Beck's medium, Sula's medium, Sauton's medium. Liquid culture systems available are: BACTEC 460 (Becton Dickinson Microbiology Systems, Sparks, MD), mycobacteria growth indicator tube (MGIT) systems, VersaTrek system (Trek Diagnostic Systems, 982 Keynote Circle, Suite 6 Cleveland, OH USA 44131) and MB/BacT Alert® system (bioMérieux, France). Liquid culture systems have a sensitivity ranging from 81 to 85% and specificity in detecting mycobacteria 99.6–99.9%.

Mycobacteria Growth Indicator Tube 960 system (Becton Dickinson)

Recently, the BACTEC MGIT 960 system, a newly developed nonradiometric, fully automated, continuously monitoring system, was introduced as an alternative to the radiometric BACTEC 460 for growth and detection of mycobacteria. The results of several comparative studies show that BACTEC 960/MGIT is a suitable tool for the detection of *Mycobacterium tuberculosis* and other mycobacterial species. Chance of contamination of the culture is seen as 12.8% with solid media, 8.6% with MGIT 960 system, and 4.4% with the BACTEC 460 system.[9]

IDENTIFICATION OF CULTURE POSITIVE MYCOBACTERIA

Biochemical Identification of *Mycobacterium*

Identification of culture is important for proper diagnosis and management of patients. Mycobacterium is identified to species level by growth characteristic and various biochemical reactions. The growth character includes growth rate, pigment production, colony morphology. The biochemical test used for identification of mycobacterium species are niacin test, nitrate test, heat-stable catalase test, semiquantitative catalase test, tellurite reduction test, urease test, tween 80 hydrolysis, growth on MacConkey media without crystal violet, growth on 5% sodium chloride media and susceptibility to para-nitrobenzoic acid. Each test done along with positive and negative control. The standard strains commonly used during the test are *Mycobacterium tuberculosis* H37Rv, *Mycobacterium chelonae* ATCC 35752, *Mycobacterium abscessus* ATCC 19977 and *Mycobacterium fortuitum* ATCC 6841 or any other ATCC mycobacterial strains.[10]

Lateral Flow Assays

Mycobacterium culture grown in solid or liquid media is identified as MTBC by immunochromatographic method using lateral flow technique. In this method MTBC are detected by observing presence of control and test bands in a lateral flow device. This assay detects the presence of the MTBC-specific protein MPT64 in culture isolates. For detection approximately 10^5 colony forming unit (CFU)/mL, bacterial growth on solid or liquid medium is required. Test provides results in 15–30 minutes and compare favorably with other conventional phenotypic or molecular methods overall sensitivity of 98.6% and specificity of 97.9%.[11]

Line Probe Assays

Line probe assay method for nontuberculous mycobacteria (NTM) detection is based on polymerase chain reaction (PCR) amplification of 16S-23S deoxyribonucleic acid (DNA) spacer region and detected by hybridization of amplified product with oligonucleotide probes present over nitrocellulose membrane. The hybridized product produces colored lines that are used for identifying NTM. The nitrocellulose membrane also contains conjugate control (CC), internal control (IC) and genus control (GC) for ensuring the correct test procedure. This procedure enables detection of 27 different NTMs, along with MTBC within 5–6 hours whereas conventional method takes 4–6 weeks time. The recent review and meta-analysis of these tests showed that the pooled sensitivity is 85% (range, 36–100%) and specificity 97% (range, 54–100%).[12]

Polymerase Chain Reaction-restriction Enzyme Analysis

The PCR restriction enzyme analysis (PCR-REA) targeting *hsp65* gene is a standardized method for identification of species of mycobacterium. It involves amplification of extracted DNA followed by REA using BstE II and Hae III enzymes. For quality control of experiment each batch has to be tested with positive control, i.e. pure mycobacterial DNA of H37Rv and negative control with deionized water.[13]

Deoxyribonucleic Acid Sequencing

While DNA sequencing of variable genomic regions offers a rapid and accurate identification of mycobacteria, this method is not yet practical for use outside academic settings in most resource-poor countries. These assays are based on the amplification of one or more genes [16S ribosomal ribonucleic acid (rRNA) genes, *rpoB*, *gyrB*, *hsp65*, *secA1*, the gene encoding the 32-kDa protein, or the 16S–23S rRNA gene spacer].[14]

Identification of *Mycobacterium* by Deoxyribonucleic Acid Probes (Accuprobe™ System)

Nucleic acid hybridization tests are based on the ability of complementary nucleic acid strands to specifically align to form double-stranded complexes. The Accuprobe™ System uses a chemiluminescent labeled, single-stranded DNA probe that is complementary to the rRNA of the target organism. After the rRNA is released from the organism, the labeled DNA probe combines with the target organism's rRNA to form a DNA-RNA hybrid. The selection reagent allows for the differentiation of nonhybridized and hybridized probes. The labeled DNA-RNA hybrids are measured in the Gen-Probe luminometer. Nucleic acid probes provide the most rapid identification of mycobacteria.[15]

Gen-Probe Amplified Mycobacterium Tuberculosis Direct Test

This is used for detection of MTBCs rRNA from clinical samples. The *Mycobacterium tuberculosis* direct (MTD) test is a two part test in which amplification and detection take place in a single tube. Initially nucleic acids are

Table 1: Sensitivity of different commercially available molecular test for diagnosis of *Mycobacterium tuberculosis*[18]

Nucleic acid amplification test	Company	Sensitivity in range (%)		
		Smear +ve	Smear –ve	Overall
Amplicor PCR	Roche Molecular System	90–100	50–95.9	91.3–100
Amplified MTD	Gen-Probe Inc.	91.7–100	65.5–92.9	92.1–100
BD ProbeTec	Becton Dickinson	98.5–100	33.3–85.7	99.9–100
GenoType Direct	Hain Lifescience	85.7–94.6	33.3–65.4	99.6–100
LAMP	Eiken Chemical Co.	97.7	48.8	99

LAMP, loop-mediated isothermal amplification; MTD, *Mycobacterium tuberculosis* direct; PCR, polymerase chain reaction.

released from mycobacterial cell by sonication and heat is used to denature the nucleic acid and disrupts the secondary structure of the rRNA. The gene probe transcription-mediated amplification (TMA) method uses a constant 42°C and then amplifies a specific mycobacterial rRNA target by transcription of DNA intermediates resulting in multiple copies of rRNA amplification. MTBCs-specific sequences are then detected in rRNA amplicon using gene probe hybridization protection assay (HPA). The *Mycobacterium tuberculosis* hybridization reagent contains a single-stranded DNA probe with chemiluminescent label. This probe is complimentary to MTBC-specific sequences. When stable RNA-DNA hybrids are formed between the probe and the specific sequence, hybridized probe is selected and measured in Gen-Probe leader luminometer.[16]

Loop-mediated Isothermal Amplification Test[17]

It is latest WHO endorsed technique for direct detection of TB from patients' specimen in three steps procedure.
- Step 1: Approximately 60 μL sputum samples are transferred into lysis tube which is incubated at 90°C for 5 minutes to extract the DNA and kill the mycobacterium
- Step 2: Deoxyribonucleic acid (DNA) is multiplied into number of copies at 67°C temperature for 40 minutes in a heating block
- Step 3: Results are visually detected using UV light. It has sensitivity of 97.7% in smear and culture positive specimen and 48.8% in smear negative and culture positive specimens (Table 1).[18]

IMMUNOLOGICAL DIAGNOSIS OF TUBERCULOSIS

At present over 40 different types of serologic TB tests are available. These serological tests produce inconsistent and imprecise estimates of sensitivity and specificity. Recently, WHO strongly recommended that these commercial tests not be used for the diagnosis of pulmonary and extrapulmonary TB.

Interferon-gamma Release Assays

The recent introduction of interferon-gamma (IFNγ) release assays (IGRAs) has provided an alternative test for the diagnosis of latent tuberculosis infection (LTBI). Currently, two commercial assays are available, (1) the Quantiferon-TB assay (Cellestis Ltd., Carnegie, Victoria, Australia) and (2) the T-SPOT.TB assay (Oxford Immunotec, Oxford, United Kingdom). These tests measure the IFNγ release from T-cells after stimulation by *M. tuberculosis*-specific antigens using a peptide cocktail ESAT-6, CFP-10 and TB 7.7 (p-4) proteins via an enzyme-linked immunosorbent assay (ELISA) or an enzyme-linked immunospot (ELISPOT) assay. However, in the absence of a true gold standard, the reliable determination of sensitivity and specificity is not accurately predicted yet.[19]

DRUG SENSITIVITY TESTING METHODS

Drug susceptibility is done by solid, liquid and molecular methods. In solid method LJ media are used for susceptibility testing through 1% proportion, resistance ratio, and absolute concentration method.

- 1% proportion method: Mycobacterial strains are said to be resistant when 1% of bacilli is resistant to drugs and can be calculated by comparing the number of bacilli grown in drug-free media and drug containing media. For example, if drug-free media contains 100 colonies and in drug containing media more than one colony tested strains are resistant strains
- Absolute concentration method: Mycobacterium strains are tested against several concentrations of drugs, resistance is determined by the lowest concentration of drug that inhibits growth, is called as minimal inhibitory concentration (MIC) of the said strain
- The resistance ratio method: The test strains are compared with standard mycobacterium strain H37Rv. Strains are called resistant when growth is seen in test strains, whereas at the given concentration of drug, no growth is seen in standard mycobacterium strains.[20]

DRUG SUSCEPTIBILITY TESTING BY LIQUID CULTURE METHOD-MGIT 960

The BACTEC MGIT 960 system is used for sensitivity testing against the 1st and 2nd line of antituberculous drugs. The commonly tested 1st line antitubercular therapy (ATT) drugs are streptomycin (S), isoniazid (I), rifampicin (R), and ethambutol (E), called SIRE. Amongst the 2nd line drugs commonly tested drugs are kanamycin, amikacin, capreomycin, ethionamide, moxifloxacin, levofloxacin, ofloxacin, pyrazinamide (PZA), and clofazimine. It is a rapid and qualitative procedure for establishing susceptibility of *M. tuberculosis* against antituberculous drugs using critical test concentrations. Critical concentration used for susceptibility testing are S 1.0 µg/mL, I 0.1 µg/mL, R 1.0 µg/mL, E 5.0 µg/mL and PZA 100.0 µg/mL, amikacin 1.0 µg/mL, capreomycin 2.5 µg/mL, kanamycin 2.5 µg/mL, ofloxacin 2.0 µg/mL, moxifloxacin 1.0 µg/mL, ethionamide 5.0 µg/mL and para-aminosalicylic acid 4.0 µg/mL.[9]

MOLECULAR METHODS FOR DRUG SUSCEPTIBILITY TESTING

Line Probe Assay for Multi-drug Resistant-TB Diagnosis

The Genotype MTBDR plus assay is based on line probe assay (LPA) technology involving PCR amplification and binding of amplicons to specific oligonucleotide probes immobilized on a membrane strip. This is a test endorsed by WHO (2008). It is capable of the simultaneous detection of rifampin (RIF) resistance-associated mutations in the 81-bp core region of *rpoB* and the presence of isoniazid (INH) resistance-associated mutations in codon 315 of katG and mutations of *inhA* gene. The test has very high sensitivity and specificity more than 90% in smear positive specimens.[21]

GeneXpert MTB/RIF Diagnostic Test

The latest introduction in the field of TB diagnosis and primary marker of multidrug-resistant (MDR)-TB, i.e. rifampicin-resistant strains is known as Xpert MTB/RIF system. It is a fully automated system developed with the help of public-private partnership consisting of Cepheid, the Foundation for Innovative New Diagnostics, the National Institutes of Health and the Bill and Melinda Gates Foundation. It demonstrated sensitivities of 98.2% in smear-positive cases, 72.5% in smear-negative specimen and specificity 99.2% in patients without TB. In this system only manual step is on the level of sample collection and its dilution and decontamination procedure at room temperature for 15 minutes with the diluting fluid provided in diagnostic kit and rest of the complete analysis is accomplished by the GeneXpert instrument in 1 hour 50 minutes. The Xpert MTB/RIF is a cartridge-based automated diagnostic test to detect DNA sequences specific for *Mycobacterium tuberculosis* and rifampicin resistance by PCR. This assay targets the *rpoB* gene, which is critical for identifying mutations associated with rifampicin resistance.

5'GCACCAGCCAGCTGAGCCAATTCATG-GACCAGAACAACCCGCTGTCGGGGTT-GACCCACAAGCGCCGACTGTCGGCGCTG 3'

3'CGTGGTCGGTCGACTCGGT-TAAGTACCTGGTCTTGTTGGGCGA-CAGCCCCAACTGGGTGTTCGCGGCTGA-CAGCCGCGAC 5'

It provides results from unprocessed sputum samples in 90 minutes.[22]

NEW TECHNOLOGY FOR DETECTION OF TUBERCULOSIS

Urinary Lipoarabinomannan Antigen Detection

This is antigen-antibody based test and determined by detecting lipoarabinomannan (LAM) antigen by antigen capture ELISA.[23]

Volatile Markers

This test is based on the recognition of organic compound produced by mycobacterium during metabolism and detected by electronic nose.[24]

Bead-based Methods for Detection and Identification

Mycobacterium is detected by using immunomagnetic beads.[25]

Simplified Smart Flow Cytometry

Mycobacterium is detected by identifying antigen-specific cellular immune response through smart flow cytometry.[26]

CONCLUSION

Accurate and rapid laboratory diagnosis of TB is essential for administering effective treatment to patients as well as restoring quality of life. In this section, contemporary as well as future methodologies of diagnosis have been discussed. Basic concept and updates would certainly help the graduate and postgraduate students in better understanding the subject.

REFERENCES

1. World Health Organization (WHO). (2014). Global Tuberculosis Report 2014. [online] Available from apps.who.int/iris/bitstream/10665/137094/1/9789241564809_eng.pdf. [Accessed April, 2017].
2. Centers for Disease Control and Prevention (CDC). (2005). Guidelines for Preventing the Transmission of Mycobacterium tuberculosis in Health-Care Settings, 2005. [online] Available from www.cdc.gov/mmwr/pdf/rr/rr5417.pdf. [Accessed April, 2017].
3. World Health Organization (WHO). (2007). Reduction of number of smears for the diagnosis of pulmonary TB. [online] Available from www.who.int/tb/dots/laboratory/policy/en/index2.html. [Accessed April, 2017].
4. Frieden T. Toman's Tuberculosis Case detection, treatment, and monitoring—questions and answers, 2nd edition. Geneva: World Health Organization. 2004.
5. Steingart KR, Henry M, Ng V, et al. Fluorescence versus conventional sputum smear microscopy for tuberculosis: a systematic review. Lancet Infect Dis. 2006;6(9):570-81.
6. Bonnet M, Gagnidze L, Guerin PJ, et al. Evaluation of combined LED-fluorescence microscopy and bleach sedimentation for diagnosis of tuberculosis at peripheral health service level. PLoS One. 2011;6(5):e20175.
7. Diagnostic Standards and Classification of Tuberculosis in Adults and Children. This official statement of the American Thoracic Society and the Centers for Disease Control and Prevention was adopted by the ATS Board of Directors, July 1999. This statement was endorsed by the Council of the Infectious Disease Society of America, September 1999. Am J Respir Crit Care Med. 2000;161(4 Pt 1):1376-95.
8. Pfyffer G. Mycobacterium: general characteristics, laboratory detection, and staining procedures. In: Murray PR, Baron EJ, Jorgensen JH, Landry ML, Pfaller MA (Eds). Manual of Clinical Microbiology, 9th edition. Washington, DC: ASM Press; 2007. pp. 543-72.
9. Cruciani M, Scarparo C, Malena M, et al. Meta-analysis of BACTEC MGIT 960 and BACTEC 460 TB, with or without solid media, for detection of mycobacteria. J Clin Microbiol. 2004;42(5):2321-5.
10. Metchock BG, Nolte FS, Wallace RJ. Mycobacterium. In: Murray PR, Baron EJ, Pfaller MA, Tenover FC, Yolken RH (Eds). Manual of Clinical Microbiology, 7th edition. Washington, DC: ASM Press; 1999. pp. 399-437.
11. Park MY, Kim YJ, Hwang SH, et al. Evaluation of an immunochromatographic assay kit for rapid identification of Mycobacterium tuberculosis complex in clinical isolates. J Clin Microbiol. 2009;47(2):481-4.
12. Padilla E, González V, Manterola JM, et al. Comparative evaluation of the new version of the INNO-LiPA Mycobacteria and GenoType Mycobacterium assays for identification of Mycobacterium species from MB/BacT liquid cultures artificially inoculated with mycobacterial strains. J Clin Microbiol. 2004;42(7):3083-8.
13. Telenti A, Marchesi F, Balz M, et al. Rapid identification of mycobacteria to the species level by polymerase chain

13. reaction and restriction enzyme analysis. J Clin Microbiol. 1993;31(2):175-8.
14. Patel JB, Leonard DG, Pan X, et al. Sequence-based identification of Mycobacterium species using the MicroSeq 500 16S rDNA bacterial identification system. J Clin Microbiol. 2000;38(1):246-51.
15. Zheng X, Pang M, Engler HD, et al. Rapid detection of Mycobacterium tuberculosis in contaminated BACTEC 12B broth cultures by testing with Amplified Mycobacterium Tuberculosis Direct Test. J Clin Microbiol. 2001;39(10):3718-20.
16. Ling DI, Flores LL, Riley LW, et al. Commercial nucleic-acid amplification tests for diagnosis of pulmonary tuberculosis in respiratory specimens: meta-analysis and meta-regression. PLoS One. 2008;3(2):e1536.
17. Boehme CC, Nabeta P, Henostroza G, et al. Operational feasibility of using loop-mediated isothermal amplification for diagnosis of pulmonary tuberculosis in microscopy centers of developing countries. J Clin Microbiol. 2007;45(6):1936-40.
18. Parsons LM, Somoskövi Á, Gutierrez C, et al. Laboratory diagnosis of tuberculosis in resource-poor countries: challenges and opportunities. Clin Microbiol Rev. 2011; 24(2):314-50.
19. Lalvani A, Richeldi L, Kunst H. Interferon gamma assays for tuberculosis. Lancet Infect Dis. 2005;5:322-4.
20. Ministry of Health and Family Welfare. (2005). Technical and Operational Guidelines for Tuberculosis Control. [online] Available from health.bih.nic.in/Docs/Guidelines/Guidelines-TB-Control.pdf. [Accessed April, 2017].
21. World Health Organization (WHO). (2008). Molecular line probe assays for rapid screening of patients at risk of multidrug-resistant tuberculosis (MDR-TB). [online] Available from www.who.int/tb/features_archive/policy_statement.pdf. [Accessed April, 2017].
22. World Health Organization (WHO). (2010). Roadmap for rolling out Xpert MTB/RIF for rapid diagnosis of TB and MDR-TB. [online] Available from www.who.int/entity/tb/laboratory/roadmap_xpert_mtb_rif rev23dec2010.pdf. [Accessed April, 2017].
23. Lawn SD, Edwards DJ, Kranzer K, et al. Urine lipoarabinomannan assay for tuberculosis screening before antiretroviral therapy: diagnostic yield and association with immune reconstitution disease. AIDS. 2009;23(14):1875-80.
24. Phillips M, Cataneo RN, Condos R, et al. Volatile biomarkers of pulmonary tuberculosis in the breath. Tuberculosis (Edinb). 2007;87(1):44-52.
25. Lee H, Yoon TJ, Weissleder R. Ultrasensitive detection of bacteria using core-shell nanoparticles and an NMR-filter system. Angew Chem Int Ed Engl. 2009;48(31):5657-60.
26. Janossy G. The changing pattern of "smart" flow cytometry (S-FC) to assist the cost-effective diagnosis of HIV, tuberculosis, and leukemias in resource-restricted conditions. Biotechnol J. 2008;3(1):32-42.

CHAPTER 4

Pathology Relevant to Radiologist

Saumya Shukla, Nuzhat Husain

INTRODUCTION

The pathology of tuberculosis (TB) like most infectious diseases is the consequence of the interplay between the bacillus and the immunity of the host.[1] Tuberculosis is classified into various clinical-pathological subtypes based on the location, site, and the sequence of events following the first exposure.[2]

CLASSIFICATION

- Classification based on location:
  - Pulmonary TB
  - Extrapulmonary TB
  - Disseminated TB.
- Classification based on the sequence of events following the first exposure to the bacillus:
  - Primary TB
  - Progressive primary TB
  - Postprimary TB.

Primary TB occurs in individuals with no previous exposure to *Mycobacterium tuberculosis* (MTB). In primary TB, there is a unit comprising of a focus of primary TB and infected draining lymph nodes. This unit is known as primary complex of Ranke.[2-4]

Progressive primary TB occurs in individuals with poor immune status. In infants, children, elderly, and individuals with low immunity the primary lesions progress giving rise to progressive primary TB.[2,5]

Postprimary TB is a disease of the adults. This occurs due to exogenous reinfection or endogenous reactivation in a person who has been previously infected by the organism but has retained substantial acquired immunity.[2,5]

Disseminated TB occurs due to hematogenous spread of bacilli from a source of active infection. This is generally characterized by tubercles involving the visceral organs and surfaces. These characteristic lesions are small, discrete nodules, grey to yellow in color. The most commonly affected organs are lung, liver, spleen, and bone marrow. Pleural and pericardial involvement is also common. The histology of the miliary tubercles has the classical features.[2,3,5]

HISTOPATHOLOGY OF TUBERCULOSIS

The histopathological hallmark of TB is the granuloma. The characteristic lesion is a confluent, necrotizing epithelioid cell granuloma along with multinucleated Langhans giant cell.[4,6] The exudative lesions are the "soft granulomas" that are loose collection of epithelioid histiocytes along with macrophages, plasma cells, neutrophils, and lymphocytes. There is minimal fibroblastic proliferation around these lesions (Fig. 1). These lesions are likely to contain acid-fast bacilli (AFB) demonstrated in histopathological sections (Fig. 2).[6,7] The proliferative lesions or the "hard granulomas" are well-demarcated, circumscribed aggregates of epithelioid histiocytes surrounded by marked fibroblastic proliferation with Langhans giant cell almost pathognomonic of TB composed of nuclei arranged around the periphery like a "horseshoe" with a clear central cytoplasmic area (Fig. 3). Acid-fast bacilli is less readily demonstrated.[6,7]

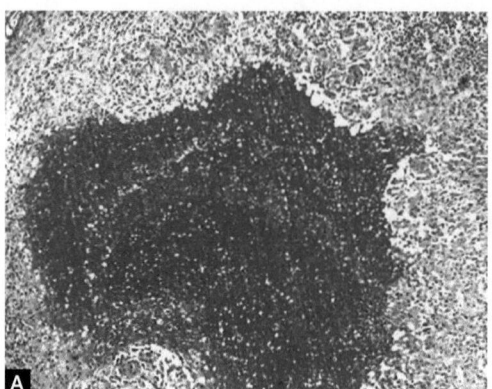 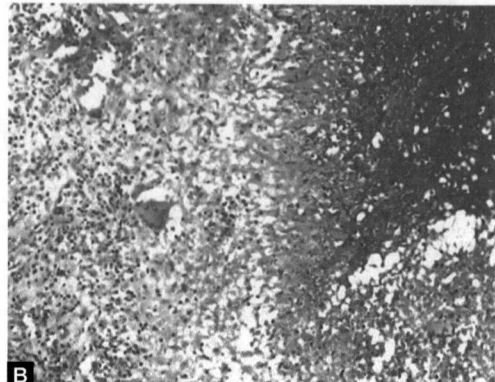

FIG. 1: Photomicrograph depicting the classical "soft granuloma" with central area of caseous necrosis surrounded by loose aggregates of epithelioid cells with Langhans type of giant cell and minimal lymphocytic cuffing (A = H&E 50x, B = H&E 100x) *(For color version, see Plate 1)*

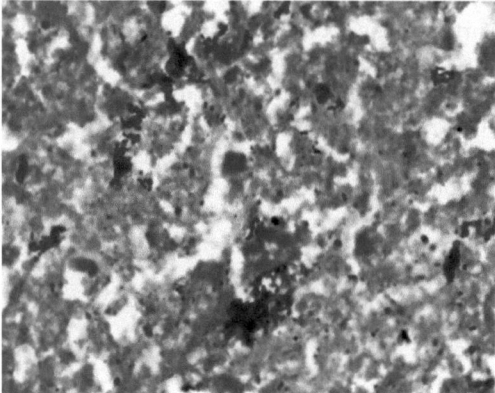

FIG. 2: Ziehl-Neelsen staining: Multiple acid-fast bacilli identified singly and in clusters within the necrotic debris (1,000x) *(For color version, see Plate 2)*

The "cheese-like" caseous necrosis of TB occurs due to permanent tissue destruction that occurs due to low pH, low oxygen tension, and accumulation of fatty acids. This phenomenon also inhibits the replication of MTB. The caseous focus may get encapsulated by fibrous tissue to form a fibrocaseous granuloma or may become organized to form a fibrous scar which is often calcified or ossified. Proteolytic enzymes derived from the neutrophils and macrophages within the granuloma may lead to liquefaction of the caseous material with cavitation.[2,7,8] Rarely tubercular lesions present as pseudotumors called "tuberculomas". These are organized granulomas with extensive fibroblastic proliferation mistaken for malignancy.[2]

PULMONARY TUBERCULOSIS

Pulmonary TB is the most common form of infection caused by MTB. Miliary TB invariably affects both the lungs bilaterally.[9] The organism enters the lungs from the inhalation of airborne droplets which have been coughed out by sputum positive individuals who have either not received any treatment or has received incomplete treatment. Initially the organism forms a localized infection in the peripheral region of the lung.[10]

Primary Pulmonary Tuberculosis

The primary complex is composed of a parenchymal lesion in the lung enlarged draining lymph nodes (Fig. 4). The location of the parenchymal lesion is usually located in the middle part of the lung. On histopathological examination, granulomatous inflammation composed of epithelioid cells and Langhans giant cells is evident. Caseous necrosis may or may not be present. The surrounding lung parenchyma shows a fibrotic reaction. The primary complex may heal or progress further. Healing of primary lung lesions occurs in about 85% cases. The caseous focus is completely replaced by reticulin and collagen which is followed by hyalinization and calcification.[7,8,9,11]

Pathology Relevant to Radiologist

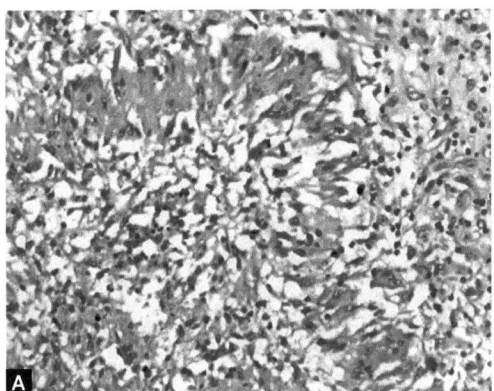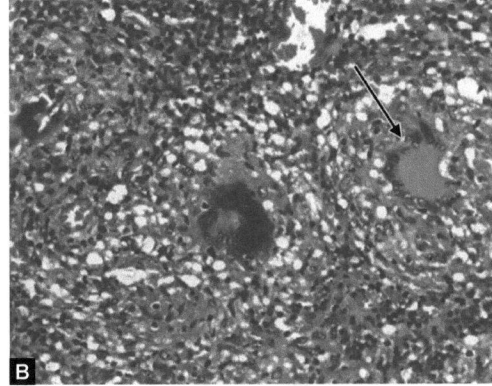

FIG. 3: A, The granuloma of tuberculosis with slipper-shaped epithelioid histiocytes; **B,** Multinucleated Langhans giant cell (arrow) having peripherally arranged nuclei with central clear cytoplasmic area (A = H&E 200x, B = H&E 200x) *(For color version, see Plate 2)*

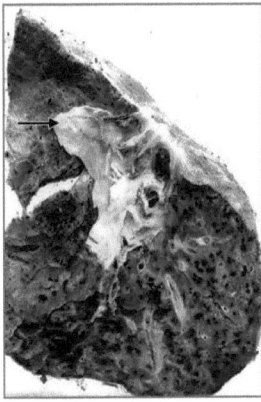

FIG. 4: Ghon's complex: Gross specimen of the lung with a minute parenchymal lesion and hilar lymphadenopathy (arrow) *(For color version, see Plate 2)*

Progressive and Postprimary Pulmonary Tuberculosis

Progressive primary TB occurs in the lung following primary TB. This is generally characterized by extension of the primary focus with cavitation or bronchopneumonia.[11-13]

The lesions of postprimary pulmonary TB have been classified into:
- Pulmonary lesions
    - Lobular pneumonia
    - Nodular TB
    - Fibrocaseous TB
    - Tuberculous bronchopneumonia
- Bronchial lesions
- Whole lung TB
- Miliary TB
- Pleural lesions.

Pulmonary Lesions

The earliest pulmonary lesion is lobular pneumonia involving the apical and subapical regions. Nodular lesions, also known as tuberculomas or coin lesions are well-defined localized areas of TB. The nodules are white to yellow in color and vary in consistency from soft form to hard. The soft lesions are generally necrotic whereas the firm to hard lesions are fibrotic or calcified. These lesions have the classical hallmark features of TB on histology. It is believed that the small nodules give rise to the larger ones which in turn form fibrocaseous lesions. Fibrocaseous TB commonly affects the apical and posterior segments of the upper lobe. The hallmark of TB that includes caseation, consolidation, liquefaction, and fibrosis are all well evident in fibrocaseous TB. One or more cavities of varying sizes are seen and the wall of the cavity is irregular and lined by tuberculous granulation tissue. The surrounding lung parenchyma is fibrotic (Fig. 5). These cavities may communicate with bronchi. The caseous necrosis may also soften the wall of the pulmonary artery leading formation of aneurysms that cause hemoptysis. Acid-fast bacilli is generally present especially in the cavitatory lesions. The healing of these lesions leads to fibrosis, scarring, and calcification.[9,10,12,13]

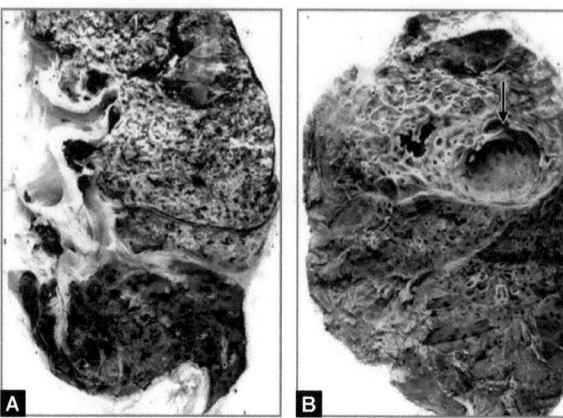

FIG. 5: Fibrocaseous tuberculosis: Gross specimen of the lung showing numerous yellow gray caseating nodules with a cavity (arrow) with an irregular wall and pleural thickening *(For color version, see Plate 2)*

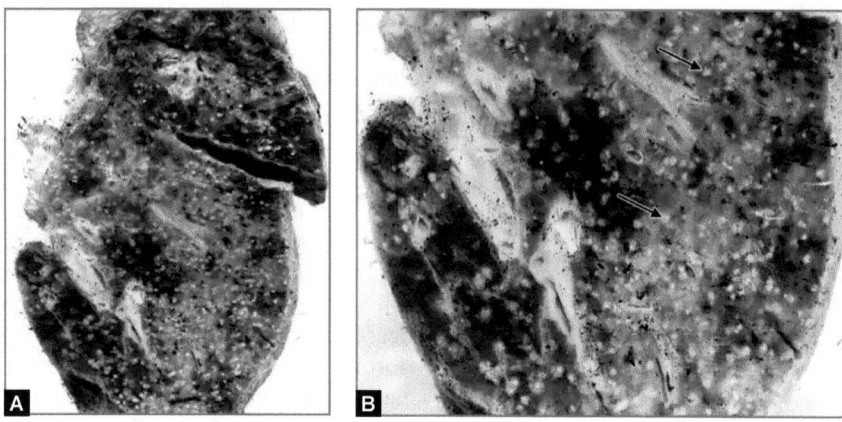

FIG. 6: Miliary tuberculosis: Gross specimen of the lung with numerous small, discrete yellow gray nodules involving the entire lung *(For color version, see Plate 3)*

Bronchial Lesions

The earliest microscopic finding of bronchial TB is small epithelioid cell granulomas with or without caseation in the subepithelial region and region of mucous glands. In advanced stages, these lesions extend to the adventitia. Rupture of these subepithelial foci leads to ulceration and destruction of the bronchial wall. Healing occurs by fibrosis and may produce stenosis.[11]

Miliary Tuberculosis

Miliary TB occurs due to hematogenous spread of virulent bacilli. This is generally characterized by tubercles involving the visceral organs and organ surfaces (Fig. 6). In most of the cases the immunity of the host is compromised.[13,14]

Whole Lung Tuberculosis

Whole lung TB is extremely rare and is associated with high mortality. This generally occurs due to hematogenous dissemination or diffuse bronchogenic spread.[13]

Pleural Lesions

Pleural and subpleural granulomas are seen both on the visceral and parietal surfaces. The examination of the pleural fluid reveals a predominance of lymphocytes. The healing occurs by focal or diffuse fibrosis.[14-17]

LYMPH NODE TUBERCULOSIS

Tubercular lymphadenitis may occur during primary tubercular infection or as a result of reactivation of a dormant focus or by direct extension from contiguous spread. Tubercular lymphadenitis most frequently involves the cervical lymph nodes followed in frequency by mediastinal, axillary, mesenteric, hepatic, portal, peripancreatic, and inguinal lymph nodes.[18-20]

The histopathological features are characterized by replacement of nodal architecture with confluent epithelioid granulomas, Langhans giant cells with or without caseous necrosis (Fig. 7).[12]

ABDOMINAL TUBERCULOSIS

The route of infection for abdominal TB include: (i) swallowing of infected sputum, (ii) hematogenous spread, (iii) ingestion of contaminated milk and milk products, (iv) contiguous spread from other organs, and (v) tuberculous peritonitis in patients undergoing long-term dialysis.[21]

Gastrointestinal TB affects the ileocecal region, jejunum/ileum, colon, anorectum, stomach, appendix, duodenum, and esophagus. The primary form of gastrointestinal TB is extremely rare and most cases of intestinal TB are due to postprimary TB.[22] The ileocecal region is most vulnerable to MTB due to the abundance of Peyer's patches, increased physiological stasis, and minimal digestive activity. The

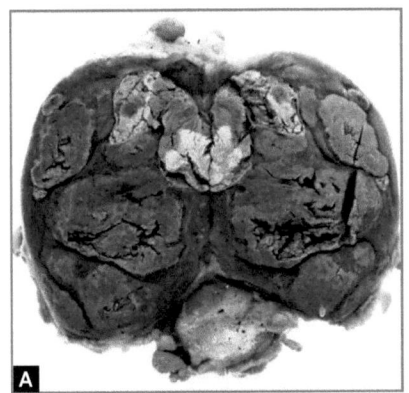

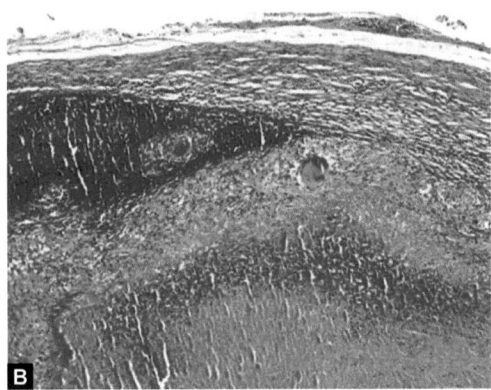

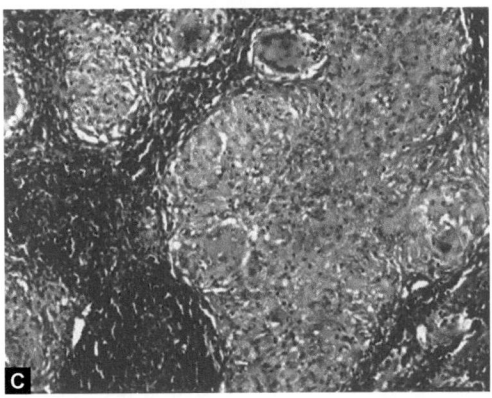

FIG. 7: Tubercular lymphadenitis. **A,** Gross specimen of a matted group of lymph nodes with caseation; **B and C,** Photomicrograph with partial effacement of nodal architecture by numerous epithelioid granulomas with central caseous necrosis and Langhans giant cell (B = H&E 50x, C = H&E 100x) *(For color version, see Plate 3)*

tubercle bacilli traverse through the mucosa and lodge in the submucosa. The presence of the bacilli elicits an inflammatory response, which includes edema, cellular infiltrates, and lymphatic hyperplasia. This is generally followed by formation of epithelioid granulomas that produce small papillary mucosal elevations. Lymphangitis, endarteritis, and fibrosis leads to mucosal ulceration, caseous necrosis, and narrowing of the intestinal lumen. Infection generally spreads to involve the mesenteric lymph nodes also. The involvement of the intestine is usually segmental; however, diffuse involvement also occurs uncommonly.[22-24]

Grossly, intestinal TB is classified into the following types:[24]

- Ulcerative lesions: These are characterized by multiple superficial ulcers. The disposition of the ulcers is the reflection of the direction of lymphatics around the intestine and the ulcers generally transverse to the long axis of the intestine. The base of the ulcer is covered by necrotic slough. Tubercles may be identified on the serosal surface (Fig. 8A)[25,26]
- Hypertrophic type: It is characterized by scarring, fibrosis, and pseudotumor formation
- Ulcerohypertrophic type: It is characterized by an inflammatory mass with thickened intestinal wall and ulcerated mucosa. The mucosa may show very superficial fissures giving rise to a cobblestone appearance of the mucosa. Small pseudopolyps may also present. This form is most commonly identified in the ileocecal region[25,26]
- Sclerotic type: It is characterized by multiple fibrous strictures produced as a result of healed ulcerations leading to luminal narrowing and intestinal obstruction.[25] Regional lymph nodes may be enlarged (Fig. 8B). Rarely, lymph nodes may assume a large size, giving rise to the condition called tabes mesenterica.[25-27]

The microscopic appearance of intestinal TB shows a mixture of patterns that include—necrotizing and noncaseating granulomas, ulceration with nonspecific granulation tissue and infiltration of polymorphs with formation of microabscesses and mucosal reparative changes. The early lesions show granulomas in the mucosa and Peyer's patches, in advanced disease any portion of the intestine may be affected. The base of ulcer is lined by inflammatory granulation tissue. Fibrosis and scarring are variable (Fig. 9). Acid-fast bacilli can be demonstrated in 6–8% of the cases.[26,27]

Hepatobiliary TB is documented in 25–50% patients who die from active pulmonary TB. Hematogenous spread of tubercle bacilli to the liver is seen in miliary TB. The presentations of TB of the liver include granulomatous hepatitis, nodular lesions, tubular lesions, and tuberculous liver abscess. Granulomatous hepatitis is characterized by irregular cheesy nodules

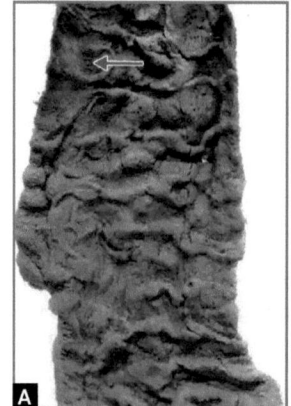 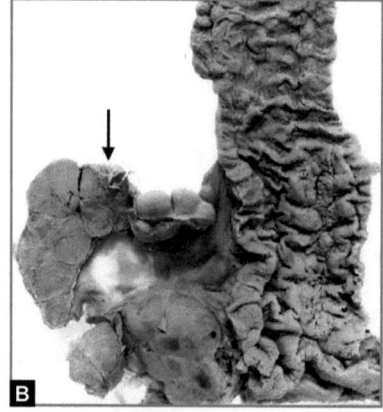

FIG. 8: Ileal tuberculosis with mesenteric lymphadenopathy: **A,** The cut open specimen of the ileum with numerous small ulcers with necrotic base (red arrow); **B,** matted group of enlarged mesenteric lymph nodes (black arrow) *(For color version, see Plate 4)*

Pathology Relevant to Radiologist

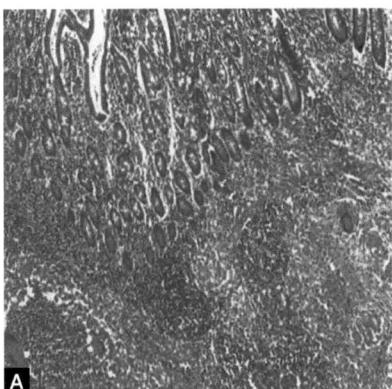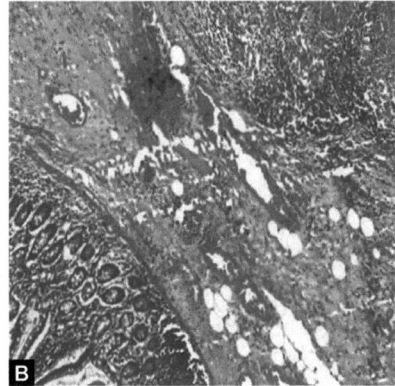

FIG. 9: Intestinal tuberculosis. Necrotizing granulomas in the mucosa and submucosa (A, B = H&E 50x) *(For color version, see Plate 4)*

on the liver surface. Bile ducts are involved by either an enlarged tuberculous lymph node or by diffuse involvement of the intrahepatic ducts by tubercle bacilli.[28] The histopathological findings reveal lesions composed of typical Kupffer cells that have a stellate rather than rounded configuration and lack characteristic epithelioid cells. Microgranulomas are also identified that are small aggregates of epithelioid cells, usually centrilobular in location and lack giant cells and caseation. In fatal form of hepatic TB, granulomatous inflammation with caseous necrosis is identified along with the nonspecific changes.[25,26,28] TB of the spleen presents as splenomegaly associated with fever, night sweats, and loss of weight. Splenic abscess may also rarely occur due to TB.[28] Pancreatic TB generally presents as a mass and is accompanied by a spectrum of symptoms that include abdominal pain, weight loss, fever, and obstructive jaundice.[28]

UROGENITAL TUBERCULOSIS

The disease involves the urinary tract and the genital tract either singly or in combination. The classification of urogenital TB[29,30] consists of:
- Urinary TB:
  - Kidney TB (nephrotuberculosis)
  - Urinary tract TB (TB of pelvis, ureters, bladder, and urethra)
- Male genital tract TB
- Female genital tract TB
- Generalized urogenital TB: Simultaneous lesion of urinary organs and genitals.

Renal Tuberculosis

Mycobacterium tuberculosis generally spreads to the kidneys by the hematogenous route. The renal cortex is the most common site of microscopic localization of granulomas as the oxygen tension is high and the blood supply is rich. Highly virulent organisms or low resistance can cause progression of the lesion and formation of a large nodule that may rupture into the renal tubules and produce medullary granulomas. The medullary lesions which can enlarge coalesce and produce papillary necrosis. Sloughing of the necrotic contents into the calyx leads to cavity formation. Tuberculosis can lead to changes of pyonephrosis with dilatation of calyces. The ureter, urinary bladder, and urethra are infected through this antegrade method and bacilli may appear in urine. Renal parenchymal healing occurs through fibrosis, scarring and calcification. Histopathological examination of these specimens reveals renal parenchymal fibrosis with calcification. In active disease, granulomatous inflammation with caseous necrosis is noted (Fig. 10). Renal amyloidosis can occur in patients with pulmonary TB of long duration.[30-33]

TB of the urinary bladder occurs secondary to renal TB. The initial lesions of vesicular TB are seen around the urethral orifices which may

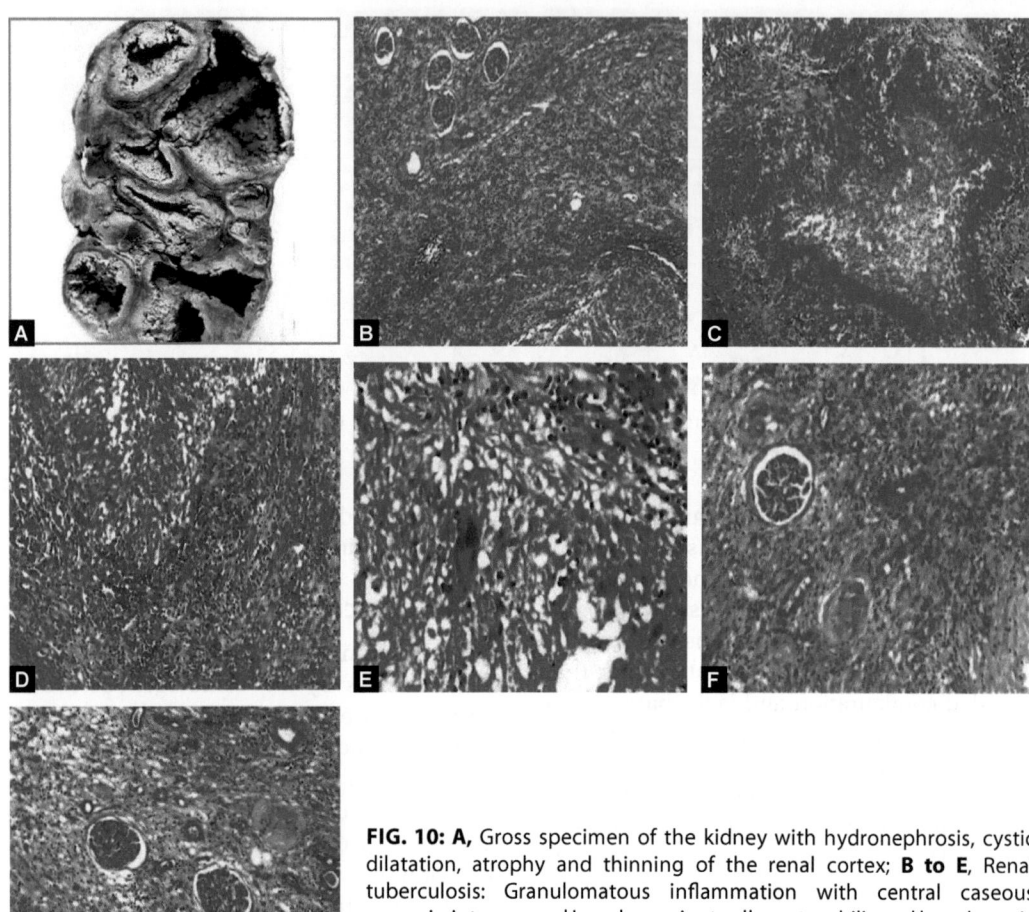

FIG. 10: A, Gross specimen of the kidney with hydronephrosis, cystic dilatation, atrophy and thinning of the renal cortex; **B to E,** Renal tuberculosis: Granulomatous inflammation with central caseous necrosis, interspersed Langhans giant cell, neutrophilic and lymphocytic infiltrate (B = H&E 50x; C, D = H&E 100x; E = H&E 200x). **F and G,** Photomicrograph showing secondary changes in renal parenchyma characterized by glomerular sclerosis and thyroidization of tubules (F,G = H&E 100x) *(For color version, see Plate 5)*

become inflamed and edematous. Progressively in advanced lesion, the whole bladder wall may be involved. There is granulomatous inflammation and ulceration of the mucosa. Due to the spread of the infection and inflammation to the deeper layer of the muscles fibrosis occurs. The fibrosis causes urethral stricture formation and reduction in bladder capacity leading to the formation of "thimble bladder."[30,32-36]

Examination of the urine in cases of urinary TB may rarely demonstrate MTB by polymerase chain reaction.[37,38]

Male Genital Tuberculosis

Tuberculosis of the male genital tract presents as painless hemospermia, scrotal pain and swelling or nodularity of the epididymis, vas deferens, seminal vesicle, or prostate. Involvement of the testis is rare. Tuberculous epididymitis presents as a painful inflamed scrotal swelling. Tuberculosis of the epididymis can lead to thickening of vas deferens by the granulomatous process. Testicular TB is always secondary to tuberculous epididymitis. Tuberculosis of the prostate presents as diffuse nodular enlargement and histopathological examination shows

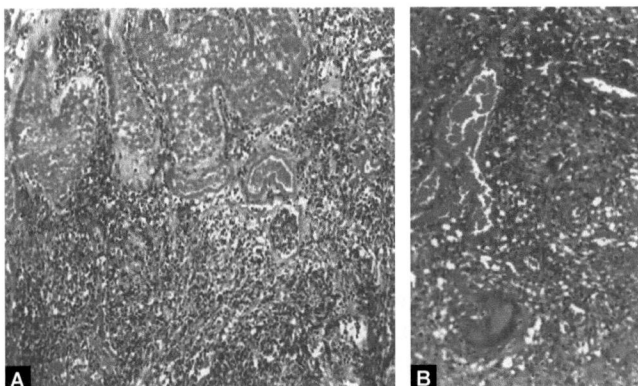

FIG. 11: Tuberculous orchitis: Tuberculous granulomatous inflammation involving the testis (A = H&E 100x, B = H&E 200x) *(For color version, see Plate 5)*

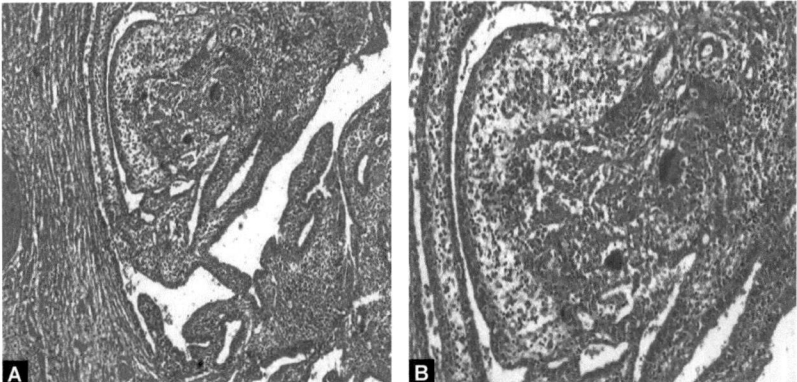

FIG. 12: Tuberculous salpingitis. Granulomatous inflammation with epithelioid granulomas, Langhans type giant cells along with lymphoplasmacytic and neutrophilic infiltrate (A = H&E 50x, B = H&E 100x) *(For color version, see Plate 6)*

chronic granulomatous inflammation with fibrosis. Primary penile TB occurs as a sexually transmitted disease, due to transmission from the female genital tract. The lesions present as penile ulcers and histopathological evaluation aids in diagnosis (Fig. 11).[39-41]

Female Genital Tuberculosis

Female genital TB is a common cause of infertility, chronic pelvic pain and menstrual irregularities. The fallopian tube is the most common site of involvement. The gross appearance of the fallopian tube depends on the stage of the disease. In the early stages, there is congestion of the tubes with mild adhesions and tiny tubercles may be evident on the surface. In severe disease, there are dense adhesions between the fallopian tube and the other organs. In healed cases, hydrosalpinx or pyosalpinx is evident. The histopathological appearance also depends on the stage of the disease. The presence of chronic inflammatory cells with or without caseation, granulomas along with Langhans giant cells is evident (Fig. 12). Fibrosis is evident in the healing phase.[42] Endometrial TB is occurs due to spread from fallopian tubes. Ovarian infection can also occur from the tubal source. In most cases the lesions present as tubo-ovarian masses formed due to excessive adhesions.[36,38,42] Less commonly, cervix and vagina are involved, as an extension from the endometrial lesion or by sexual transmission.

Ulcerations or small nodular masses are evident on gross examination. Microscopic examination reveals granulomatous inflammation associated with reactive atypia in the surrounding epithelium.[42]

EXTRASPINAL SKELETAL TUBERCULOSIS

Skeletal TB occurs due to hematogenous spread and affects almost all bones.[43] Typically, an active focus forms in the metaphysis (in children) or epiphysis (in adults) and the inflammation extends peripherally along the shaft to reach the subperiosteal space. The inflammatory exudates may extend outwards through the soft tissue to form cold abscess and sinuses. The granulation tissue can invade the area of calcified cartilage and interfere with longitudinal growth (Fig. 13).[43,44] Two classical forms of the disease have been described, granular and exudative (caseous) that involves the bone and synovium.[45]

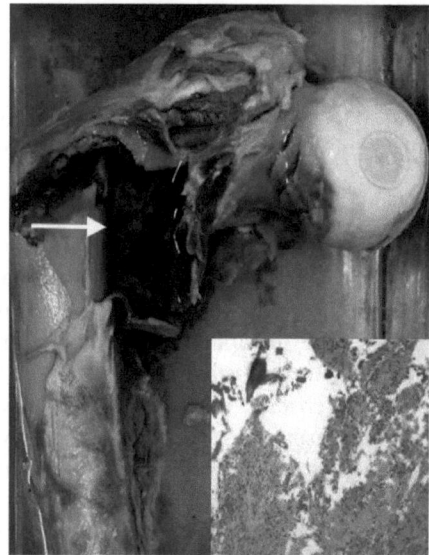

FIG. 13: Gross specimen of the femur with a cavity (arrow) near the head indicative of osteomyelitis. Inset: The microscopic evaluation revealed necrotizing granulomatous inflammation composed of epithelioid granulomas, Langhans giant cell, and caseous necrosis along with destruction of the bone (H&E 100x) *(For color version, see Plate 6)*

Types of Osteoarticular Tuberculosis[43-45]

- Osseous granular type: In this type the bone involvement occurs at metaphysis or epiphysis often following trauma. The onset is insidious. Constitutional symptoms are rare. Overlying soft tissue is slightly warm and tender. Muscle atrophy occurs rapidly
- Osseous exudative (caseating) type: The onset in this type is more rapid. Constitutional symptoms, muscle pain and spasm are more marked. The overlying soft tissue is warm, swollen, and tender. When the caseous material penetrates into the joint, severe destructive arthritis ensures
- Synovial granular type: It is characterized by intermittent joint effusion with little or no pain. Constitutional symptoms are mild and muscle atrophy gradually sets in this form of synovitis can continue for a long time without involving the bone
- Synovial exudative (caseous) type: This type has acute onset with marked local and constitutional symptoms. Overlying soft tissue is very tender. Abscess and sinuses formation is common.

CENTRAL NERVOUS SYSTEM AND SPINAL TUBERCULOSIS

Classification of TB of the central nervous system:[46,47]
- Intracranial TB:
    - Tuberculous meningitis (TBM)
    - Tuberculous encephalopathy
    - Tuberculous vasculopathy
    - Central nervous system tuberculoma
    - Tuberculous brain abscess
- Spinal TB:
    - Pott's spine and Pott's paraplegia
    - Tuberculous arachnoiditis/myeloradiculopathy
    - Nonosseous spinal tuberculoma
    - Spinal meningitis.

Tubercular Meningitis

The commonly involved sites are interpeduncular fossa, pontine cistern, and perimesencephalic and suprasellar cisterns.[48] Histologic

Pathology Relevant to Radiologist

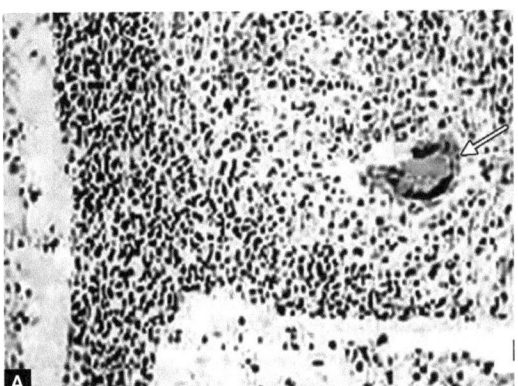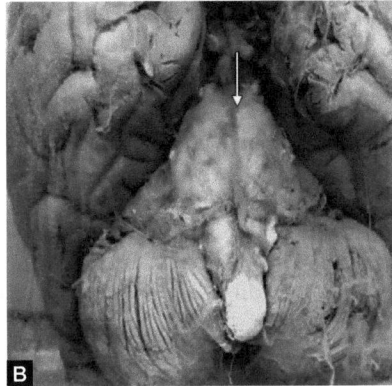

FIG. 14: Tubercular meningitis. **A,** The histology revealed inflammation of the meninges along with lymphocytic infiltration and scattered Langhans giant cell (arrow) (H&E 100x); **B,** Gross specimen of the brain with exudates at the basal meninges (arrow) *(For color version, see Plate 6)*

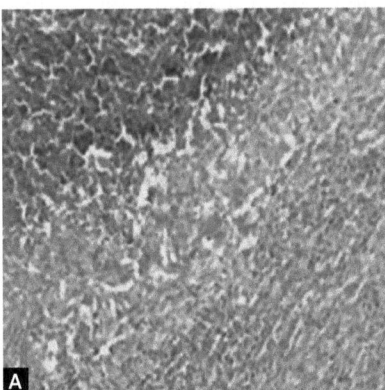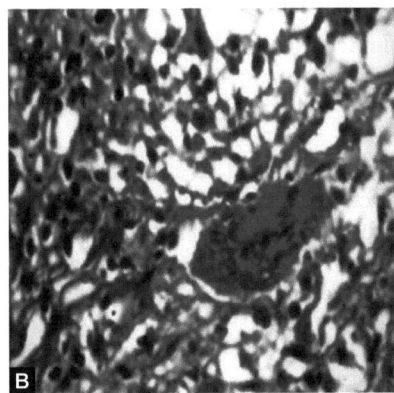

FIG. 15: Tuberculoma. **A,** Photomicrograph showing necrosis surrounded by a thin layer of granulomatous infiltrate, fibrosis, and gliosis; **B,** A cellular region of the same lesion with Langhans giant cell (A = H&E 50x, B = H&E 200x) *(For color version, see Plate 7)*

findings in TBM consist of epithelioid cell granulomas with Langhans giant cells, lymphocytic infiltrates, and caseous necrosis (Fig. 14A). These changes involve the arachnoid membrane and subarachnoid space diffusely. Acid-fast organisms can be shown in necrotic tissue and in the granulomas.[49-51] The sequelae associated with TBM include hydrocephalus and vasculitis.[52-54] In TB vasculitis, the adventitial layer of the vessels develops changes similar to those of the adjacent tubercular exudates. The intima of the vessels may eventually be affected or eroded by a fibrinoid degeneration. In later stages, the lumen of the vessel may be completely occluded by reactive subendothelial cellular proliferation resulting in infarction (Fig. 14B).[52,53]

Brain tuberculoma on histopathology has been divided into an initial nonspecific focal cerebritis followed by noncaseating granulomas that evolve into tuberculomas with solid caseation and subsequently into tuberculomas with liquefaction of caseation.[50,55-57] Bacilli are scarce. Liquefaction commences from the center. Astrocytic gliosis and fibrosis is evident in the surrounding brain parenchyma (Fig. 15).[48,50,52]

Molecular Pathology of Tuberculosis

Vascular endothelial growth factor (VEGF) expression and microvascular density in tuberculomas is comparable with that in grade 2 gliomas. Vascular endothelial growth factor is strongly expressed in the Langhans cells, epithelioid cells, and also in the surrounding fibrocytes and astrocytes.[57-60]

Tuberculous brain abscess consists of pus filled cavities containing tubercle bacilli. The wall of TB abscess cavity shows granulation tissue with inflammatory cells. There is usually a paucity of epithelioid cells or giant cells. The content of the cavity usually shows numerous AFB. In long-standing healed cases there is gliosis of the brain with focal calcification.[58,59,61]

Tuberculous encephalopathy is pathologically characterized by diffuse cerebral white matter edema with loss of neurons in grey matter.[58,59]

Spinal Tuberculosis

Histopathological examination may reveal tuberculous granulomatous inflammation with caseous necrosis, osteomyelitis, and sequestrum formation.[62,63]

Nonosseous spinal cord TB can occur in the form of tuberculomas. Such tuberculomas can be multiple. These lesions can be extramedullary or intramedullary. Intramedullary tuberculomas are extremely rare and occur frequently in the thoracic region.[64]

OCULAR TUBERCULOSIS

The ocular manifestations of TB are caused by active infection or by an immunological reaction. Manifestations of primary ocular TB are limited to conjunctival and corneal disease.[65] These lesions generally present as ulceration, tumor mass, phlyctenulosis or interstitial keratitis.[66] Tuberculosis of the eyelid may present as a tumor or as an abscess associated with erythema and focal or diffuse swelling of the eyelid.[67]

Conjunctival lesions of tuberculosis have been classified into five groups: (i) ulceration, (ii) miliary tubercle, (iii) hypertrophic granulation, (iv) lupus, and (v) pedunculated tumors. Conjunctival involvement is generally unilateral and commonly involves the upper palpebral conjunctiva.[66,67] Phlyctenulosis are small nodules that arise in the conjunctiva or limbus. These lesions usually ulcerate. These lesions generally arise due to hypersensitivity to the tuberculoprotein.[68] Corneal manifestations of TB include infiltrates, ulceration, and interstitial keratitis. Sclera involvement in TB is rare and may present as sclera ulceration or scleritis.[69] Tuberculosis-associated uveitis is usually granulomatous with mutton fat keratic precipitates iris granulomas and posterior synechiae. Choroiditis is the most common ocular manifestation of intraocular TB. Choroidal tubercles are generally unilateral and have indistinct borders. The involvement of the retina with endophthalmitis and optic neuropathy is extremely rare.[66,67] Phlyctenules are characterized by dense accumulation of lymphocytes, histiocytes, and plasma cells. There is generally an absence of giant cells and eosinophils. Choroidal tubercles demonstrate the classical histopathological features of TB. Tuberculosis endophthalmitis is characterized by necrosis and caseation.[69]

TUBERCULOSIS OF THE HEAD AND NECK

The mucosa of the oral cavity is relatively resistant to the invasive by MTB and presence of saliva further inhibits its replication. The tongue is the most common site affected. The lesions generally begin as nodules or plaques that later ulcerate. Involvement of the other parts like floor of mouth, soft palate uvula is extremely rare. The histopathological features are classical.[70,71]

Laryngeal TB occurs either due to direct spread from infected sputum or by lymphohematogenous spread. The gross examination of the larynx reveals edema, hyperemia, nodularity with ulceration, and formation of pseudotumors. There is thickening of the vocal cords with obliteration of the anatomical landmarks. There is marked edema of the epiglottis (turban epiglottis). The histopathological examination generally reveals tubercular granulation tissue. Caseation is evident in the advanced stages. Fibrosis is identified in cases undergoing resolution that leads to formation of turban epiglottis.[72] Tuberculous sialadenitis on histopathology vary from nonspecific reactive changes to the characteristic granulomatous inflammation.[73,74] Tuberculosis of the pharynx and tonsils is uncommon. The lesions may present as ulcers or neck abscesses.[74]

Tuberculosis of the nasopharynx is rare. Endoscopic examination revels irregularity of the nasopharyngeal mucosa with the presence of a pseudotumorous mass.[74] Tuberculosis of the paranasal sinuses involves the maxillary and the ethmoid sinuses. The presentations include irregularity of the sinus mucosa with formation of polyps. In advanced cases, there is bony involvement leading to tubercular osteomyelitis associated with sequestrum and fistula formation.[75] Nasal tuberculosis manifests as nasal obstruction and catarrh. The gross examination of the nasal mucosa reveals multiple minute nodules that characteristic of tubercles. The microscopic examination generally reveals tuberculous granulation tissue.[76]

CARDIOVASCULAR TUBERCULOSIS

Tuberculosis mainly affects the pericardium but rarely the myocardium and the endocardium may also be involved. The heart and the pericardium can be infected by MTB via the hematogenous route during pulmonary TB or by direct, peribronchial or lymphatic dissemination.[77] Clinically, TB pericarditis presents as acute pericarditis, pericardial effusion, cardiac tamponade, and constrictive pericarditis (Fig. 16).[77,78] Tuberculous endocarditis is extremely rare. It involves the valvular surface or the endothelial surface of the cardiac chambers and the great vessels. The valvular involvement generally leads to regurgitation and aneurysm formation.[79,80] Myocardial involvement in TB can be associated with pseudomasses causing obstruction of the chambers that reveal granulomatous inflammation on histopathological examination.[81,82]

CONCLUSION

The histopathological findings in TB are pathognomonic. Till date, no other disease in history matches the sheer magnitude of the misery inflicted by TB on the human race in terms of morbidity and mortality. The current newer improved modalities of treatment have an impact on the overall morbitidity of the disease. However, TB remains as a formidable foe threatening to annihilate the human race.

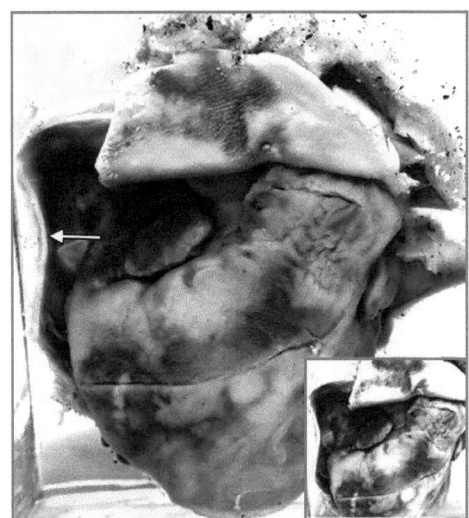

FIG. 16: Tuberculous pericarditis: The gross specimen of the heart with thickening of the pericardium (arrow) along with fibrinous exudates. Inset: Closer view of the thickened wall with the classical bread and butter appearance *(For color version, see Plate 7)*

REFERENCES

1. Sharma SK, Mohanan S, Sharma A. Relevance of latent TB infection in areas of high TB prevalence. Chest. 2012;142(3):761-73.
2. Gupta SD, Roy R, Gill SS. Pulmonary pathology. In: Sharma SK, Mohan A (Eds). Tuberculosis, 2nd edition. New Delhi: Jaypee Brothers Medical Publishers (P) Ltd; 2009. pp. 66-101.
3. Davis JM, Ramakrishnan L. The role of the granuloma in expansion and dissemination of early tuberculous infection. Cell. 2009;136(1):37-49.
4. Rich AR. The Pathogenesis of Tuberculosis, 2nd edition. Illinois: Charles C Thomas Publisher; 1951.
5. Hunter RL. Pathology of post primary tuberculosis of the lung: an illustrated critical review. Tuberculosis (Edinb). 2011;91(6):497-509.
6. Sakula A. Robert Koch: centenary of the discovery of the tubercle bacillus, 1882. Thorax. 1982;37(4):246-51.
7. Akhtar M, Al Mana H. Pathology of tuberculosis. In: Madkour MM (Ed). Tuberculosis, 1st edition. Germany: Springer-Verlag; 2004. pp. 153-61.
8. McAdam AJ, Sharpe AH. Infectious disease. In: Kumar V, Abbas A, Fausto N (Eds). Robbins and Cotran Pathologic Basis of Disease, 7th edition. Philadelphia: Saunders Elsevier; 2004. pp. 343-414.
9. Madkour MM, Abusabaah Y, Mousa AB, et al. Post-primary pulmonary tuberculosis. In: Madkour MM (Ed). Tuberculosis, 1st edition. Germany: Springer-Verlag; 2004. pp. 313-27.

10. Leong FJ, Dartois V, Dick T. A Color Atlas of Comparative Pathology of Pulmonary Tuberculosis. New York: CRC Press; 2016.
11. Chung HS. Endobronchial tuberculosis. In: Madkour MM (Ed). Tuberculosis, 1st edition. Germany: Springer-Verlag; 2004. pp. 329-48.
12. Kim WS, Moon WK, Kim IO, et al. Pulmonary tuberculosis in children: evaluation with CT. AJR Am J Roentgenol. 1997;168(4):1005-9.
13. Cardona PJ. The key role of exudative lesions and their encapsulation: lessons learned from the pathology of human pulmonary tuberculosis. Front Microbiol. 2015; 6:612.
14. Curvo-Semedo L, Teixeira L, Caseiro-Alves F. Tuberculosis of the chest. Eur J Radiol. 2005;55(2):158-72.
15. Gadkowski LB, Stout JE. Cavitary pulmonary disease. Clin Microbiol Rev. 2008;21(2):305-33.
16. Vijayan VK, Sajal D. Pulmonary tuberculosis. In: Sharma SK, Mohan A (Eds). Tuberculosis, 2nd edition. New Delhi: Jaypee Brothers Medical Publishers (P) Ltd; 2009. pp. 217-26.
17. Madkour MM, Idrees M, Al Shahed M. Pleural tuberculosis. In: Madkour MM (Ed). Tuberculosis, 1st edition. Germany: Springer-Verlag; 2004. pp. 349-57.
18. Popescu MR, Călin G, Strâmbu I, et al. Lymph node tuberculosis - an attempt of clinico-morphological study and review of the literature. Rom J Morphol Embryol. 2014;55(2 Suppl):553-67.
19. Baskota DK, Prasad R, Kumar Sinha B, Amatya RC. Distribution of lymph nodes in the neck in cases of tuberculous cervical lymphadenitis. Acta Otolaryngol. 2004;124(9):1095-8.
20. Ramanathan VD, Jawahar MS, Paramasivan CN, et al. A histological spectrum of host responses in tuberculous lymphadenitis. Indian J Med Res. 1999;109:212-20.
21. Tiwari M, Sahoo SP, Shukla HS. Abdominal tuberculosis. In: Sharma SK, Mohan A (Eds). Tuberculosis, 2nd edition. New Delhi: Jaypee Brothers Medical Publishers (P) Ltd; 2009. pp. 275-93.
22. Debi U, Ravisankar V, Prasad KK, Sinha SK, Sharma AK. Abdominal tuberculosis of the gastrointestinal tract: Revisited. World J Gastroenterol. 2014;20(40):14831-40.
23. Khuroo MS, Khuroo NS. Abdominal tuberculosis. In: Madkour MM (Ed). Tuberculosis, 1st edition. Germany: Springer-Verlag; 2004. pp. 659-78.
24. de Araujo AL. Relevance of imaging in the evaluation of abdominal tuberculosis. Radiol Bras. 2015;48(3):VII.
25. Marshall JB. Tuberculosis of the gastrointestinal tract and peritoneum. Am J Gastroenterol. 1993;88(7):989-99.
26. Yoon HJ, Song YG, Park WI, et al. Clinical manifestations and diagnosis of extrapulmonary tuberculosis. Yonsei Med J. 2004;45(3):453-61.
27. Sharma MP, Bhatia V. Abdominal tuberculosis. Indian J Med Res. 2004;120(4):305-15.
28. Chaudhary P. Hepatobiliary tuberculosis. Ann Gastroenterol. 2014;27(3):207-11.
29. Kulchavenya E. Urogenital tuberculosis: definition and classification. Ther Adv Infect Dis. 2014;2(5-6):117-22.
30. Kulchavenya E. Best practice in the diagnosis and management of urogenital tuberculosis. Ther Adv Urol. 2013;5(3):143-51.
31. Colbert G, Richey D, Schwartz JC. Widespread tuberculosis including renal involvement. Proc (Bayl Univ Med Cent). 2012;25(3):236-9.
32. Hemal AK. Genitourinary tuberculosis. In: Sharma SK, Mohan A (Eds). Tuberculosis, 2nd edition. New Delhi: Jaypee Brothers Medical Publishers (P) Ltd; 2009. pp. 463-78.
33. Madkour MM. Genitourinary tuberculosis. In: Madkour MM (Ed). Tuberculosis, 1st edition. Germany: Springer-Verlag; 2004. pp. 699-729.
34. Fekak H, Rabii R, Moufid K, et al. A rare cause of urinary obstruction: urogenital tuberculosis. Ann Urol (Paris). 2003;37(2):71-4.
35. Figueiredo AA, Lucon AM. Urogenital tuberculosis: update and review of 8961 cases from the world literature. Rev Urol. 2008;10(3):207-17.
36. Kulchavenya E. Some aspects of urogenital tuberculosis. Int J Nephrol Urol. 2010;2:351-60.
37. Wise GJ, Shteynshlyuger A. An update on lower urinary tract tuberculosis. Curr Urol Rep. 2008;9(4):305-13.
38. Wise GJ, Marella VK. Genitourinary manifestations of tuberculosis. Urol Clin North Am. 2003;30(1):111-21.
39. Muttarak M, Peh WCG, Lojanapiwat B, Chaiwun B. Tuberculous epididymitis and epididymo-orchitis sonographic appearances. AJR Am J Roentgenol. 2001;176(6):1459-66.
40. Gupta N, Mandal AK, Singh SK. Tuberculosis of the prostate and urethra: A review. Indian J Urol. 2008;24(3):388-91.
41. Kulchavenya E, Khomyakov V. Male genital tuberculosis in Siberians. World J Urol. 2006;24(1):74-8.
42. Arora VK, Gupta R, Arora R. Female genital tuberculosis-Need for more research. Indian J Tuberculosis. 2003;50:9-11.
43. Madkour MM, Kudwah AJ, El Bagi MA. Extraspinal musculoskeletal tuberculosis. In: Madkour MM (Ed). Tuberculosis, 1st edition. Germany: Springer-Verlag; 2004. pp. 587-604.
44. Kumar A, Malaviya AN. Musculoskeletal manifestations of tuberculosis. In: Sharma SK, Mohan A (Eds). Tuberculosis, 2nd edition. New Delhi: Jaypee Brothers Medical Publishers (P) Ltd; 2009. pp. 373-83.
45. Pigrau-Serrallach C, Rodríguez-Pardo D. Bone and joint tuberculosis. Eur Spine J. 2013;22(Suppl 4):556-66.
46. Rock BR, Olin M, Baker CA, et al. Central Nervous System Tuberculosis: Pathogenesis and Clinical Aspects. Clin Microbial Rev. 2008;21(2):243-61.
47. Garg RK. Tuberculosis of the central nervous system. Postgrad Med J. 1999;75(881):133-40.
48. Garcia-Monco JC. Central nervous system tuberculosis. Neurol Clin. 1999;17(4):737-59.
49. Dastur DK, Manghani DK, Udani PM. Pathology and pathogenetic mechanisms in neurotuberculosis. Radiol Clin North Am. 1995;33(4):733-52.
50. Tandon PN, Pathak SN. Tuberculosis of the central nervous system. In: Spillane JD (Ed). Tropical Neurology. New York: Oxford University Press; 1973. pp. 37-62.

51. Bernaerts A, Vanhoenacker FM, Parizel PM, et al. Tuberculosis of the central nervous system: overview of neuroradiological findings. Eur Radiol. 2003;13(8):1876-90.
52. Dastur DK, Lalitha VS, Udani PM, Parekh U. The brain and meninges in tuberculous meningitis-gross pathology in 100 cases and pathogenesis. Neurol India. 1970;18(2):86-100.
53. Kioumehr F, Dadsetan MR, Rooholamini SA, et al. Central nervous system tuberculosis: MRI. Neuroradiology. 1994; 36(2):93-6.
54. Murthy JM. Tuberculous meningitis: the challenges. Neurol India. 2010;58(5):716-22.
55. Galimi R. Extrapulmonary tuberculosis: tuberculous meningitis new developments. Eur Rev Med Pharmacol Sci. 2011;15(4):365-86.
56. Bidstrup C, Andersen PH, Skinhøj P, et al. Tuberculous meningitis in a country with a low incidence of tuberculosis: still a serious disease and a diagnostic challenge. Scand J Infect Dis. 2002;34(11):811-4.
57. Sütlaş PN, Unal A, Forta H, et al. Tuberculous meningitis in adults: review of 61 cases. Infection. 2003;31(6):387-91.
58. Kumar R, Singh SN, Kohli N. A diagnostic rule for tuberculous meningitis. Arch Dis Child. 1999;81(3):221-4.
59. Youssef FG, Afifi SA, Azab AM, et al. Differentiation of tuberculous meningitis from acute bacterial meningitis using simple clinical and laboratory parameters. Diagn Microbiol Infect Dis. 2006;55(4):275-8.
60. Trivedi R, Saksena S, Gupta RK. Magnetic resonance imaging in central nervous system tuberculosis. Indian J Radiol Imaging. 2009;19(4):256-65.
61. Thwaites GE, Chau TT, Stepniewska K, et al. Diagnosis of adult tuberculous meningitis by use of clinical and laboratory features. Lancet. 2002;360(9342):1287-92.
62. Jain AK. Tuberculosis of the spine: a fresh look at an old disease. J Bone Joint Surg Br. 2010;92(7):905-13.
63. Polley P, Dunn R. Noncontiguous spinal tuberculosis: incidence and management. Eur Spine J. 2009;18(8):1096-101.
64. Garg RK, Sharma R, Kar AM, et al. Neurological complications of miliary tuberculosis. Clin Neurol Neurosurg. 2010;112(3):188-92.
65. Shwu-Jiuan Sheu. Ocular manifestations of tuberculosis. In: Madkour MM (Ed). Tuberculosis, 1st edition. Germany: Springer-Verlag; 2004. pp. 731-40.
66. Garg SP, Chawla R, Venkatesh P. Ocular tuberculosis. In: Sharma SK, Mohan A (Eds). Tuberculosis, 2nd edition. New Delhi: Jaypee Brothers Medical Publishers (P) Ltd; 2009. pp. 420-33.
67. Akal A, Goncu T, Boyaci FN, et al. Primary tubercular chorioretinitis. Ann Med Health Sci Res. 2014;4(6):965-7.
68. Sheu SJ, Shyu JS, Chen LM, et al. Ocular manifestations of tuberculosis. Ophthalmology. 2001;108(9):1580-5.
69. Gupta V, Gupta A, Arora S, et al. Presumed tubercular serpiginouslike choroiditis: clinical presentations and management. Ophthalmology. 2003;110(9):1744-9.
70. Muranjan S. Otorhinolaryngeal aspects of tuberculosis. In: Madkour MM (Ed). Tuberculosis, 1st edition. Germany: Springer-Verlag; 2004. pp. 741-49.
71. Nalini B, Vinayak S. Tuberculosis in ear, nose, and throat practice: its presentation and diagnosis. Am J Otolaryngol. 2006;27(1):39-45.
72. Rizzo PB, Da Mosto MC, Clari M, et al. Laryngeal tuberculosis: an often forgotten diagnosis. Int J Infect Dis. 2003;7(2):129-31.
73. Michalak A, Wojtas G, Kidawa I, Tylzanowska-Nitek K. Tuberculosis of the tongue in a patient with disseminated pulmonary tuberculosis. Pneumonol Alergol Pol. 2004; 72(1-2):28-31.
74. Sethi A, Sareen D, Sabherwal A, Malhotra V. Primary parotid tuberculosis: varied clinical presentations. Oral Dis. 2006;12(2):213-5.
75. Meher R, Singh I, Yadav SP, Gathwala G. Tubercular otitis media in children. Otolaryngol Head Neck Surg. 2006;135(4):650-2.
76. Vaamonde P, Castro C, Garcia-Soto N, et al. Tuberculous otitis media: a significant diagnostic challenge. Otolaryngol Head Neck Surg. 2004;130(6):759-66.
77. Fowler NO. Tuberculous pericarditis. JAMA. 1991;266(1): 99-103.
78. Salcedo EE, Omran AS. Tuberculosis of the heart and pericardium. In: Madkour MM (Ed). Tuberculosis, 1st edition. Germany: Springer-Verlag; 2004. pp. 431-43.
79. Licht J, Diefenbach C, Stang A, et al. Tuberculoma of the myocardium: a rare case of intra-vitam diagnosis. Clin Res Cardiol. 2009;98(5):331-3.
80. Jagia P, Gulati GS, Sharma S, et al. MRI features of tuberculoma of the right atrial myocardium. Pediatr Radiol. 2004;34(11):904-7.
81. Gulati GS, Singh S, Arepalli CD, et al. Superior vena caval obstruction after complete resolution of cardiac tuberculoma. Clin Radiol. 2008;63(5):605-9.
82. Chang BC, Ha JW, Kim JT, et al. Intracardiac tuberculoma. Ann Thorac Surg. 1999;67(1):226-8.

CHAPTER 5

Basics of Antitubercular Therapy

Randeep Guleria, Ashesh Dhungana

INTRODUCTION

Tuberculosis (TB), caused by *Mycobacterium tuberculosis*, is a leading cause of death by an infectious disease worldwide. India contributes significantly to the global burden of the disease with an estimated 2 million new infections and 276,000 deaths annually.[1] This translates to an estimated loss in economic well-being amounting to approximately US$ 23.7 billion every year. Early diagnosis by sputum smear microscopy or cultures and early initiation of treatment with combination chemotherapy remains the cornerstone in the management, thereby preventing person to person transmission and reducing the disease burden. All patients having a cough of more than 2 weeks duration with or without other symptoms should be evaluated for TB by Ziehl-Neelsen (ZN) staining of the sputum, with or without culture. Sputum smear examination has a sensitivity of about 50% and a specificity of greater than 99% with a positive predictive value of 91–98.5%.[2] Radiography is an important supportive tool which assists primarily in the diagnosis of sputum smear-negative and extrapulmonary disease. Major limitations of radiology in contrast to sputum examination in the diagnosis of TB are high intra and interreader variation, absence of radiologic sign with 100% specificity, and both underreading (10–15% culture-positive cases remain undiagnosed) and overreading (40% patients diagnosed as having TB by radiograph alone may not have active TB disease).[3]

However, radiology [chest radiograph, computed tomography (CT) scan and magnetic resonance imaging (MRI)] continues to be important to assist in the diagnosis and management of pulmonary and extrapulmonary TB. Recently, there has been an attempt to formulate radiological guidelines to assist a physician in a more valid way to diagnose and assess treatment response in TB.[4] Other investigations like fine-needle aspiration cytology (FNAC), biopsy, biochemical analysis of fluids, and immunological tests (Mantoux test) may also assist in the diagnosis of the disease.

The resurgence of TB in conjunction with human immunodeficiency virus (HIV) has caused more deaths and morbidity, and warrants timely and appropriate therapy. The spread of multidrug-resistant TB (MDR-TB) strains and the advent of extensively drug-resistant TB (XDR-TB) forms add new challenges in management. More recently, rapid culture methods using liquid broth and molecular methods like line probe assays and GeneXpert have enabled rapid detection of drug resistance and aid in the early institution of appropriate second-line therapy. The Revised National Tuberculosis Control Programme (RNTCP) recommends the use of directly observed treatment short-course (DOTS) strategy, where a health worker or a trained volunteer watches and supports the patient in taking the drug (DOT). The drugs are given for 6 or 8 months depending on the disease category. MDR-TB is treated with combination of oral and injectable second-line drugs, for 18–24 months.

ANTITUBERCULAR DRUGS: BASIS OF CURRENT TREATMENT STRATEGY

Treatment of TB was revolutionized after the discovery of streptomycin in 1944, but it was soon realized that streptomycin monotherapy caused emergence of resistance and subsequent deterioration after initial improvement. Later, streptomycin was combined with para-aminosalicylic acid (PAS) or isoniazid (INH) which prevented emergence of drug resistance to a large extent. However, the duration of chemotherapy required for complete cure was almost up to 2 years. The discovery of rifampicin and pyrazinamide in the 70s reduced the duration of therapy to less than a year and subsequently to 6–8 months.

Currently, the antitubercular agents are classified into two groups: (i) first-line agents are primarily used to treat the newly diagnosed cases and retreatment cases whose bacilli are drug susceptible and (ii) second-line agents are reserved for the treatment of multidrug-resistant (MDR) disease. Other drugs like macrolide antibiotics, oxazolidinones (linezolid) and clofazimine may be used for treatment of difficult to treat cases and extensively drug-resistant cases. After 40 years two newer antitubercular drugs have been approved recently by World Health Organization (WHO) for treatment of resistant cases. These are bedaquiline and delamanid. Other newer drugs in the pipeline are being evaluated in clinical trials, and may be available in the recent future. Search is still on for effective drugs which will further shorten the duration of therapy and at the same time prevent drug resistance. Table 1 lists the available antitubercular drugs.[5]

The presence of four distinct types of bacterial population has been suggested in patients with TB. One is an actively multiplying bacillary population present in large numbers in the extracellular liquefied caseous area. These organisms are killed mainly by INH. Rifampicin and streptomycin also have some action against these organisms. Ethambutol is bacteriostatic against these metabolically active bacilli. The second population consists of a small number of organisms present outside the cell and in the solid caseous material. These organisms are slow growing with intermittent spurts of growth. Rifampicin is effective against these organisms. The third population is that of bacilli living in low pH environment. These organisms are present within the macrophages and pyrazinamide is the only drug effective against these pathogens. The fourth population is that of dormant bacilli and none of the currently available drugs are effective against this population. The current strategy of short-course chemotherapy in TB is to give drugs which will act simultaneously against the first three populations so as to

Table 1: Classification of antitubercular drugs		
First-line agents	Second-line agents	Other drugs

• Isoniazid (H)
• Rifampicin (R)
• Pyrazinamide (Z)
• Ethambutol (E)
• Streptomycin (S)
	• Aminoglycosides: Kanamycin (Km), capreomycin (Cm) and amikacin (Am)
	• Fluoroquinolones: Ciprofloxacin (Cfx), ofloxacin (Ofx), levofloxacin (Lvx) and moxifloxacin (Mfx)
	• Ethionamide (Eto)
	• Prothionamide (Pto)
	• Cycloserine (Cs)
	• Para-aminosalicylic acid (PAS)
	• Thioacetazone (TH)
		• Macrolides: Azithromycin, clarithromycin
		• Rifamycins*: Rifabutin, rifapentine
		• Linezolid
		• Clofazimine
		• Thalidomide
		• Newer drugs [approved by World Health Organization (WHO)]:
		  ○ Bedaquiline
		  ○ Delamanid
		• Other drugs in the pipeline:
		  ○ Pretomanid
		  ○ Sutezolid
		  ○ SQ109 (ethylenediamine)
		  ○ TBA-354 (nitroimidazole)

*Rifamycins other than rifampicin.

ensure rapid sterilization of the tubercular lesion. Aminoglycosides, fluoroquinolones, and cycloserine are the most important second-line agents as they have broad spectrum of activity and are used more frequently in MDR regimens.

Chemotherapy is therefore, given to achieve bactericidal action, sterilizing action, and to prevent the emergence of drug-resistant organisms. Bactericidal drugs are those which are rapidly able to kill rapidly growing bacteria. INH has the highest bactericidal activity followed by rifampicin and streptomycin. Sterilizing drugs are those which can kill some dormant organisms. Both rifampicin and pyrazinamide have a sterilizing activity. Combinations of drugs are used to prevent emergence of resistance. Hence, combination of rifampicin, INH, streptomycin, and ethambutol are effective in preventing resistance.

ADVERSE REACTIONS

Adverse drug reactions are common with most antitubercular drugs. Monitoring for the adverse reactions and their timely management ensures adherence to the drugs and improves the cure rate. This is more important while prescribing second-line agents which are notorious to cause a myriad of adverse effects. Most of them are minor and require only symptomatic management. However, serious adverse events like hepatotoxicity and acute liver failure do occur and require discontinuation of antitubercular treatment (ATT) temporarily.[6] Sputum-positive patients and those who are critically ill should be put on alternate nonhepatotoxic drugs (usually aminoglycoside, fluoroquinolone, and ethambutol) while the hepatotoxicity resolves. Antitubercular treatment should be reintroduced one by one, once liver functions return to baseline and jaundice disappears starting with INH then rifampicin. Pyrazinamide should be reintroduced the last as it is the most hepatotoxic. Hepatotoxicity does not reoccur on reintroduction of the drugs and more than 90% of patients who develop hepatotoxicity tolerate all the drugs after reintroduction. Rise in transaminases after reintroduction should help in identifying the culprit drug and this drug should be avoided. Hearing loss caused by aminoglycosides is irreversible and warrants permanent discontinuation of the drug. Neuropathy caused by INH can be prevented by supplementing pyridoxine during the course of therapy. Assessment of liver function may be done at baseline and after first 2 weeks of therapy while initiating an antitubercular regimen especially in the high-risk group. Monitoring the hemoglobin, thyroid function tests and audiometry is also recommended while using second-line drugs. Some common adverse effects of antitubercular drugs are listed in Table 2.

Table 2: Adverse reactions of common antitubercular drugs

Drug	Adverse reactions
Isoniazid	Neuropathy, rash, hepatitis, and neuropsychiatric manifestations
Rifampicin	Hepatitis and gastrointestinal (vomiting or epigastric discomfort)
Pyrazinamide	Hepatitis and hyperuricemia
Ethambutol	Visual disturbance, hyperuricemia, and renal toxicity
Aminoglycosides	Ototoxicity, nephrotoxicity, vertigo, and electrolyte imbalance
Fluoroquinolones	Gastrointestinal symptoms, dizziness, convulsions, phototoxicity, photosensitivity, and tendinopathy
Cycloserine	Dizziness, convulsions, tremor, depression, suicidal tendency, and hypersensitivity reaction
Ehionamide/ Prothionamide	Epigastric discomfort, anorexia, nausea, hallucination, depression, hepatitis, hypothyroidism, and menstrual disturbances
Para-aminosalicylic acid (PAS)	Anorexia, nausea, vomiting, skin rash hepatitis, hypokalemia, and hypothyroidism

SHORT-COURSE CHEMOTHERAPY (DOTS)[3,7]

Antitubercular drugs are prescribed in combination in a predefined dose and duration. Combination chemotherapy prevents transmission, achieves cure and prevents relapse of the disease. The entire duration of chemotherapy is divided into two phases: (i) the intensive phase (IP) and (ii) the continuation

Basics of Antitubercular Therapy

Table 3: DOTS regimen recommended by RNTCP[3]			
Treatment groups	Type of patients	Regimen*	
		Intensive phase	Continuation phase
New case	• Sputum smear-positive • Sputum smear-negative • Extrapulmonary TB	$2H_3R_3Z_3E_3$	$4H_3R_3$
Previously treated case	• Smear-positive relapse • Smear-positive failure • Smear-positive treatment after default	$2H_3R_3Z_3E_3S_3/1H_3R_3Z_3E_3$	$5H_3R_3$

DOTS, directly observed treatment short-course; RNTCP, Revised National Tuberculosis Control Programme
*The number before the letters refers to the number of months of treatment. The subscript after the letters refers to the number of doses per week.
Drug dose (For adults): H = 600 mg, R = 450 mg (extra 150 mg if weight >60 kg), Z = 1,500 mg, E = 1,200 mg, S = 750 mg for less than 50 years and 500 mg for more than 50 years.

phase (CP). Intensive phase in a new case of TB and for retreatment is for 2 and 3 months, respectively. Continuation phase for a new case and retreatment case are 4 and 5 months, respectively. After the failure of the National Tuberculosis Program (NTP), the RNTCP was launched in 1992 with incorporation of the globally recommended DOTS strategy which has now achieved coverage in all states.[8] The five components of DOTS are: (i) political commitment, (ii) good quality diagnosis, (iii) uninterrupted supply of quality drugs, (iv) directly observed treatment and (v) systematic monitoring. Each of the five components is equally important and is critical to the success of the TB control program. DOTS shifts the responsibility for TB cure from patient to healthcare system. The DOT provider ensures that the patient ingests the drugs under direct supervision. All the doses in the IP are supervised, whereas the first dose of the week in the CP is supervised. Currently in India drugs are given thrice weekly, i.e., intermittent dosing. The relapse rate with intermittent dosing is comparable to daily dosing and the adverse effects are less.[9] However, intermittent dosing is not recommended for HIV-positive patients and in regions where INH resistance is high. Recently, the Government of India has introduced daily DOTS therapy and the plan is to rollout daily therapy for treatment of all cases of TB (new and retreatment).[10] Monitoring for response is done by sputum smear microscopy in sputum-positive cases, whereas in sputum-negative and extrapulmonary disease monitoring for clinical response and radiological resolution is of paramount importance. Sputum is usually rendered negative in more than 90% patients by 3 months of treatment. Failure of ATT regimen is defined as persistence of sputum positivity past 5 months of ATT. Failure to respond should warrant evaluation for MDR-TB. Defaulters are those who after taking the ATT for at least 1 month and have discontinued the medications for 2 or more months. The treatment categories for treatment of TB under RNTCP are given in Table 3.

TREATMENT OF MULTIDRUG-RESISTANT TUBERCULOSIS[11,12]

Multidrug-resistant TB is defined as TB caused by *Mycobacteria* which is resistant in vitro to both rifampicin and INH with or without resistance to other drugs. Those with resistance to rifampicin alone even if INH resistance is not tested should also be treated with MDR regimen. The prevalence of MDR-TB is approximately 3% in new cases and 12–17% in retreatment cases.[13] Prevention of MDR-TB is given priority by RNTCP and can be achieved by strengthening the DOTS programme to treat the newly diagnosed cases. Programmatic management of drug-resistant TB (PMDT) includes aspects of MDR-TB diagnosis, management and treatment. All patients who continue to remain sputum sputum-positive treatment by first-line drugs and contacts of MDR-TB should be evaluated for drug resistance. Currently all HIV-positive patients and all retreatment cases are also offered drug susceptibility testing (DST). Drug susceptibility testing can be done by culture on egg or agar-based Lowenstein-Jensen (LJ) media which takes about 6–8 weeks. Alternatively, liquid broth based media [automated mycobacteria growth indicator tube (MGIT) 960] can give results by 2 weeks. Line probe assay and cartridge-based nucleic acid amplification test (CBNAAT), i.e., GeneXpert can demonstrate drug resistance gene mutation within hours and are highly sensitive for sputum-positive samples.[14-16] Multidrug-resistant-TB should be treated by at least six drugs of which one should be aminoglycoside, one fluoroquinolone, and four other oral drugs which are thought to be active against the *Mycobacteria*. MDR guidelines recommend an IP of 6–9 months with six drugs and 16–18 months of CP with four oral drugs. All doses are directly observed. Drugs are given in single daily doses but in case of intolerance they can be given in divided doses. Treatment monitoring is done by sputum culture starting from 4th month of treatment till 7th month and every 3 monthly. The most important objective evidence of improvement is the conversion of sputum smear and culture to negative. Hence, provision for quality assured culture and DST laboratory remains the backbone of any MDR-TB program. Response to treatment in extrapulmonary MDR-TB is clinico-radiological. The MDR-TB treatment schedule under RNTCP is given in Table 4.

Table 4: DOTS plus regimen recommended by RNTCP		
Category	Intensive phase	Continuation phase
MDR-TB	6 (9*) Km Lvx Eto Z E Cs	18 Lvx Eto E Cs

Cs, cycloserine; DOTS, directly observed treatment short-course; E, ethambutol; Eto, ethionamide; Km, kanamycin; Lvx, levofloxacin; RNTCP, Revised National Tuberculosis Control Programme; Z, pyrazinamide.
Para-aminosalicylic acid (PAS) is included in the regimen as a substitute drug if any bactericidal drug (Km, Lvx, Z and Eto) or two bacteriostatic (E and Cs) drugs are not tolerated.
*Intensive phase (IP) is extended to 9 month if 4th month culture is positive.
Drugs dosage is based on body weight. For body weight (BW) more than 45 kg; Km = 750 mg, Lvx = 750 mg, Eto = 750 mg, Z = 1,500 mg, E = 1,000 mg, Cs = 750 mg, PAS = 12 gm.

TREATMENT OF EXTENSIVELY DRUG-RESISTANT TUBERCULOSIS[17]

Extensively drug-resistant strains are those MDR-TB isolates which are found to be resistant to both fluoroquinolone and one of the aminoglycosides. The treatment of XDR-TB is of 24–30 months duration, with 6–12 months IP and 18 months CP.
Seven drugs are given during IP:
1. Capreomycin (Cm)
2. Para-aminosalicylic acid
3. Moxifloxacin (Mfx)
4. High-dose isoniazid (INH)
5. Clofazimine
6. Linezolid
7. Amoxiclav.

The continuation phase consists of six drugs:
1. Para-aminosalicylic acid
2. Moxifloxacin (Mfx)
3. High-dose isoniazid (INH)
4. Clofazimine
5. Linezolid
6. Amoxiclav.

Evaluation for surgery is imperative in all cases.

TREATMENT OF TUBERCULOSIS IN SPECIAL SITUATIONS

Human immunodeficiency virus prevalence among TB cases in India is reported to be 6.7%. All newly diagnosed TB patients should be offered HIV testing. TB is one of the leading causes of death in "people living with HIV/AIDS (PLHA)", hence early diagnosis and effective treatment is imperative in this group.[18] Treatment is similar to HIV-negative patients except that they should not be given alternate day regimen. Prompt referral for antiretroviral therapy (ART) is also indicated. Drug interactions should be considered while prescribing both ATT and ART. The treatment for extrapulmonary TB is similar to pulmonary TB. Central nervous system (CNS) and bone TB require longer duration of treatment. Streptomycin is preferred to be added to CNS TB regimens due to its better CNS penetration.

Tuberculosis in pregnancy is treated similarly except that streptomycin is contraindicated and the newborn should receive chemoprophylaxis with INH. Antitubercular treatment is not a contraindication to breastfeeding. Diabetics are treated with the same regimen as nondiabetics. Some studies have shown that prolonging the treatment to 9 months in a newly diagnosed case may prevent recurrence in diabetic population. Dose modification in renal insufficiency is not warranted unless the renal failure is advanced. Aminoglycosides are contraindicated whereas ethambutol requires dose adjustment based on creatinine clearance. Many of the antitubercular drugs are hepatotoxic and should be used cautiously in those with pre-existing liver disease with regular monitoring of the liver function tests.

CONCLUSION

The treatment of TB is prolonged, expensive and requires close monitoring of the patient during the course of treatment. The advent of DOTS has enabled the treatment to be provided to the underprivileged and the poor, free of cost, thus reducing the disease burden to the family and the country. Emergence of multidrug and extensively drug-resistant disease has added to the challenge in TB treatment. Adequate treatment of drug-sensitive TB is central to preventing emergence of drug resistance. MDR-TB control program needs expansion and should be accessible to all TB patients with drug-resistant TB. There are many drugs in the pipeline being tried for reduction of duration of TB treatment. Future research should be directed towards designing regimens which can reduce the duration of treatment, and at the same time can prevent both recurrence and emergence of resistance.

REFERENCES

1. World Health Organization (WHO). (2007). Improving the diagnosis and treatment of smear-negative pulmonary and extrapulmonary tuberculosis among adults and adolescents: recommendations for HIV-prevalent and resource-constrained settings. [online] Available from: apps.who.int/iris/bitstream/10665/69463/1/WHO_HTM_TB_2007.379_eng.pdf. [Accessed April, 2017].
2. Leitch AG. Pulmonary tuberculosis: clinical features. In: Seaton A, Seaton D, Leitch AG (Eds). Crofton and Douglas's Respiratory Diseases, 5th edition. United States: Wiley-Blackwell; 2008. pp. 507-27.
3. Ministry of Health and Family Welfare. (2010). Revised National Tuberculosis Control Programme (RNTCP) – Training Module for Medical Practitioners. [online] Available from: tbcindia.nic.in/WriteReadData/l892s/5949760355Training%20Module%20for%20Medical%20Practitioners.pdf. [Accessed April, 2017].
4. Bhalla AS, Goyal A, Guleria R, Gupta AK. Chest tuberculosis: Radiological review and imaging recommendations. Indian J Radiol Imaging. 2015;25(3):213-25.
5. Blumberg HM, Burman WJ, Chaisson RE, et al. American Thoracic Society/Centers for Disease Control and Prevention/Infectious Diseases Society of America: treatment of tuberculosis. Am J Respir Crit Care Med. 2003;167(4):603-62.
6. Saukkonen JJ, Cohn DL, Jasmer RM, et al. An official ATS statement: hepatotoxicity of antituberculosis therapy. Am J Respir Crit Care Med. 2006;174(8):935-52.
7. World Health Organization (WHO). (2010). Guidelines for treatment of tuberculosis. [online] Available from: www.who.int/tb/publications/2010/9789241547833/en/. [Accessed April, 2017].
8. Volmink J, Garner P. Directly observed therapy for treating tuberculosis. Cochrane Database Syst Rev. 2006;(2): CD003343.
9. Menzies D, Benedetti A, Paydar A, et al. Effect of duration and intermittency of rifampin on tuberculosis treatment outcomes: a systematic review and meta-analysis. PLoS Med. 2009;6(9):e1000146.
10. Sachdeva KS, Shah A, Rade K, et al. Transitioning to daily treatment for drug-sensitive TB in India. Indian J Tuberc. 2015;62(4):239-42.
11. Ministry of Health and Family Welfare. (2012). Revised National Tuberculosis Control Programme (RNTCP): Guidelines on Programmatic Management of Drug-resistant TB (PMDT) in India. [online] Available from: http://tbcindia.gov.in/WriteReadData/l892s/8320929355Guidelines%20for%20PMDT%20in%20India%20-%20May%202012.pdf. [Accessed April, 2017].
12. World Health Organization (WHO). (2011). Companion handbook to the WHO guidelines for the programmatic management of drug-resistant tuberculosis. [online] Available from: www.who.int/tb/publications/pmdt_companionhandbook/en/. [Accessed April, 2017].
13. Ramachandran R, Nalini S, Chandrasekar V, et al. Surveillance of drug-resistant tuberculosis in the state of Gujarat, India. Int J Tuberc Lung Dis. 2009;13(9):1154-60.
14. Raizada N, Sachdeva KS, Sreenivas A, et al. Feasibility of decentralised deployment of Xpert MTB/RIF test at lower level of health system in India. PLoS One. 2014;9(2):e89301.
15. Sam IC, Drobniewski F, More P, et al. Mycobacterium tuberculosis and rifampin resistance, United Kingdom. Emerg Infect Dis. 2006;12(5):752-9.
16. Barnard M, Albert H, Coetzee G, et al. Rapid molecular screening for multidrug-resistant tuberculosis in a high-volume public health laboratory in South Africa. Am J Respir Crit Care Med. 2008;177(7):787-92.
17. Michael JS, John TJ. Extensively drug-resistant tuberculosis in India: a review. Indian J Med Res. 2012;136(4):599-604.
18. World Health Organization (WHO). (2008). Anti-tuberculosis Drug Resistance in the World: Fourth Global Report. [online] Available from: www.who.int/tb/publications/2008/drs_report4_26feb08.pdf. [Accessed April, 2017].

CHAPTER 6

Multidrug-resistant Tuberculosis

GC Khilnani, Raju P Dungeni

INTRODUCTION

Despite the fact that tuberculosis (TB) is potentially a preventable and curable disease, it still remains a major cause of global morbidity and mortality affecting one-third of the world's population. India shares the largest burden with 2.3 million new cases including an estimated 320,000 deaths annually.[1] Since the introduction of streptomycin in early 1940s, significant progress has been made in improving the diagnosis and treatment of this disease, leading to reduction of incidence and mortality in the recent years. However, drug-resistant TB has posed a constant threat to global efforts for TB control.

DEFINITION

The term "multidrug-resistant TB (MDR-TB)" refers to TB caused by strains of *Mycobacterium tuberculosis* (MTB) that are resistant to at least rifampicin and isoniazid, the two agents that currently form the backbone of first-line anti-TB regimen. "Extensively drug-resistant TB (XDR-TB)" is due to MDR-TB strains that are additionally resistant to one of the second-line injectable agents (i.e., amikacin, kanamycin or capreomycin) and any of the fluoroquinolones (i.e., levofloxacin, ofloxacin or moxifloxacin). This distinction is important since drug-resistant TB requires prolonged therapy with drugs which are costly, less effective, and more toxic than the first-line agents, which further contribute to poor compliance and treatment failure.

BURDEN OF MULTIDRUG-RESISTANT TUBERCULOSIS

Multidrug-resistant TB is essentially a man-made problem; inadequate treatment, ineffective drugs and poor adherence contribute to the development of drug resistance. The advent of powerful drugs like isoniazid and rifampicin during 1960s and subsequent short-course combination regimens had raised hope that this disease could potentially be eradicated. However, the emergence of drug resistance soon came into picture, further complicated by the increasing incidence of MDR-TB in human immunodeficiency virus (HIV)-infected patients and the emergence of XDR-TB since the last decade. According to the global TB report in 2015, an estimated 3.3% of the newly diagnosed TB cases and 20% of previously treated cases have MDR-TB. Approximately 9.7% of the patients with MDR-TB harbor XDR-TB. In India, prevalence of MDR-TB is estimated to be about 2.2% in new cases and 15% in retreatment cases.[1] Under-reporting (missing patients) is another major issue in assessing the burden of TB in India because of limited access to universal drug susceptibility testing especially in the rural areas and private sectors. The problem of increasing coinfection of TB and HIV is making the TB control activities more complex and demanding.

DIAGNOSIS

Clinical Diagnosis

The clinical manifestations of MDR-TB are similar with those of drug susceptible disease. However, a careful history and review of the medical records may provide important clues raising the suspicion for the presence of MDR-TB in any patient as outlined in Box 1.[2] All patients with these risk factors should undergo laboratory testing to confirm the presence of MDR-TB bacilli.

Laboratory Diagnosis

Currently, the diagnosis of MDR-TB is based upon the detection of causative organism which is resistant to isoniazid and rifampicin in a clinical sample (usually sputum, affected body tissues or fluid).[3] The techniques that are used for this purpose are summarized in table 1.[4]

Culture-based Techniques

The diagnosis of MDR-TB is based upon standardized drug susceptibility testing procedures using solid or liquid media. By conventional methods using solid media (e.g., Lowenstein-Jensen medium), 6 to 12 weeks are required to identify drug-resistant organisms. The automated liquid culture-based detection systems such as 'BACTEC 460' and modern mycobacteria growth indicator tube (MGIT) are more sensitive than the solid cultures with reduced turnaround time of 2-4 weeks.

Molecular Techniques

The novel rapid molecular tools for the identification of TB have revolutionized the diagnosis of TB and drug resistance. It utilizes the nucleic acid amplification technique to simultaneously identify the TB bacilli and detect specific mutation responsible for the drug resistance. The Xpert MTB/RIF (GeneXpert) assay is a cartridge-based automated nucleic acid amplification test that can simultaneously identify TB bacilli and resistance to rifampicin within 2 hours. This information is clinically important since more than 90% of the patients with rifampicin resistance also have resistance to isoniazid (MDR-TB). This test has been endorsed by the World Health Organization for initial diagnostic test in adults and children presumed to have MDR-TB or HIV-associated TB.[5] GeneXpert has sensitivity of 98% and 72% for smear positive and negative pulmonary TB respectively with specificity of 99%.[6] It has also been used in the identification of TB from other sources such as pleural, cerebrospinal, and ascitic fluids with variable sensitivity and specificity. Similarly, the line probe assay (LPA) is a molecular probe capable of detecting both rifampicin and isoniazid resistance mutations. The sensitivity and specificity in sputum-positive patients using MGIT as a gold standard is around 97% and 94% respectively.[7] LPAs for the detection of resistance to second-line anti-TB drugs are also available. In India, the programmatic management of drug-resistant TB (PMDT) has recommended LPA as a preferred diagnostic method for drug sensitivity testing if available, followed by liquid culture and solid culture in order of preference.

Radiological Diagnosis

Imaging findings of MDR-TB do not basically differ from those of drug-sensitive TB. Patients exhibit a wide range of radiological signs, some of them showing extensive pattern of involvement of the affected organs. The pulmonary imaging may reveal extensive bilateral consolidation,

---

Box 1: Risk factors for MDR-TB

- Residence in a region with known high MDR prevalence
- Contact with a patient with drug-resistant TB
- HIV/AIDS
- Previous TB therapy
- Relapse or recurrence after previous successful treatment
- Nonadherence or default
- Substance abuse
- Malabsorption
- Use of medications that interact with anti-TB drugs, e.g., antifungals
- History of fluoroquinolone therapy

AIDS, acquired immunodeficiency syndrome; HIV, human immunodeficiency virus; MDR-TB, multidrug-resistant tuberculosis.

Table 1: Diagnostic tests for multidrug-resistant-tuberculosis	
Diagnostic tests	**Turnaround time**

• Solid culture:
  ○ Lowenstein-Jensen media (egg-based)
  ○ Middlebrook 7H10 media (agar-based)
• Liquid culture: Growth in liquid media (Middlebrook 7H12) visualized using automated machines, e.g., BACTEC, MGIT, etc.
• Molecular tests:
  ○ Line probe assay: Detects resistance to isoniazid and rifampicin
  ○ Xpert MTB/RIF (GeneXpert)
	• Smear positive: 3 weeks
	• Smear negative: 6–12 weeks
	• Smear positive: 8 days
	• Smear negative: 2–6 weeks
	• Smear positive: 3 days
	• Smear negative: Culture should be done first 2 hours

MGIT, mycobacteria growth indicator tube.

cavitation, and interstitial infiltrates including miliary and reticular opacities, lymphadenopathy, and/or pleural effusion.[8] Features of chronicity, such as bronchiectasis and calcified granulomas are more common in patients with MDR-TB.[9] A suspicion of MDR-TB in patients who are receiving treatment or those with risk factors may be raised based on the activity of TB by imaging, such as the presence of cavitation or evidence of endobronchial spread, e.g., centrilobular nodules or a tree-in-bud pattern.[10-12] CT may also help to localize the lesions for appropriate sampling (such as lung segments for bronchoalveolar lavage, lymph nodes, abscesses, etc. for aspiration) and also in locating the site of activity for surgical management.

MULTIDRUG-RESISTANT EXTRAPULMONARY TUBERCULOSIS

Extrapulmonary TB among the immunocompetent individuals constitutes about 15% to 20% of all cases of TB and accounts for more than 50% in HIV-infected individuals.[13,14] Though multidrug-resistant extrapulmonary TB (MDR-EPTB) is an uncommon form of presentation, it is predicted that due to an increasing magnitude of drug-resistant TB around the world, its incidence is also on the rise.[15,16] The exact incidence of MDR-EPTB is difficult to determine given the difficulty in diagnosing such cases. As with drug-sensitive TB, MDR-TB can also involve several extrapulmonary sites such as lymph nodes, pleura, peritoneum, meninges, genitourinary system, pericardium, skin, and skeletal system (bones, joints, and spine), etc.[3,5-7] Some of these diseases such as MDR-TB involving spine, joints or meninges may cause significant long-term sequelae and morbidity, highlighting diagnostic and therapeutic challenges while managing these patients.[15]

Definitive diagnosis of extrapulmonary TB involves demonstration of resistant MTB in appropriate tissue specimens and body fluids by microbiological and histopathological methods. The need for multiple invasive tests including image-guided needle aspirations and biopsies along with poor yield of the conventional histopathological and microbiological diagnostic methods make a diagnosis of MDR extrapulmonary tuberculosis difficult. Sometimes the diagnosis is made based upon clinical, radiographic, pathological features, and response to treatment, even without the microbiological evidence.

TREATMENT

Medical Therapy

The currently available drugs for the treatment of TB are summarized in the table 2. In general, the intensive phase of MDR-TB treatment should be given for 6 to 9 months and consists of at least four second-line anti-TB drugs that are likely to be effective (including an injectable such as kanamycin) along with the first-line agents such as pyrazinamide and ethambutol. The intensive phase may be extended to further 3 months if patient has persistently positive-

Table 2: Currently available antituberculosis drugs

Group: One (first-line)	Group: Two (fluoroquinolones)	Group: Three (injectables)	Group: Four (bacteriostatic)	Group: Five (unclear role)
• Isoniazid (INH) • Rifampicin • Pyrazinamide • Ethambutol	• Levofloxacin • Moxifloxacin • Gatifloxacin • Ofloxacin	• Capreomycin • Amikacin • Kanamycin • Streptomycin	• Ethionamide • Prothionamide • Cycloserine • Terizidone • Para-aminosalicylic acid	• Bedaquiline* • Delamanid* • High-dose INH • Clofazimine • Co-amoxiclav • Linezolid • Imipenem/cilastatin • Meropenem • Clarithromycin • Thioacetazone

*New drugs with promising results.

sputum cultures. During the continuation phase, at least four drugs from different groups (except the injectables) are given for another 18 months (e.g., ethambutol, levofloxacin, ethionamide, and cycloserine).[14,17] Sputum examination should be conducted monthly during the intensive phase and at least quarterly during the continuation phase. Sputum for acid-fast bacilli cultures are sent at regular intervals. Sputum conversion is said to be achieved after two consecutive cultures taken a month apart are negative.[16]

Every effort should be made to ensure drug compliance and clinical response during regular follow-up visits. Early identification and management of side effects is equally important. They include gastrointestinal (nausea and vomiting), hepatitis, allergic reactions, neuropathy, joint pains, visual and auditory disturbances, psychosis, and abnormal thyroid functions.

Role of Surgery

Surgical resection of the affected lobe or the segment as an adjunct to medical therapy is considered to play a useful role in selected cases of MDR-TB. The potential candidates for surgical treatment are: (i) Patients with persistent infection despite extended treatment, (ii) Extensive patterns of drug resistance with risk of treatment failure and (iii) Localized parenchymal destruction in which surgical resection is amenable without causing respiratory insufficiency. In experienced hands, this looks promising with reported success rates of more than 90% with perioperative mortality below 4%. It should be performed after minimum of 2 months of intensive chemotherapeutic regimen, achieving sputum-negative status, if possible.

PROGNOSIS

Despite WHO's treatment success target of 75% by 2015 for MDR-TB, only 50% global success rate could be achieved during 2015, with 16% mortality and the remaining contributed by patients who were lost to follow-up (16%), failed treatment (10%), or had no outcome information (8%).[18] Patients with XDR-TB have substantially worse outcome with only 40% cure rate and mortality rate of 30-50%. Factors associated with poor outcomes include male gender, alcohol abuse, immunosuppression, malnutrition, delay in diagnosis, and extent of resistance pattern.[18]

PREVENTION

The top priority for the control and ultimately, elimination of MDR-TB is to prevent its emergence. It is a well-known fact that MDR-TB is largely related to poor treatment practices. The areas with poor control of TB have higher rates of drug-resistant TB. Hence, a good quality directly observed treatment short-course (DOTS) program is essential for its prevention and control. Similarly rational use of drugs, proper infection control measures, and improved diagnostic facilities with regular monitoring are essential components to prevent MDR-TB and to stop TB transmission.

REFERENCES

1. Ministry of Health and Family Welfare. (2014). Annual Reports. [online] Available from: www.tbcindia.nic.in/index1.php?lang=1&level=1&sublinkid=4160&lid=2807. [Accessed April, 2017].
2. Shao Y, Yang D, Xu W, et al. Epidemiology of anti-tuberculosis drug resistance in a Chinese population: current situation and challenges ahead. BMC Public Health. 2011;11:110.
3. Millard J, Ugarte-Gil C, Moore DA. Multidrug resistant tuberculosis. BMJ. 2015;350:h882.
4. World Health Organization (WHO). (2014). Companion handbook to the WHO guidelines for the programmatic management of drug-resistant tuberculosis. [online] Available from: apps.who.int/iris/bitstream/10665/130918/1/9789241548809_eng.pdf?ua=1&ua=1. [Accessed April, 2017].
5. World Health Organization (WHO). (2017). TB diagnostics and laboratory strengthening. [online] Available from: www.who.int/tb/areas-of-work/laboratory/mtbrifrollout/en/. [Accessed April, 2017].
6. Boehme CC, Nabeta P, Hillemann D, et al. Rapid molecular detection of tuberculosis and rifampin resistance. N Engl J Med. 2010;363:1005-15.
7. Singhal R, Arora J, Lal P, et al. Comparison of line probe assay with liquid culture for rapid detection of multi-drug resistance in Mycobacterium tuberculosis. Indian J Med Res. 2012;136(6):1044-7.
8. Yeom JA, Jeong YJ, Jeon D, et al. Imaging findings of primary multidrug-resistant tuberculosis: a comparison with findings of drug-sensitive tuberculosis. J Comput Assist Tomogr. 2009;33(6):956-60.
9. Jeong YJ, Lee KS. Pulmonary tuberculosis: up-to-date imaging and management. AJR Am J Roentgenol. 2008;191(3):834-44.
10. Lee KS, Hwang JW, Chung MP, et al. Utility of CT in the evaluation of pulmonary tuberculosis in patients without AIDS. Chest. 1996;110(4):977-84.
11. Sharma SK, Mohan A, Gupta R, et al. Clinical presentation of tuberculosis in patients with AIDS: an Indian experience. Indian J Chest Dis Allied Sci. 1997;39(4):213-20.
12. Pablos-Méndez A, Raviglione MC, Laszlo A, et al. Global surveillance for antituberculosis-drug resistance, 1994-1997. World Health Organization-International Union against Tuberculosis and Lung Disease Working Group on Anti-Tuberculosis Drug Resistance Surveillance. N Engl J Med. 1998;338(23):1641-9.
13. Mirsaeidi SM, Tabarsi P, Edrissian MO, et al. Primary multi-drug resistant tuberculosis presented as lymphadenitis in a patient without HIV infection. Monaldi Arch Chest Dis. 2004;61(4):244-7.
14. Golden MP, Vikram HR. Extrapulmonary tuberculosis: an overview. Am Fam Physician. 2005;72(9):1761-8.
15. Pawar UM, Kundnani V, Agashe V, Nene A, Nene A. Multidrug-resistant tuberculosis of the spine--is it the beginning of the end? A study of twenty-five culture proven multidrug-resistant tuberculosis spine patients. Spine (Phila Pa 1976). 2009;34(22):E806-10.
16. Ministry of Health and Family Welfare. (2012). Revised National Tuberculosis Control Programme: Guidelines on Programmatic Management of Drug-resistant TB (PMDT) in India. [online] Available from: www.tbcindia.nic.in/showfile.php?lid=3155. [Accessed April, 2017].
17. Joseph P, Desai VBR, Mohan NS, et al. Outcome of standardized treatment for patients with MDR-TB from Tamil Nadu, India. Indian J Med Res. 2011;133(5):529-34.
18. World Health Organization. Global tuberculosis report 2015. Geneva: World Health Organization; 2015.

CHAPTER 7

Central Nervous System Tuberculosis

Rakesh K Gupta, Mudit Gupta

INTRODUCTION

Tuberculosis (TB) accounts for 8 million deaths annually in the world.[1] Involvement of the central nervous system (CNS) is one of the most serious forms of this infection and is a prominent cause of sickness and death in developing countries.[2] In India alone, active TB has been reported in about 200 million people. In developed countries, there has been a rise in the number of CNS TB cases which may be attributed to the pandemic of acquired immunodeficiency syndrome.[3] *Mycobacterium tuberculosis* is responsible for almost all cases of the tubercular infection in CNS.[2] Tubercular bacilli evoke granulomatous inflammatory reaction in CNS involving the meninges, brain, spinal cord, bones covering the brain, and spinal cord. They manifest in a variety of forms, both tuberculous meningitis and its complications like hydrocephalous, focal infarction, and parenchymal atrophy, and focal cerebritis, tuberculoma, and tubercular abscess. Spinal cord infection is less common; it results in either arachnoiditis or focal intramedullary tuberculomas.

Early diagnosis of CNS TB is necessary for early institution of appropriate treatment to reduce the morbidity and mortality. Noninvasive imaging modalities such as computed tomography (CT) and magnetic resonance imaging (MRI) are routinely used in the diagnosis of CNS TB; however, MRI is known to offer greater inherent sensitivity and specificity over CT. In this chapter, the various forms of CNS TB including its complications along with imaging features are discussed.

PATHOPHYSIOLOGY

The tubercular bacilli reach the brain and its coverings by bloodstream from a distant active focus located in the rest of the body. In the brain, the bacilli lodge in the areas rich in vascularity and hence a predilection for the cortical and subcortical region and/or meninges.[4] Direct spread of infection to the brain from adjacent paranasal sinuses or mastoid air cells is rare.[5] Infection starts in a subpial or subependymal cortical focus evoke a nonspecific inflammatory reaction that may be termed as tuberculous cerebritis. Once sensitized, the inflammatory response results in a granuloma that erodes into the subarachnoid space and CSF causing basal leptomeningitis. Vasculitis involving the lenticulostriate and thalamoperforating arteries may occur and cause small infarcts in the deep gray-matter nuclei and deep white matter.[4]

The initial lesion is a tubercle consisting of a central area of incipient or frank necrosis surrounded by layers of inflammatory cells, lymphocytes, epithelioid, and Langerhans' giant cells with an encircling zone of rich vascularity.[4] These lesions originate as a conglomerate of microgranulomata in an area of tuberculous cerebritis that join to form a noncaseating tuberculoma. In most cases, subsequent central caseous necrosis develops that is initially solid but in some instances may eventually liquefy. A capsule of collagenous tissue, epithelioid cells, multinucleated giant cells, and mononuclear inflammatory cells surround this solid caseation. The may contain a few bacilli. Liquefaction then usually begins from the center in the caseation. The capsule contains granulation tissue and compressed glial tissue. Tubercular abscess shows central cavitation with chronic inflammatory reaction with fibrosis in the wall. Aspirate from the pus stains positive for acid fast bacilli. All these different types of lesions are usually accompanied by edema and some proliferation of astrocytes in the surrounding brain parenchyma.

CLINICAL FEATURES

Central nervous system TB is common in children and older persons because their immune systems are less robust than those of adults. Tubercular meningitis (TBM) is also common in patients who are immunesuppressed, such patients with human immunodeficiency virus (HIV) or diabetes, and patients taking steroids or cytotoxic drugs. The prodrome of TBM is insidious and characterized by persistent low-grade fever, malaise, headache, and confusion. The most common clinical features of TBM are fever with nausea, vomiting, headache, neck stiffness and photophobia.[6] Cranial nerve palsies especially of third, fourth, and sixth nerves are common. The signs and symptoms of intracranial tuberculomas are essentially those of a space occupying lesions of the brain. For the definitive diagnosis, isolation of *M. tuberculosis* from the tissue on smear or culture is possible only in a small number of patients. Hence the index of suspicion is mostly indirect, i.e., concomitant tubercular involvement elsewhere (only 10% of cases may show disease elsewhere in the body), malaise, low grade fever, loss of weight, positive tuberculin test, raised sedimentation rate, history of contact, etc.[7]

Cerebrospinal fluid (CSF) analysis is usually used to diagnose TBM that characteristically shows a lymphocytosis, increased CSF protein and decreased sugar concentration.[8] Cerebrospinal fluid culture and polymerase chain reaction examination for acid-fast bacilli are confirmatory tests, with higher sensitivity of the latter.[9]

CRANIAL TUBERCULOSIS

Tubercular Meningitis

Tubercular meningitis is the commonest cause of chronic meningitis in developing countries. The infection may occur either by haematogenous seeding of the meninges or direct introduction into the meningeal space.

The common findings on imaging are meningeal thickening and marked enhancement of the basal cisterns, hydrocephalus, and vascular sequelae. Magnetic resonance imaging is more sensitive than CT for early detection of meningeal pathologies, including swelling of the affected subarachnoid spaces occurs and abnormal meningeal enhancement on post contrast study.[10] The commonly involved sites are interpeduncular fossa, pontine cistern, perimesencephalic, and suprasellar cisterns (Fig. 1); however, involvement of sulci over the convexities can also be seen.[11]

Magnetization transfer (MT) imaging is considered superior to routine imaging to demonstrate abnormal meninges, which are seen as hyperintense on precontrast MT-T1 images and further enhances on postcontrast T1-weighted MT images.[12] In addition, MT ratio (MTR) quantification helps in predicting the etiology of meningitis.[11,12] Visibility of the inflamed meninges on precontrast MT-T1 images with low MTR is fairly specific of TBM, which differentiates it from other non-tuberculous chronic meningitis.[11] The complications and sequelae of TBM are discussed as as follows.

Hydrocephalus

Hydrocephalus is usually communicating type, which is secondary to the blockage of the basal cisterns by the inflammatory exudates. Obstructive hydrocephalus is due to a focal parenchymal lesion with mass effect or secondary to entrapment of the ventricle by granulomatous ependymitis.[13] Periventricular hyperintensity on proton density and T2W and FLAIR images usually suggest hydrocephalus under pressure. It is due to the transventricular seepage of the CSF fluid across the white matter. Chronic

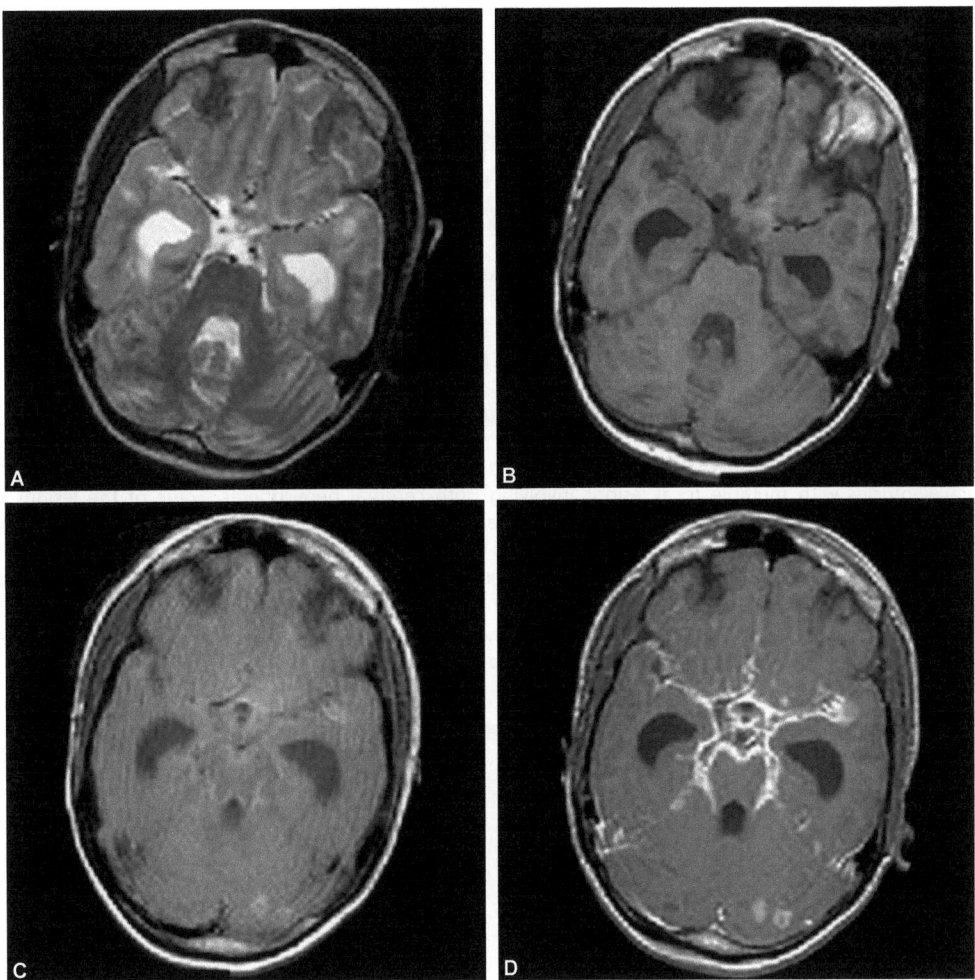

FIG. 1: Tuberculous meningitis: **A**, Axial T2-weighted and **B**, T1-weighted images show no apparent signal abnormality in basal brain parenchyma. **C**, Corresponding MT T-1 weighted image shows hyperintensity in perimesencephalic and supraseller cisterns. **D**, On PC T1-weighted image, abnormal enhancement is seen along perimesencephalic and supraseller cisterns

hydrocephalus may result in atrophy of brain parenchyma. Endoscopic third ventriculostomy is gaining acceptance in its management and patency of the stoma can be demonstrated by CSF flow dynamics.[14]

The choroid plexus is an important CNS structure that may serve as a portal of entry for the pathogens into the CNS. Sometimes choroid plexus involvement is the only sign of meningitis on imaging, however, it is usually associated with ependymitis, ventriculitis, and meningitis. Contrast enhanced MRI usually shows prominent enhancement of the choroid plexus and is described as choroid plexitis (Fig. 2).

Vasculitis

It is a common complication, next to hydrocephalus, seen at autopsy in cranial TBM.[13] Small and medium sized vessels are commonly involved. The adventitial layer of the vessels develops changes similar to those of the adjacent tuberculous exudates. The intima of the vessels may eventually be affected or eroded by a fibrinoid-hyaline degeneration. In later stages, the lumen of the vessel may get completely occluded by reactive subendothelial cellular proliferation.[15] Ischemic cerebral infarction is a common sequelae of tuberculous arteritis (Fig. 3) and is usually associated with

Imaging in Tuberculosis: Clinicopathological Correlation

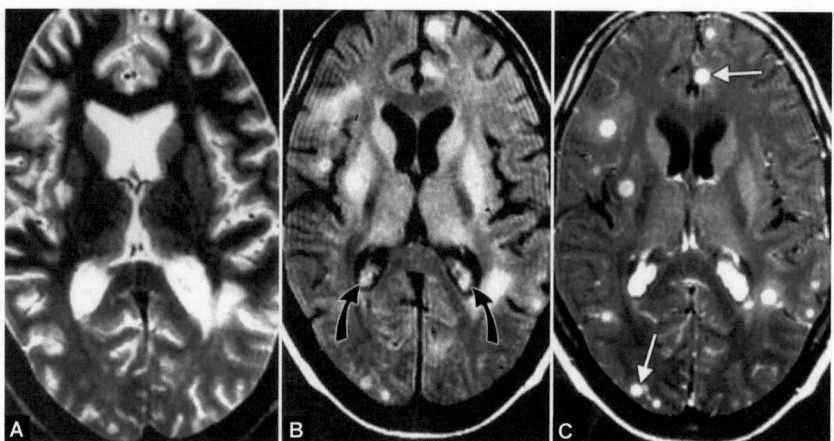

FIG. 2: Tuberculous choroid plexitis with multiple tuberculomas: **A**, Axial T2WI shows mild dilatation of lateral ventricles with multiple focal lesions involving both cerebral hemispheres. Some of the lesions are hyperintense while others are hypointense with peripheral hyperintensity along with perifocal edema. **B**, Magnetization transfer (MT) T1WI shows thickened choroid plexus with hyperintense foci within (curved arrows). More lesions are visible in **B** and **C** (arrows). **C**, Postcontrast MT T1WI shows intense enhancement of the choroid plexus along with rim and nodular enhancement of the tuberculomas

With permission from: Gupta RK. Tuberculosis and other non tuberculous bacterial granulomatous infections. In: Gupta RK, Lufkin RB, editors. MR imaging and spectroscopy of central nervous system infection. Springer Nature; 2001. pp. 95-145

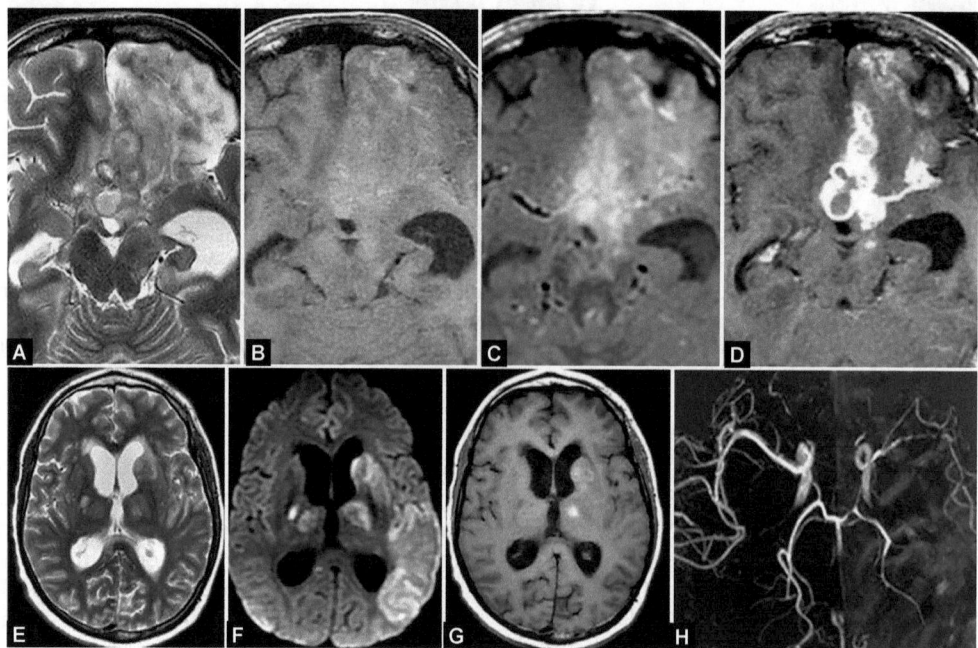

FIG. 3: Tuberculoma with vasculitis and hemorrhagic infarction: **A** and **B**, T2-weighted image shows mixed intensity loculations in the suprasellar cistern appearing isointense on T1-weighted image. **C**, Corresponding MT-T1weighted image shows hyperintensity in the margins of the lesion. **D**, Postcontrast T1 weighted image shows intense enhancement of the margins of the loculation. **E** to **G**, Axial magnetic resonance imaging sequences at higher level show hyperintensities on T2-weighted image (E) in the bilateral thalami, head of left caudate nucleus and left temporal region with restricted diffusion on diffusion-weighted imaging (F) and an area of hyperintensity on T1-weighted image (G), suggesting hemorrhagic infarct. In the same patient 3D-TOF sequence (H) shows irregular narrowing of the left M1 and M2 MCA and attenuation of the left MCA branches suggesting vasculitis

a poor outcome.[16] Middle cerebral artery and the lenticulostriate arteries penetrate the base of the brain are most commonly affected.[15,17] Conventional angiography shows hydrocephalic pattern, and narrowing of the arteries at the skull base.[18] Magnetic resonance angiography (MRA) may help in the detection of the vascular occlusion. Magnetic resonance imaging detects more number of hemorrhagic as well as nonhemorrhagic infarcts than CT.[19] Majority of the infarcts are in the basal ganglia and internal capsule regions due to the involvement of the lenticulostriate arteries, however, we may observe involvement of large vascular territory like middle cerebral artery.[17,20]

Diffusion-weighted imaging (DWI) helps in early detection of this complication (Fig. 4).[20] The vascular complications are usually seen following initiation of specific therapy. This is due to the healing and fibrosis of meninges resulting in the occlusion of vasculature embedded in the inflamed meninges. Arterial spin labelling techniques is now increasing being used in evaluation of brain ischemia.[21]

Focal or Diffuse Pachymeningitis

An unusual presentation of CNS TB is isolated involvement of the duramater known as pachymeningitis. It is an entity distinct from the inflammation of the duramater adjacent to an intraparenchymal tuberculoma.[22,23] It consists of either isolated dural involvement or a pial or parenchymal involvement secondary to dural-based lesion. Pachymeningitis may exist as focal or diffuse involvement of the duramater.[22,23] Focal pachymeningitis appear isointense on T1, iso to hypointense on T2WI and enhances on postcontrast images. In

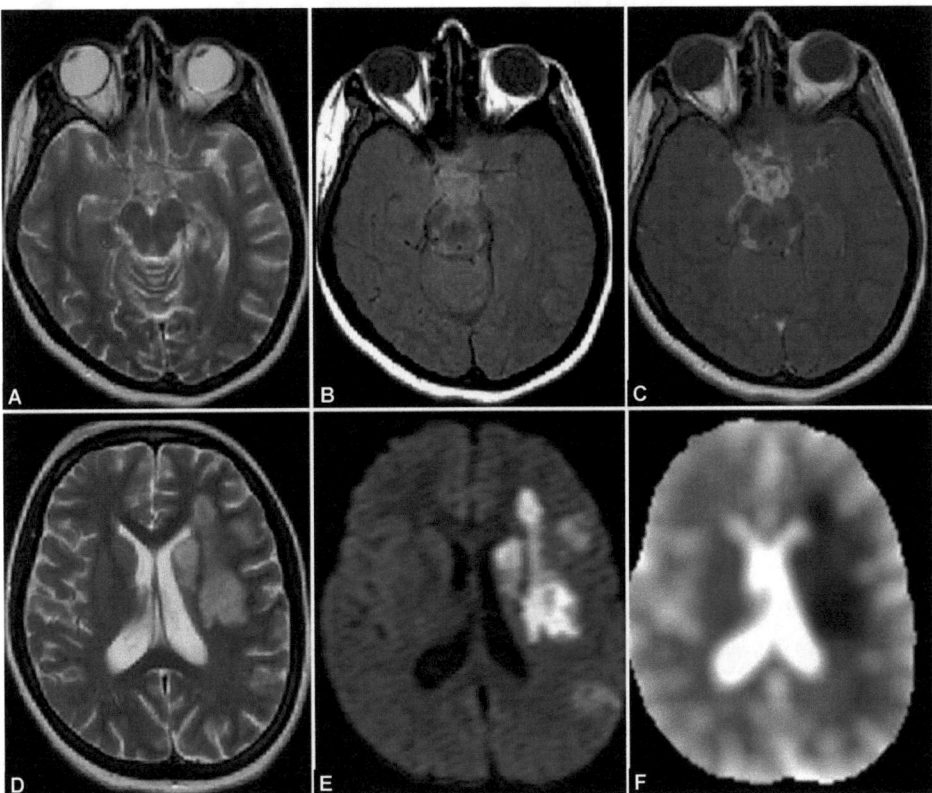

FIG. 4: Tuberculous meningitis with vasculitis: **A**, T2-weighted image shows no apparent signal abnormality in basal brain parenchyma. Corresponding magnetization transfer T-1 weighted image shows hyperintensity in perimesencephalic and suprasellar cisterns. **C**, On PC T1-weighted image, abnormal enhancement is seen along perimesencephalic and suprasellar cisterns. **D** to **F**, In the same patient, axial sections at higher level shows hyperintensity on T2-weighted image (D) in the left basal ganglia and frontal region with hyperintensity on DWI (E) and low ADC values on ADC map (F) suggesting left MCA territory infarct

contrast to focal lesions, diffuse involvement may appear hyperintense on T2WI. Magnetic resonance imaging appearance of focal and diffuse pachymeningitis is nonspecific and may be seen in a large number of inflammatory and noninflammatory conditions. It may be associated with hyperintensity in the adjoining parenchyma on T2WI.[23]

Cranial Nerve Neuropathy

Clinical involvement of the cranial nerves is seen in 17.4–40% of the patients with TB meningitis. Cranial nerve palsies are considered the most important neurological predictor to differentiate TBM from acute bacterial meningitis.[24] Cranial nerve neuropathies are thought to be partly due to vascular compromise resulting in ischemia of the nerve and/or may be due to entrapment of the nerves by the exudates (Figs 5 and 6).[25]

Intracranial Tuberculoma

Brain tuberculoma, a space-occupying mass of granulomatous tissue, forms a large percentage of intracranial mass lesions in the developing countries and is responsible for high morbidity and mortality.[2-4] Early recognition and treat-

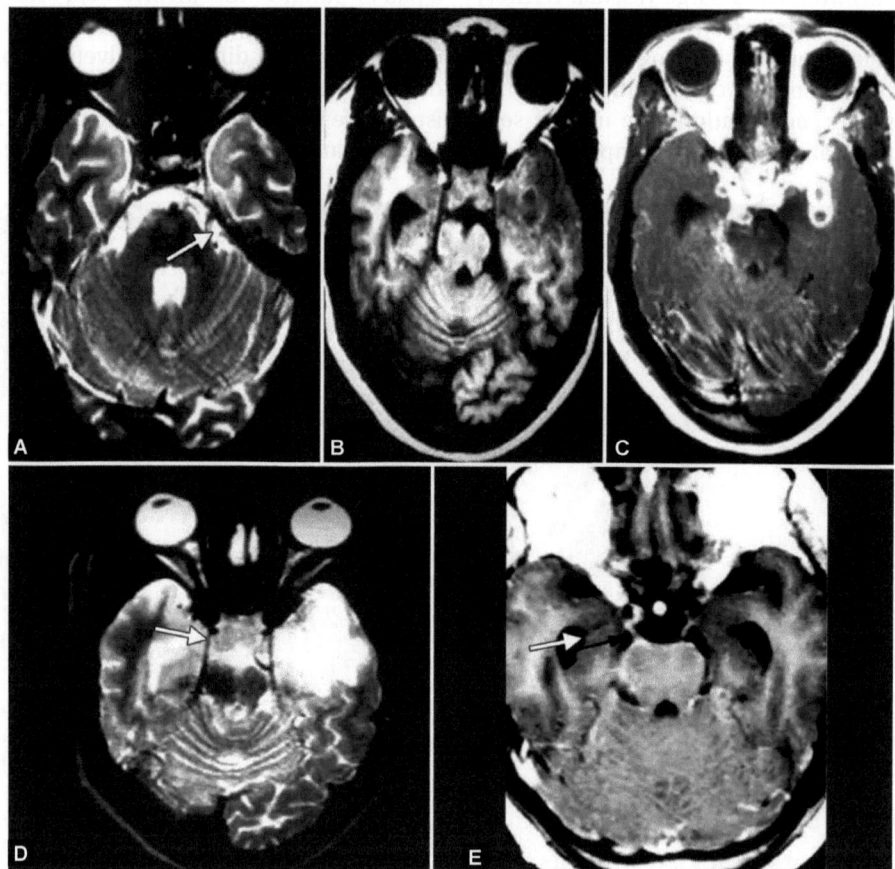

FIG. 5: Cranial neuropathies: **A**, T2 weighted axial image at the level of optic chiasm shows thickening and heterogeneous signal intensity of the chiasm (arrow). **B**, Thickened optic chiasm is seen well on T1 weighted image. **C**, Postcontrast T1 weighted image shows enhancement of the chiasm along with basal meninges and multiple tuberculomas. **D**, In another patient, postcontrast T1 weighted axial image at the level of midbrain shows thickening (black arrow) of the right third nerve along with meningeal enhancement. **E**, T2 weighted image through the lower pons shows focal hyperintensity (arrow) in the center of the left fifth nerve consistent with neuritis in another patient with tuberculous meningitis

With permission from: Gupta RK. Tuberculosis and other non tuberculous bacterial granulomatous infections. In: Gupta RK, Lufkin RB, editors. MR imaging and spectroscopy of central nervous system infection. Springer Nature; 2001. pp. 95-145.

ment on imaging may play a critical role in patient management.

Intracranial tuberculomas usually vary in size between 1 mm and 12 cm. The common locations of tuberculomas include cerebral hemispheres, basal ganglia, cerebellum, and brainstem (Fig. 6). Rarely, ventricular system is involved.[26,27]

Intracranial tuberculoma sometimes cause adjacent intracerebral inflammatory aneurysms that may be detected on MRA (Fig. 7).[25]

Tuberculoma of the Meckel's cave and cavernous sinus region may extend into the infratemporal fossa causing widening of the foramen ovale and adjacent bone destruction.[28] Tuberculoma in the hypophyseal region is

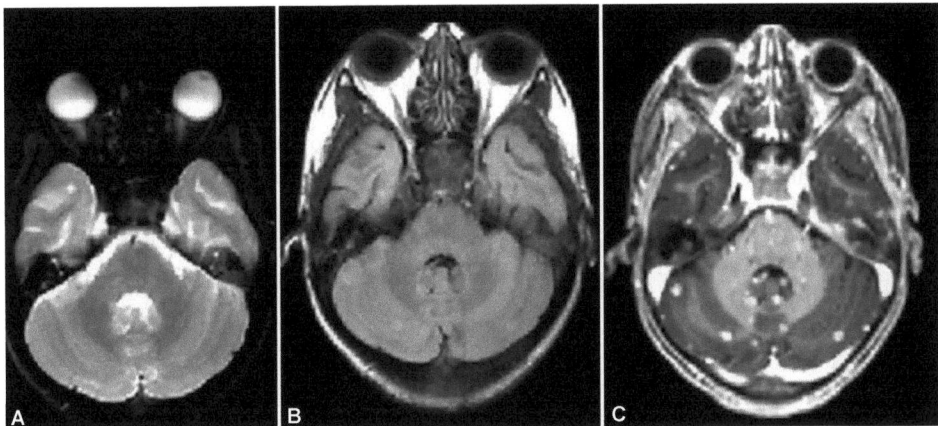

FIG. 6: A, The left facial nerve appears mildly thickened on T2WI; **B**, isointense on T1WI; and **C**, homogeneously enhancing on post-contrast T1WI. Cerebellum shows multiple nodular enhancing lesions, suggestive of miliary tuberculomas

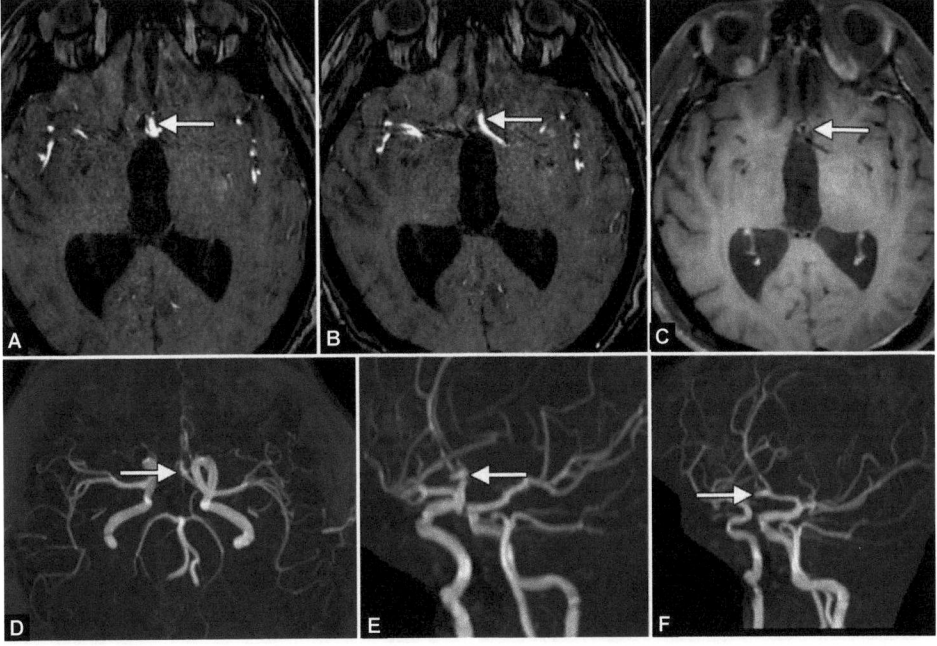

FIG. 7: A and **B**, Solitary saccular aneurysm of A1 segment of left anterior cerebral artery demonstrated by arrows on time of flight MR angiogram; **C**, isointense intact wall on T1WI; and **D** to **F**, three-dimensional magnetic resonance angiography. This aneurysm developed after the patients recovered from tuberculous meningitis following treatment

extremely rare and difficult to diagnose without a clearly suggestive context. Its radiologic features are nonspecific and are better recognized on MRI with a mass of a variable signal related to the percentage of caseous necrosis. A frequently associated thickening of the pituitary stalk suggests TB, requiring the search for another TB location.[29]

The authors propose a classification of intra-axial tuberculomas on the basis of T2 appearance on MRI as:[30]
- T2 hyperintense lesion
- T2 hypointense lesion
- T2 hyperintense centre with peripheral hypointense rim
- Lesion with mixed/heterogeneous signal intensity.

T2 Hyperintense Lesion

These lesions are noncaseating tuberculomas which appear hyperintense on T2WI. This appearance is nonspecific and may resemble metastases, lymphomas, demyelinating plaques, and other infective granulomas. T2 hyperintense lesions are usually <1.5 cm. These lesions appear iso to hypointense on T1, hyperintense on MT-T1, and FLAIR and show nodular or ring enhancement on postcontrast study.[12] These lesions may be a part of military tuberculosis or sometimes observed in patients with tuberculous meningitis. Low MTR, and enhancement pattern help in its differentiation from other lesions (Fig. 8). These lesions may show restriction of diffusion imaging with low ADC.[25]

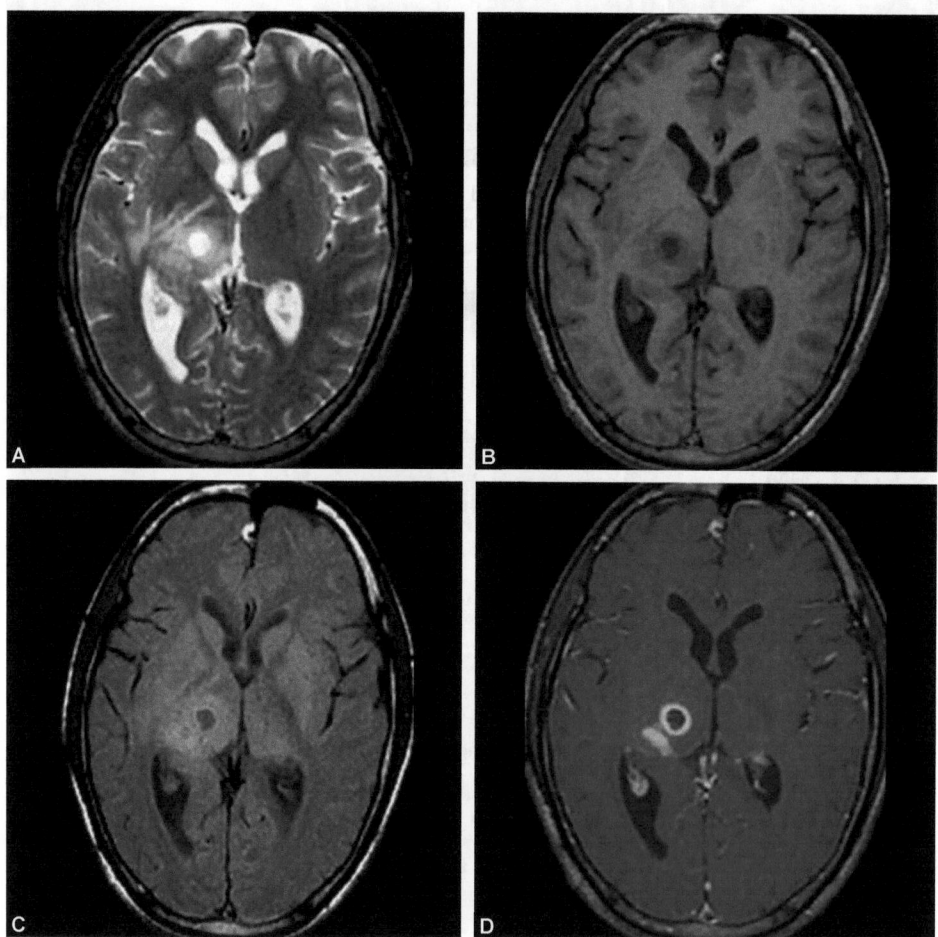

FIG. 8: T2 hyperintense tuberculoma with meningitis. **A**, Magnetic resonance imaging shows a lesion in the right thalamic region appearing hyperintense on T2; **B**, hypointense on T1 with isointense rim; **C**, the rim appears more prominent on MTT1, which enhances on **D**, postcontrast T1-weighted images consistent with tuberculoma. Abnormal leptomeningeal nhancement is also seen suggesting associated meningitis

T2 Hypointense Lesion

Tuberculomas with solid caseation are usually iso to hypointense on both T2- and T1WI. Hemorrhage, hemorrhagic tumor, occult cerebrovascular malformation, and calcification may appear as T2-hypointense lesion. This can also be seen in some lymphomas, glioblastoma, metastases from colonic carcinoma or melanoma, fungal granulomas, or cysticerci lesions. The imaging protocol for such lesions should include T2, T1, MT-T1, SWI, and post contrast (PC) T1WI for lesion <2.5 cm and inclusion of MR spectroscopy (MRS) for larger lesions. SWI with phase imaging is useful in differentiating haemorrhage and calcification from other T2 hypointense lesions. There is a rim of variable thickness seen around the solid caseating tubercular lesions which may appear hyperintense on T1 and sometimes also on T2WI in the absence of edema. This rim shows enhancement on PC-T1WI with no enhancement of the solid caseation. On MT-T1 images, the centre of tuberculomas with solid caseation shows hypointensity and the rim shows hyperintensity (Fig. 9). This rim is composed of variable amounts of cellular infiltrates, Langerhans' giant cells, and gliosis/fibrosis. The cellular wall contains fragmented portions of the cell wall of MTB that contains lipids. Lipids are known to have no MT effect, hence the rim has lower MT ratio compared to the core. This core has solid caseation, a cheesy material high in lipid contents, with macrophage infiltration, regional fibrosis/gliosis, macrophage by-products (free-radicals), and perileisonal cellular infiltrates, which are possibly responsible for the hypointensity seen on T2WI.[31] Biochemically, the core contains some amino acids due to breakdown of proteins in the bacteria and cellular infiltrates and the macromolecules of these amino acids are responsible for higher MT ratio compared to the

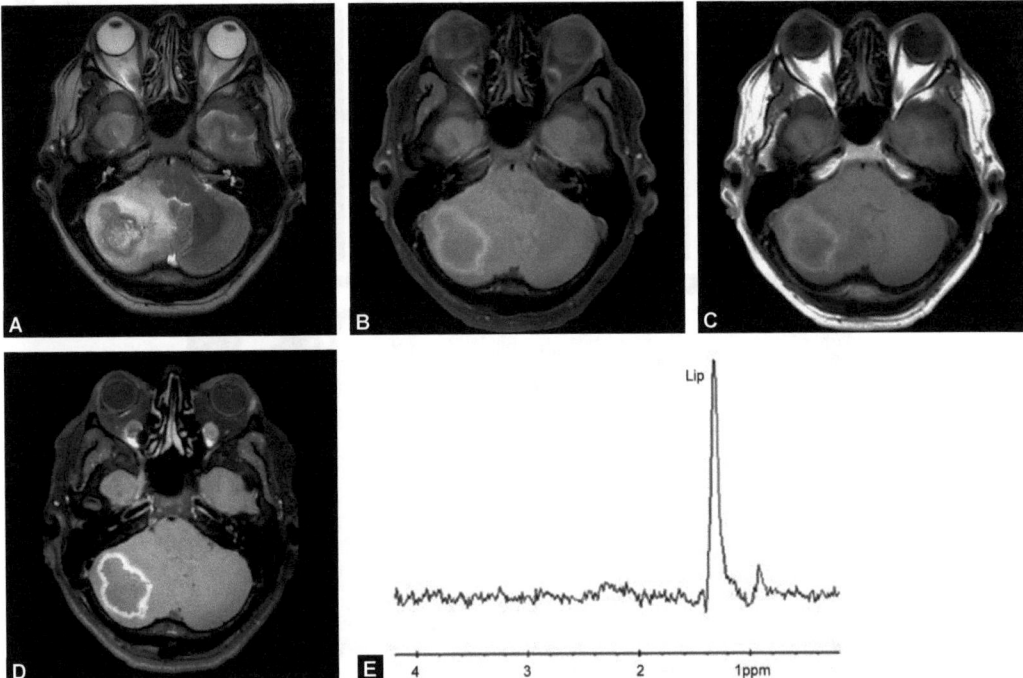

FIG. 9: Right cerebellar tuberculoma with minimal mass effect on 4th ventricle: **A**, T2 weighted axial image through cerebellum shows a large well-defined predominantly hypointense mass in right cerebellum with perifocal edema. **B** to **D**, Fat suppressed T1 and MT-T1 weighted image showing the hypointense mass with peripheral hyperintense rim that enhances on post contrast T1 image. **E**, Proton magnetic resonance spectroscopy from the center of the lesion with a voxel size of 1 mL shows predominant lipid peak (Lip, 1.3 ppm)

rim. The MTR of the core is around 24%, much lower than similar appearing cysticercal lesions (Fig. 10).[12] *In vivo* MRS of these lesions indicated the presence of lactate/lipid peaks.[32] Presence of serine at 3.7–3.9 ppm on *ex vivo/in vitro* MRS of the tuberculoma sample suggest the presence of *M. tuberculosis* as serine is found in abundance in the wall of this bacterium.[31] On DWI, there is no restriction seen in the solid caseation of the tuberculoma with high ADC.

T2 Hyperintense Center with Peripheral Hypointense Rim

T2 hyperintense lesion with peripheral hypointense rim is noted when liquefaction of the caseation occurs in the centre of tuberculoma (Fig. 11). This appearance may also be seen in certain other conditions such as pyogenic or tubercular abscesses, cysticercosis, toxoplasmosis, and metastases. Here, the imaging protocol should include T2, T1 MT-T1, steady-state free precession imaging, SW with phase imaging and PC T1W images. On T1 and MT-T1WI, the centers of these lesions are hypointense. There is a rim enhancement on postcontrast studies. The MTR of cysticercous lesions is higher than these lesions. Steady state free precession sequence provides images of fluid filled structures with very short acquisition times and helps demonstrate scolex in cysticercosis which differentiates it from tuberculoma.[33] The SWI sequence is helpful in differentiating these lesions from calcified neurocysticercosis. Magnetic resonance spectroscopy may

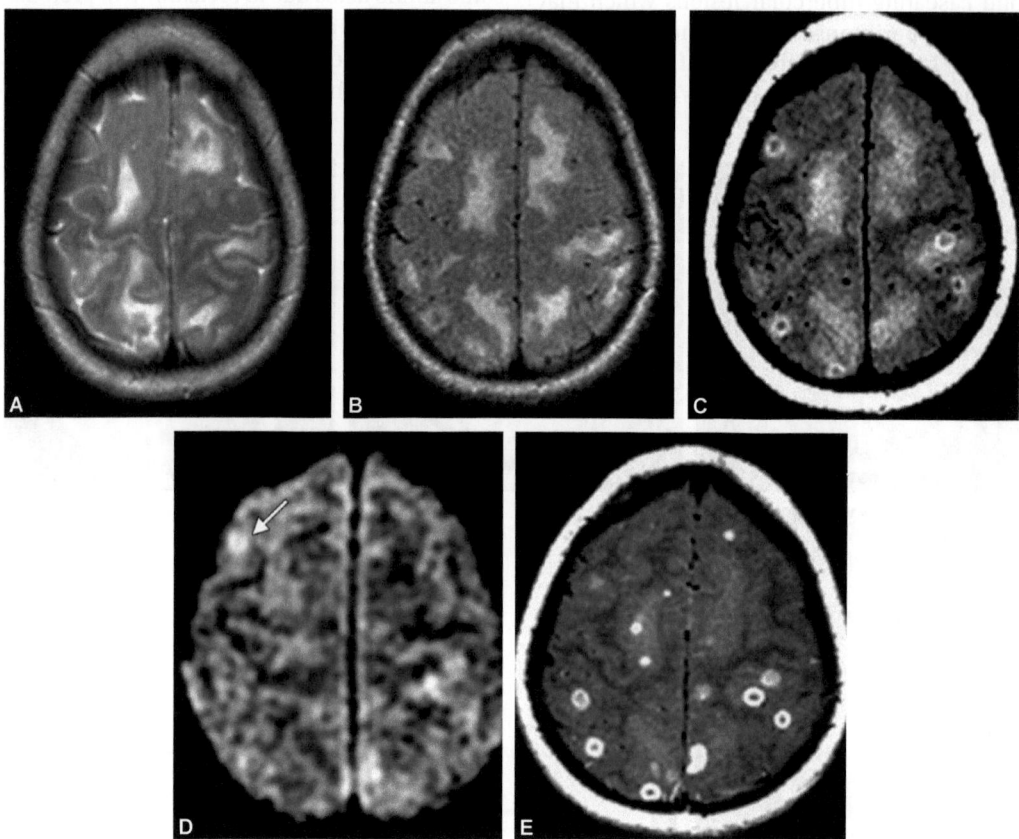

FIG. 10: Multiple tuberculomas with perilesional edema exhibiting better definition of the wall on T1-weighted MT imaging, in a 20-year-old man. **A**, T2-weighted and **B**, FLAIR images showing areas of central hypointensity surrounded by edema. **C**, T1-weighted MT image shows conspicuous hyperintense walls in all lesions. **D**, Diffusion-weighted imaging image shows restriction in the core of some of the lesions (arrow). **E**, Postcontrast T1-weighted MT image shows ring as well as disc enhancement of all lesions

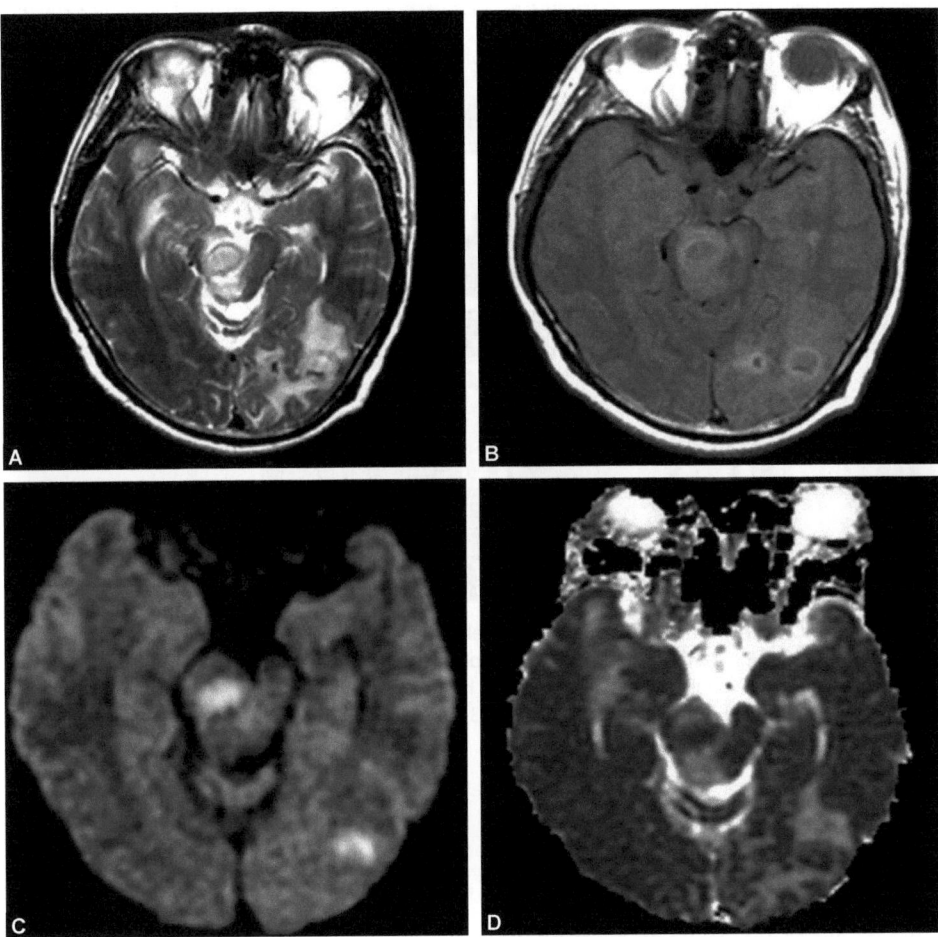

FIG. 11: Tuberculomas in the right half of midbrain and left posterior temporal region. **A,** Few hyperintense lesions are seen with hypointense wall on T2-weighted image. **B,** On MT T1-weighted image the lesions show hypo to iso-intensity with hyper-intense wall. **C** and **D,** Diffusion-weighted image show restrictions in the lesions with low ADC on ADC map

differentiate this stage of tuberculomas from pyogenic abscesses by demonstrating amino acids in the latter. Tuberculomas with liquid caseation show restriction on DWI.

Lesion with Mixed/ Heterogeneous Signal Intensity

The lesions show mixed intensity on T2WI with a rim of variable thickness which may appear minimally hyperintense on T1 and show variegated enhancement on contrast enhanced T1WI. The differential diagnoses include lymphomas, glioblastoma, metastases, fungal granulomas, and toxoplasmosis. The lesions demonstrate large choline, variable creatine resonance along with lipids on proton MR spectroscopy (PMRS) simulating neoplastic lesions and correlate with high cellularity and small areas of solid caseation on histopathology.[34] It is believed that the presence of choline in this kind of tuberculous granuloma is due to the contribution from cellular component of tuberculomas.[34] On MT images, the center of these tuberculomas shows heterogenous hypointensity and the rim shows hyperintensity (Fig. 12).

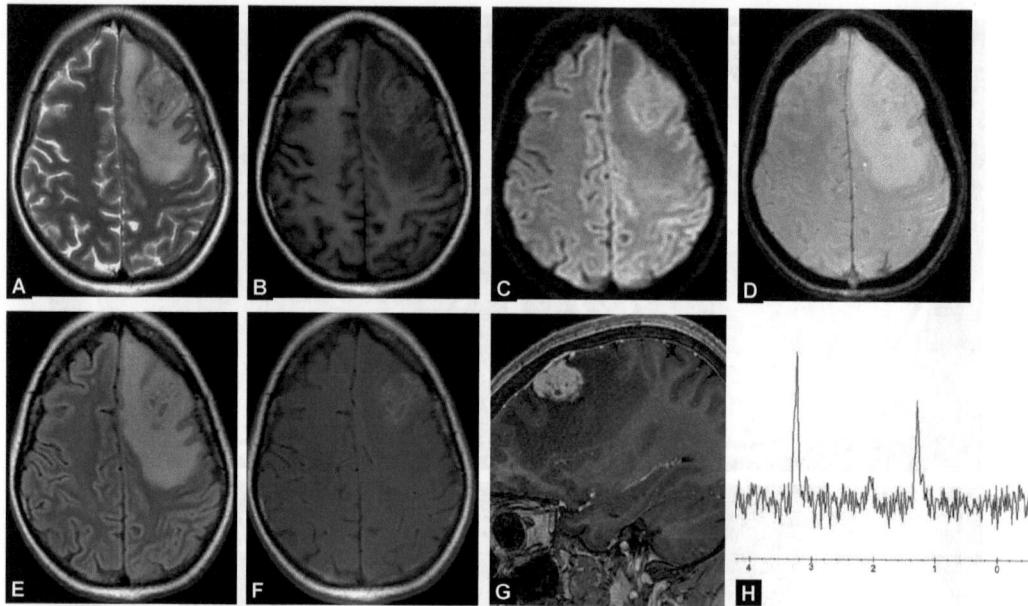

FIG. 12: Variegated tuberculoma: Well-defined, cortical-based intraparenchymal lesion in the left frontal lobe demonstrating mild **A**, T2 hyperintensity and **B**, T1 hypointensity, **C**, nodiffusion restriction or **D**, susceptibility aritfact, **E**, extensive perilesional edema on T2-FLAIR, **F**, hyperintense rim on MT-T1, **G**, variegated enhancement on postcontrast T1WI, and **H**, lipid peak resonance at 1.3 ppm and choline at 3.22 ppm

MILIARY TUBERCULOSIS

Miliary brain TB usually is associated with tuberculous meningitis. Miliary tubercles are <2 mm and are either not visible on conventional MR images or show tiny foci of hyperintensity on T2WI. T1WI after gadolinium administration show numerous small, homogeneous enhancing lesions. The spin echo invisible lesions, which may or may not enhance after intravenous injection of contrast, are clearly visible on MT-T1WI (Figs 7–13).[25]

Role of Advanced Imaging Techniques

In general, the cerebral blood volume (CBV) provides information about the angiogenic activity of pathological tissue while the permeability (k^{trans}) and leakage (v_e) give information related to the blood brain barrier integrity and changes in extravascular-extracellular space (Fig. 14).[35,36] Dynamic contrast enhanced derived relative CBV values have been studied in 13 cases of tuberculoma and have shown significant correlation of cellular fraction volume, microvascular density and vascular endothelial growth factor to suggest that rCBV is a measure of angiogenesis in the cellular fraction of the brain tuberculoma.[37,38]

These parameters may find its utility in assessment of therapeutic response in tuberculomas.

Tuberculous Brain Abscess

Tuberculous brain abscesses constitutes about 4–7% of the total CNS TB in developing countries. It show macroscopic evidence of abscess formation within the brain parenchyma and its histological confirmation that the abscess wall is composed of vascular granulation tissue containing both acute and chronic inflammatory cells and isolation of *M. tuberculosis*.[39]

The neuroimaging study is usually nonspecific for the detection of tuberculous abscesses however, on MRI these appear large, solitary/multiloculated ring-enhancing lesions with surrounding edema and mass effect.[40]

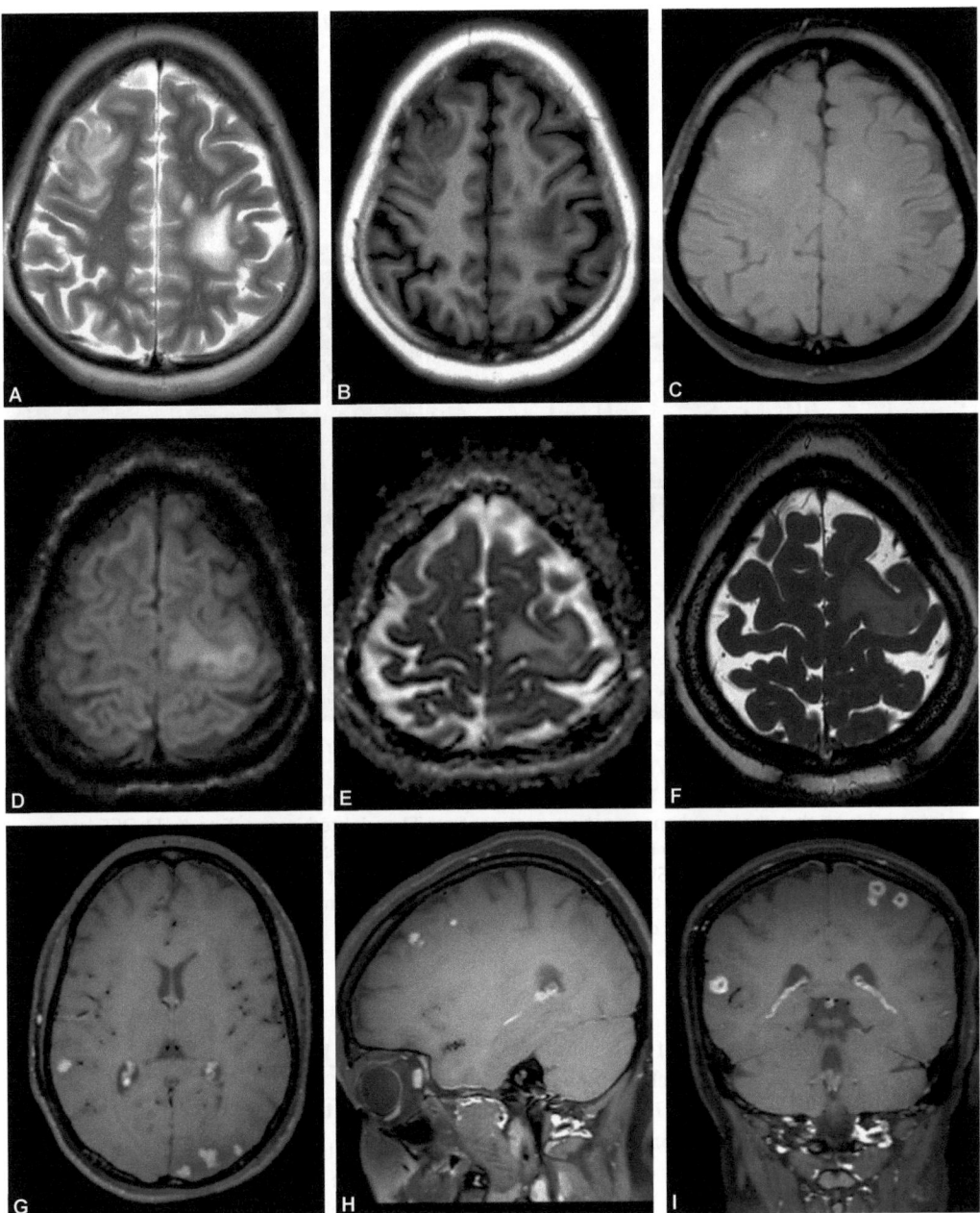

FIG. 13: Multiple Miliary tuberculomas: **A** and **B**, T2-weighted image shows few small hypo- and hyperintensities involving the left frontal region which were barely visible on T1 weighted image. **C** to **F**, Corresponding MT-T1 weighted image demonstrates more number of lesions with peripheral hyperintense rim and diffusion restriction and peripheral edema. **G** to **I**, Multiple rim and nodular enhancement is seen on PC T1-weighted image

Magnetization transfer ratio quantification from the rim of the abscess has helped in the differentiation of tuberculous abscess from the pyogenic abscesses.[41]

Diffusion-weighted imaging in tuberculous abscesses has shown restricted diffusion with low ADC values which is due to the presence of intact inflammatory cells in the pus[42–45] (Fig. 15).

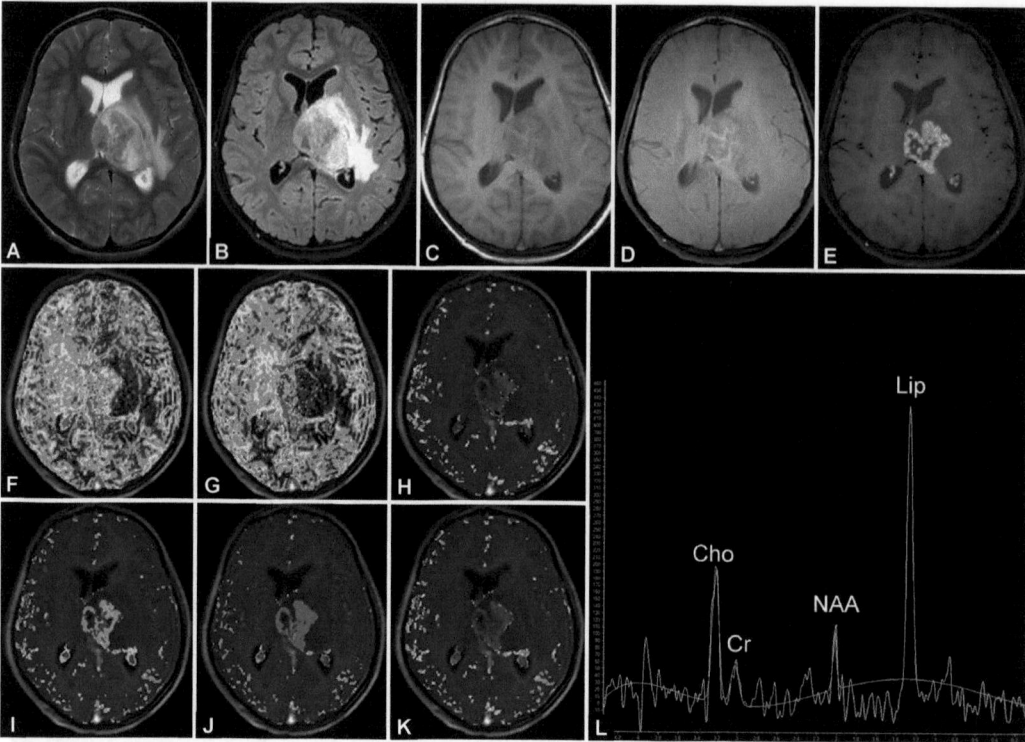

FIG. 14: Heterogeneous tuberculoma. A 13-year-old boy presented with right sided weakness. **A** and **B**, Axial T2 weighted and FLAIR images show a central hypointense lesion with surrounding peripheral hyperintensity which appears **C**, heterogeneous on T1 weighed image. **D** and **E**, MTT1 image shows a bright rim around T2 hypointense lesion that shows enhancement on post contrast T1 weighted image. **F** to **K**, T1-DCE images of rCBF, rCBV, Vp, Ve, leakage, and Kep demonstrate poor perfusion in the capsule with contrast pooling in the extra-vascular extra-cellular space. **L**, SVS at 135 ms demonstrates dominant lipid peak at 1.3 ppm. Note marginal increase in Cho at 3.2ppm to indicate cellularity of tuberculoma; and contamination of NAA at 2.0 ppm and Cr at 3.0 ppm from surrounding tissue *(For color version, see Plate 8)*

For the differentiation of tuberculous abscesses from other lesions such as pyogenic abscesses, and fungal lesions, *in vivo* PMRS has also been used. *In vivo* proton spectra in tuberculous abscesses show only Lac and lipid signals (at 0.9 and 1.3 ppm), without any evidence of cytosolic amino acids (Fig. 18). However, MRS alone may not be sufficient to differentiate tubercular from pyogenic abscess as staphylococcal abscess may show only lipid with no amino acids. It is advisable to use multiparametric quantitative imaging like MT, and diffusion imaging to help in its differentiation.

SPINAL TUBERCULOSIS

Intraspinal Tuberculosis

The inflammatory spinal diseases caused by *M. tuberculosis* are known as spinal meningitis and spinal arachnoiditis.[46] The pathophysiology of the spinal meningitis is similar to that of tuberculous meningitis.[46]

The unenhanced MR features of arachnoiditis include CSF loculation and loss of outline of the spinal cord in the cervicothoracic spine and clumping of the nerve roots in the lumbar region vis-à-vis nodular, thick, linear intradural enhancement, often completely

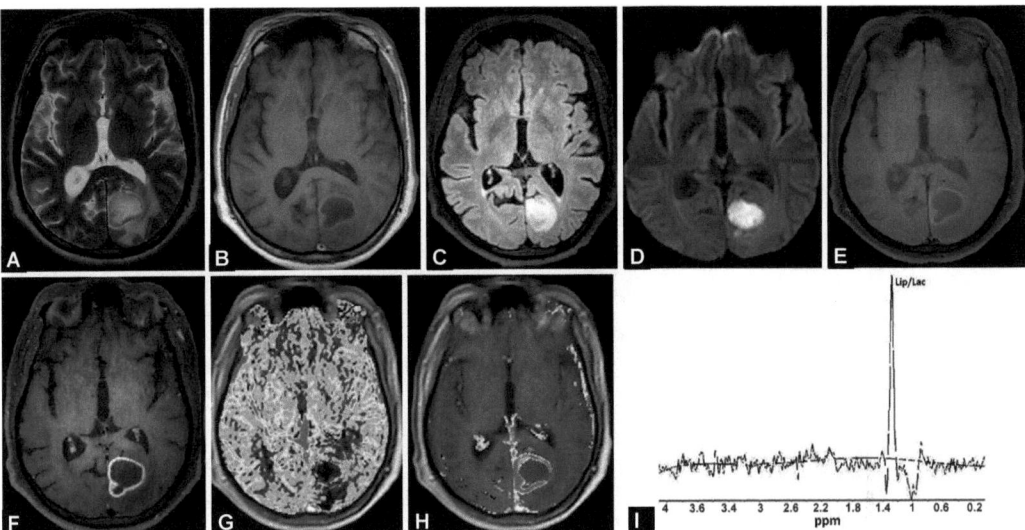

FIG. 15: Tubercular abscess in the left occipital region of a 65-year-old man. **A**, A well-defined hyperintense lesion is seen with a hypointense wall on T2-weighted image. **B**, T1-weighted image shows hypointense lesion with minimally hyperintense wall. **C**, On FLAIR images it appears hyperintense. **D**, Diffusion-weighted image shows homogeneous hyperintensity in the cavity. **E**, On MT T1-weighted image shows increased brightness of the T2 hypointense wall compared to image **B**. **F**, Postcontrast T1-weighted image shows rim enhancement. **G**, On DCE perfusion magnetic resonance imaging there is decreased CBV on corrected CBV map. **H**, Note the leakage of contrast suggesting break in blood brain barrier on leakage map. **I**, Proton magnetic resonance spectroscopy from the center of the lesion with a voxel size of 1.2 mL shows predominant lipid/lactate peak (Lip/Lac, 1.3 ppm) *(For color version, see Plate 9)*

filling the subarachnoid space on postcontrast MR images. On the other hand, in chronic stages of disease, postcontrast images may be noncontributory even when unenhanced images show signs of arachnoiditis. Spinal cord infarction and syringomyelia may be sequelae of arachnoiditis. It may also be complicated by parenchymal TB myelitis and tuberculoma formation (Fig. 16).[47,48] On T1 and T2WI, syringomyelia is seen as cavitation that demonstrates CSF like intensity and it does not enhance on postcontrast images.[47,48]

Tuberculosis Myelitis

Magnetic resonance imaging features of TB myelitis is similar to cerebritis. After 1 week of the initiation of treatment, the region of myelitis becomes less diffusely hyperintense on T2WI, with progressively delineated marginal enhancement on postcontrast T1WI.[48,49] The surrounding edema continues to be more extensive compared to the region of enhancement. These findings suggest an evolving intramedullary abscess. The central portions of the intra-axial necrotic areas are seen hypointense on T1WI and hyperintense on T2WI, respectively, which subside in several weeks, however, the contrast-enhancing foci may persist for several months.[49]

Dural and Subdural Pathology

Intradural tubercular abscess appears hyperintense on T2WI and iso- to hypointense on T1WI. The dural-based granulomas stand out in contrast, and appear hypo- to isointense on T2WI, isointense on T1WI and may demonstrate rim enhancement on post contrast images (Fig. 17).[48]

On T1WI, epidural TB lesions generally are isointense to the spinal cord and have mixed intensity on T2WI. On postcontrast study, uniform enhancement may be seen with suppurative inflammatory process or peripheral enhancement if caseation has developed.

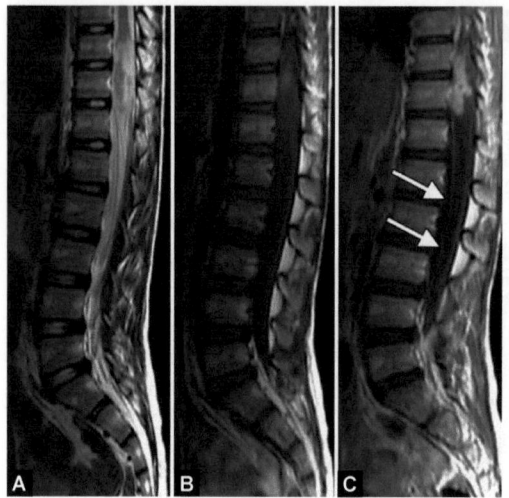

FIG. 16: Intramedullary tuberculoma with arachnoiditis. Heterogeneous hyperintensity seen at conus on **A**, T2-weighted image which appearing hypo-iso intense on **B**,T1-weighted and **C**,shows intense enhancement on post contrast T1-weighted image. Note the nerve roots as well dural enhancement consistent with arachnoiditis (arrows)

Epidural tubercular abscess may be primary in origin or may be associated with arachnoiditis, myelitis, spondylitis, and intramedullary and dural tuberculomas.[48,49]

Tuberculous Spondylitis

Tuberculous spondylitis is an important cause of spinal disease in developing countries. To avoid permanent damage or deformity in spine, early diagnosis and prompt treatment is essential (Fig. 18).

It involves one or more extradural components of the spine. Instead of involvement of the vertebral bodies which are most frequently affected, the involvement of posterior osseous elements, epidural space, paraspinal soft tissue, and inter-vertebral disks can be seen primarily or secondarily.[50] The most commonly involved sites in skeletal TB are dorsal and lumbar spine, especially the thoracolumbar junction (Fig. 19), however, sacrum and cervical spine are least affected (Fig. 20).

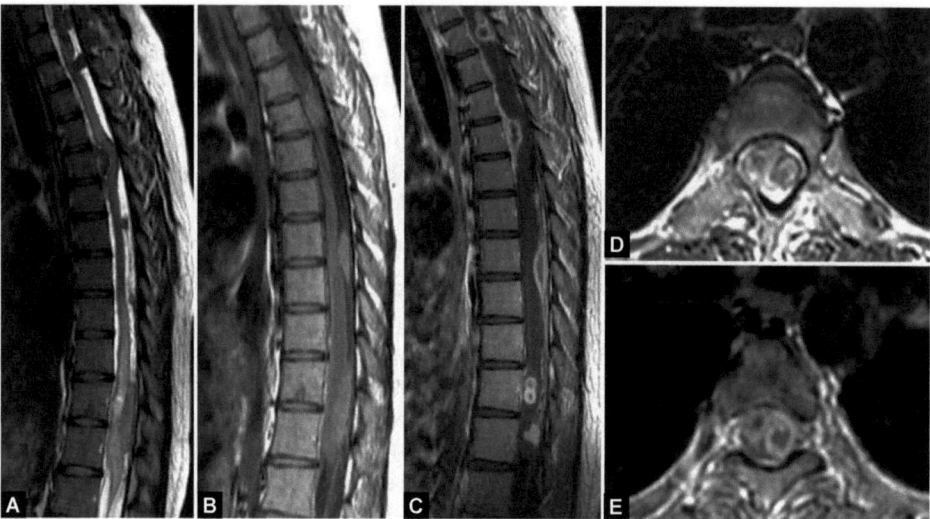

FIG. 17: Intramedullary and dural based tuberculoma: **A**, T2 weighted sagittal image of the thoracic spine shows multiple irregular predominantly hypointense round to oval lesions on the dorsal as well as ventralaspects of the cord with intrinsic hyperintensity in the distal thoracic cord and conus. **B**, On T1 weighted image the lesions are isointense. **C**, Postcontrast T1 weighted sagittal image shows thick peripheral enhancement of the lesions along with the adjacent dura. **D** and **E**, Axial T2 and post contrast T1 weighted images clearly define these T2 hypointense and peripherally enhancing lesions

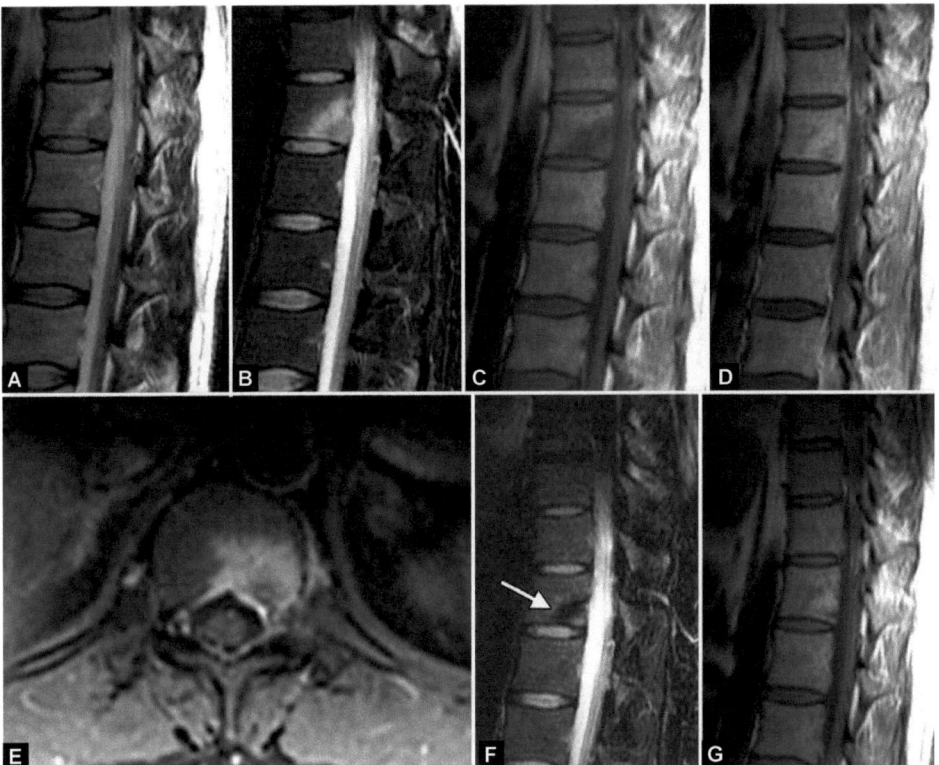

FIG. 18: Early tuberculous spondylitis in a young adult male: **A** and **B**, T2 weighted sagittal image with and without fat suppression of dorso-lumbar spine shows hyperintense lesion in the posteromedial part of the 12th dorsal vertebra clearly visible on. **C** and **D**, The lesion appears hypointense on T1 weighted image and shows enhancement on post contrast T1 weighted image. **E**, The axial postcontrast T1 weighted fat suppressed images clearly define the enhancing lesion. **F** and **G**, A repeat study after 4 months of anti-tubercular therapy shows resolution of the hyperintensity and replacement of the hypointense lesion by fat (arrow) on T1 weighted image consistent with healing

Magnetic resonance imaging is sensitive in early detection of tuberculous spondylitis even in patients with normal radiographs. In majority of cases, tuberculous spondylitis appears hyperintense on T2WI and hypointense on T1WI.[50,51] With the progression of disease classical discovertebral involvement can be noted. Vertebral intraosseous abscesses, paraspinal abscesses, discitis, skip lesions, and spinal canal encroachment, are all readily seen on MRI (Figs 19, and 21). Reduction in disk height and morphologic alteration of the paraspinal soft tissue becomes apparent during the later stages of infection.

Rim enhancing intraosseous and paraspinal soft tissue abscesses or caseating tuberculomas is characteristic of tuberculous spondylitis.[51] Following specific chemotherapy in previously affected vertebrae, progressive increase in signal intensity on T1WI suggests fatty marrow replacement and indicates healing.[50] Sometimes brachial plexuses may be primarily involved by tuberculous process which may result in plexopathy (Fig. 22).

THERAPEUTIC RESPONSE ASSESSMENT

Magnetic resonance imaging is the modality of choice for monitoring progress of disease on treatment. Several treatment regimens of antituberculosis treatment (ATT) are practiced.[52,53] Serial imaging in patients on ATT may show a decrease in lesion size between 3

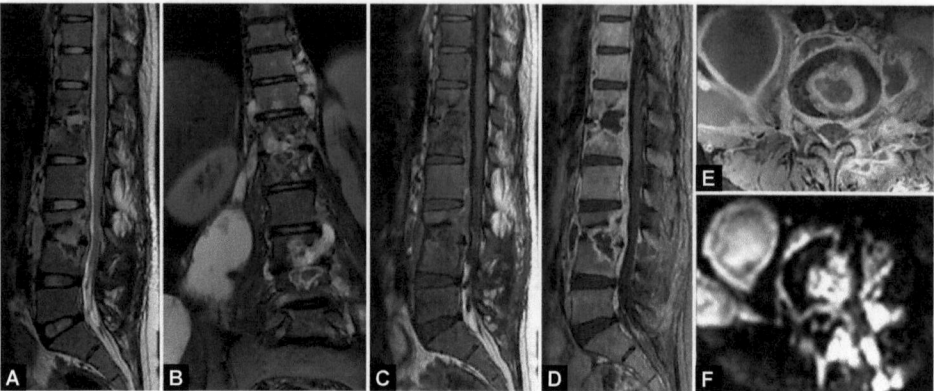

FIG. 19: Tuberculous spondylitis: T2-weighted **A,** sagittal and **B,** coronal images show hyperintense destructive process involving the D12-L1 and L3-L4 vertebrae and the intervening discs. There is evidence of a hyperintense collection with prevertebral sub-ligamentous extension, paravertebral extension along the right psoas muscle and extension into the spinal canal causing extradural compression. **C,** The vertebrae and collection appear hypointense on T1-weighted image and the rim of the collection is slightly hyperintense. Post contrast T1-weighted **D,** sagittal and **E,** axial images show peripheral enhancement of the lesion along with rim enhancement of the pre- and paravertebral collections. **F,** On DWI hyperintensity noted within the collections with low ADC value.

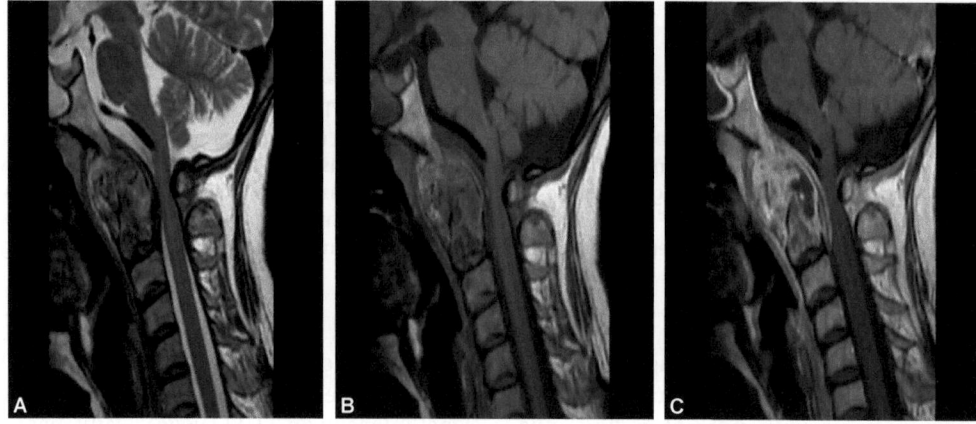

FIG. 20: Skeletal tuberculosis involving cranio-vertebral (CV) junction: **A,** T2 weighted sagittal image of the CV junction shows a hyperintense collection anterior to and around the anterior arch of atlas, atlanto-axial dislocation with compression over cervical spinal cord at cervico-medullary junction. **B,** Corresponding T1 weighted image shows cortical discontinuity of posterior aspect of dens. **C,** Postcontrast T1 weighted image shows peripheral rim enhancement of the collection along with enhancement of the granulation tissue around the anterior arch

and 4 months and complete disappearance by 12 months of therapy (Fig. 23).[53] The paradoxical progression of intracranial tuberculomas or development of new lesions during the treatment of CNS TB has been recognized as a rare response to ATT.[54] By using dynamic contrast enhanced MRI, it has been shown that changes in k^{trans} and v_e are associated with therapeutic response in follow-up of brain tuberculoma patients even in the presence of a paradoxical increase in the lesion volume.[38] In patients of TBM on ATT, resolving meningeal enhancement is indicative of response to treatment. A recent serial DTI study in TBM demonstrated progressively

Central Nervous System Tuberculosis

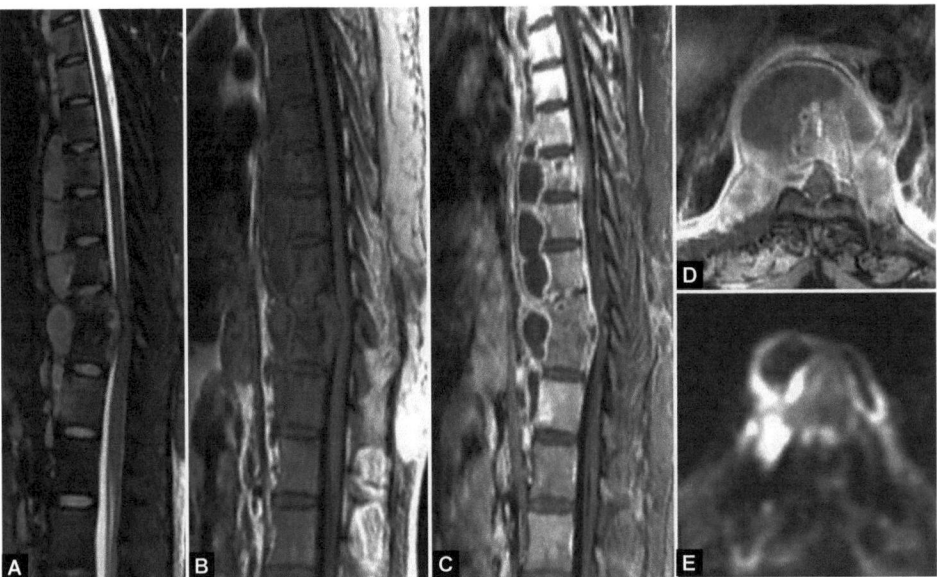

FIG. 21: Tuberculous spondylitis: **A,** T2 weighted sagittal image shows hyperintense destructive process involving the tenth and eleventh thoracic vertebrae and the intervening disc. There is evidence of a hyperintense collection with prevertebral subligamentous extension from D6 to L1 vertebrae and extension into the spinal canal causing extradural compression. **B,** The vertebrae and collection appear hypointense on T1 weighted image and the rim of the collection is slightly hyperintense. **C,** Postcontrast T1 weighted sagittal and **D,** axial images show peripheral enhancement of the lesion along with rim enhancement of the pre- and paravertebral collections. **E,** On DWI restriction noted in the periphery of the collection with low ADC value

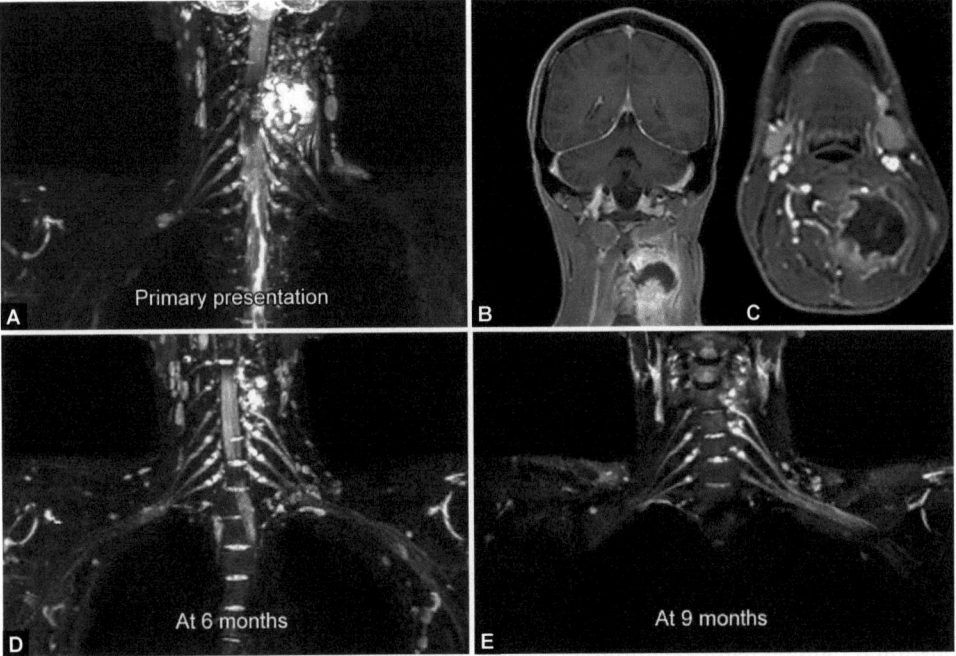

FIG. 22: Brachial plexopathy: **A,** T2W-neurography shows mass lesion with central T2-hyperintensity and rim hypointensity involving, **B** and **C,** the left brachial roots, postcontrast images show rim enhancement—suggestive of central necrosis; **D** and **E,** T2W-neurography on follow up show lesion resolution

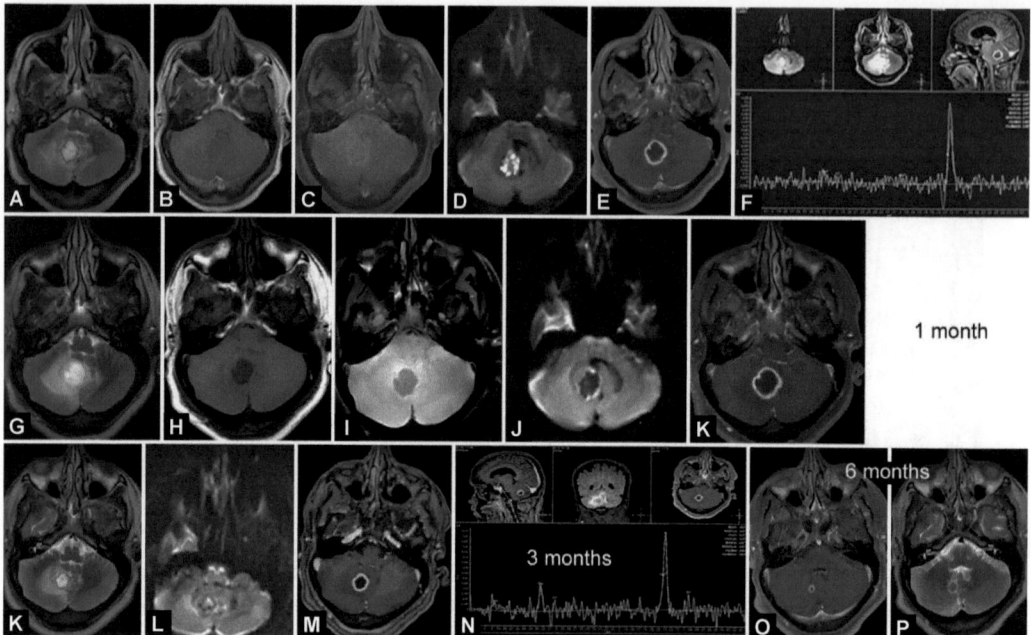

FIG. 23: Tubercular abscess on treatment. **A,** Well-defined paramedian cerebellar abscess with hyperintense contents and hypointense rim on T2WI, **B,** hypointense contents on T1WI, **C,** hyperintense rim on MT, **D,** restricting contents on DWI, **E,** rim-enhancement on post-contrast T1WI, **F,** lipid/lactate peak resonating at 1.3 ppm with single voxel spectroscopy with RoI in the contents. Lesion showed gradual resolution on ATT **G-K,** at month, **K-N,** three months and **O, P,** at 6 months *(For color version, see Plate 9)*

decreasing FA values in cerebral cortical region and basal meninges compared to elevated baseline reading over 3 months of ATT to suggest that these may be used in therapeutic response assessment in these patients.[38]

It has been shown that the patients with TBM on follow up have smaller volumes in the right thalamus, right caudate nucleus, right superior and middle temporal gyrus, right precuneus, and left putamen. This may result in multiple domain cognitive impairment which may persist in patients with chronic TBM even after appropriate treatment.[55]

Calcification of the meninges and parenchymal tuberculoma is seen as sequelae of TBM which may be best shown on SWI. The inhomogeneous ring-like high signal in the T1-weighted image suggests peripheral gliotic changes in calcification.[56] Immune reconstitution inflammatory syndrome results from the immune system's restored ability to mount an inflammatory response following antiretroviral therapy in HIV patients with and without TBM.[57] It has also been described in tuberculous meningitis even in the absence of co existing HIV infection with no differences in imaging.[58] We should be aware of this entity, where imaging may show deterioration on follow-up even when the patient is on continued anti tubercular treatment.

CONCLUSION

We conclude that CNS tuberculosis is a devastating clinical condition which needs immediate diagnosis and treatment to prevent the complications associated with this condition. Various MRI techniques help in early diagnosis of this condition and detect complications like vasculitis, tuberculoma, and hydrocephalus those develop during the course of the disease. Imaging also helps in treatment response assessment. Appropriate use of various imaging features also help in differentiation of similar imaging appearing lesions like nontuberculous granulomas, and neoplasm which will influence the treatment strategies.

REFERENCES

1. Raviglione MC, Snider DE, Kochi A. Global epidemiology of tuberculosis. Morbidity and mortality of a worldwide epidemic. JAMA. 1995;273(3):220-6.
2. Tandon PN, Pathak SN. Tuberculosis of the central nervous system. In: Spillane JD, editor. Tropical neurology. London: Oxford University Press; 1973. pp. 37-62.
3. Hopewell PC. Overview of clinical tuberculosis. In: Bloom BB, editor Tuberculosis: Pathogenesis, protection, and control. Washington DC: American Society for Microbiology; 1994. pp. 25-46.
4. Dastur DK, Manghani DK, Udani PM. Pathology and pathogenetic mechanisms in neurotuberculosis. Radiol Clin North Am. 1995;33(4):733-52.
5. Shah GV, Desai SB, Malde HM, et al. Tuberculosis of sphenoidal sinus: CT findings. Am J Roentgenol. 1993; 161(3):681-2.
6. Leonard JM, Des Prez RM. Tuberculous meningitis. Infect Dis Clin North Am. 1990;4(4):769-87.
7. Dott NM, Levine E. Intracranial tuberculoma. Edin Medical J. 1939;46:36-41.
8. Kennedy DH, Fallon RJ. Tuberculous meningitis. JAMA. 1979;241(3):264-8.
9. Zuger A, Lowy FD. Tuberculosis of the brain, meninges, and spinal cord. Boston: Little Brown; 1996. pp. 541-56.
10. Kioumehr F, Dadsetan MR, Rooholamini SA, et al. Central nervous system tuberculosis: MRI. Neuroradiology. 1994;36(2):93-6.
11. Kamra P, Azad R, Prasad KN, et al. Infectious meningitis: Prospective evaluation with magnetization transfer MRI. Br J Radiol. 2004;77(917):387-94.
12. Gupta RK, Kathuria MK, Pradhan S. Magnetization transfer MR imaging in CNS tuberculosis. AJNR Am J Neuroradiol. 1999;20(5):867-75.
13. Tandon PN, Bhatia R, Bhargava S. Tuberculous meningitis. In: Harris AA, editor. Handbook of Clinical Neurology. Amsterdam: Elsevier Health Sciences; 1988. pp. 195-226.
14. Singh I, Haris M, Husain M, et al. Role of endoscopic third ventriculostomy in patients with communicating hydrocephalus: an evaluation by MR ventriculography. Neurosurg Rev. 2008;31(3):319-25.
15. Dastur DK, Lalitha VS, Udani PM, et al. The brain and meninges in tuberculous meningitis-gross pathology in 100 cases and pathogenesis. Neurol India. 1970;18(2):86-100.
16. Andronikou S, Wilmshurst J, Hatherill M, et al. Distribution of brain infarction in children with tuberculous meningitis and correlation with outcome score at 6 months. Pediatr Radiol. 2006;36(12):1289-94.
17. Gupta RK, Gupta S, Singh D, et al. MR imaging and angiography in tuberculous meningitis. Neuroradiology. 1994;36(2):87-92.
18. Mathew NT, Abraham J, Chandy J. Cerebral angiographic features in tuberculous meningitis. Neurology. 1970; 20(10):1015-23.
19. Chang KH, Han MH, Roh JK, et al. Gd-DTPA enhanced MR imaging in intracranial tuberculosis. Neuroradiology. 1990;32(1):19-25.
20. Shukla R, Abbas A, Kumar P, et al. Evaluation of cerebral infarction in tuberculous meningitis by diffusion weighted imaging. J Infect. 2008;57(4):298-306.
21. Bulder MM, Bokkers RP, Hendrikse J, et al. Arterial spin labeling perfusion MRI in children and young adults with previous ischemic stroke and unilateral intracranial arteriopathy. Cerebrovasc Dis. 2014;37(1):14-21.
22. Brismar J, Hugosson C, Larsson SG, et al. Imaging of tuberculosis: III. Tuberculosis as a mimicker of brain tumour. Acta Radiol. 1996;37(4):496-505.
23. Goyal M, Sharma A, Mishra NK, et al. Imaging appearance of pachymeningeal tuberculosis. Am J Roentgenol. 1997;169(5):1421-4.
24. Moghtaderi A, Alavi-Naini R, Rashki S. Cranial nerve palsy as a factor to differentiate tuberculous meningitis from acute bacterial meningitis. Acta Medica Iranica. 2013;51(2):113-8.
25. Gupta RK. Tuberculosis and other non tuberculous bacterial granulomatous infections. In: Gupta RK, Lufkin RB (Eds). MR Imaging and Spectroscopy of Central Nervous System Infection. USA: Springer; 2001. pp. 95-145.
26. Gupta RK, Jena A, Sharma A, et al. MR imaging of intracranial tuberculomas. J Comput Assist Tomogr. 1988; 12(2):280-5.
27. Whelan MA, Stern J. Intracranial tuberculoma. Radiology. 1981;138(1):75-81.
28. Kesavadas C, Somasundaram S, Rao RM, et al. Meckel's cave tuberculoma with unusual infratemporal extension. J Neuroimaging. 2007;17(3):264-8.
29. Salem R, Khochtali I, Jellali MA, et al. Isolated hypophyseal tuberculoma: Often mistaken. Neurochirurgie. 2009;55(6): 603-6.
30. Gupta RK, Kumar S. Magnetic Resonance Imaging of Neurological Diseases in Tropics, 1st edition. New Delhi: Jaypee Brothers Medical Publishers (P) Ltd; 2013.
31. Gupta RK, Roy R, Dev R, et al. Finger printing of Mycobacterium tuberculosis in patients with intracranial tuberculomas by using in vivo, ex vivo, and in vitro magnetic resonance spectroscopy. Magn Reson Med. 1996;36(6):829-33.
32. Venkatesh SK, Gupta RK, Pal L, Husain N, et al. Spectroscopic increase in choline signal is a nonspecific marker for differentiation of infective/inflammatory from neoplastic lesions of the brain. J Magn Reson Imaging. 2001;14(1):8-15.
33. Padhani AR, Husband JE. Dynamic contrast-enhanced MRI studies in oncology with an emphasis on quantification, validation and human studies. Clin Radiol. 2001;56(8):607-20.
34. Jackson A. Imaging microvascular structure with contrast enhanced MRI. Br J Radiol. 2003;76 Spec No 2:S159-73.

35. Haris M, Gupta RK, Husain M, et al. Assessment of therapeutic response in brain tuberculomas using serial dynamic contrast-enhanced MRI. Clin Radiol. 2008;63(5):562-74.
36. Gupta RK, Haris M, Husain N, et al. Relative cerebral blood volume is a measure of angiogenesis in brain tuberculoma. J Comput Assist Tomogr. 2007;31(3):335-41.
37. Hasan KM, Gupta RK, Santos RM, et al. Diffusion tensor fractional anisotropy of the normal-appearing seven segments of the corpus callosum in healthy adults and relapsing-remitting multiple sclerosis patients. J Magn Reson Imaging. 2005;21(6):735-43.
38. Thomalla G, Glauche V, Weiller C, et al. Time course of Wallerian degeneration after ischaemic stroke revealed by diffusion tensor imaging. J Neurol Neurosurg Psychiatry. 2005;76(2):266-8.
39. Gupta RK, Vatsal DK, Husain N, et al. Differentiation of tuberculous from pyogenic brain abscesses with in vivo proton MR spectroscopy and magnetization transfer MR imaging. AJNR Am J Neuroradiol. 2001;22(8):1503-9.
40. Gupta RK, Prakash M, Mishra AM, et al. Role of diffusion weighted imaging in differentiation of intracranial tuberculoma and tuberculous abscess from cysticercus granulomas-a report of more than 100 lesions. Eur J Radiol. 2005;55(3):384-92.
41. Mishra AM, Gupta RK, Saksena S, et al. Biological correlates of diffusivity in brain abscess. Magn Reson Med. 2005;54(4):878-85.
42. Luthra G, Parihar A, Nath K, et al. Comparative evaluation of fungal, tubercular, and pyogenic brain abscesses with conventional and diffusion MR imaging and proton MR spectroscopy. AJNR Am J Neuroradiol. 2007;28(7):1332-8.
43. Reddy JS, Mishra AM, Behari S, et al. The role of diffusion-weighted imaging in the differential diagnosis of intracranial cystic mass lesions: a report of 147 lesions. Surg Neurol. 2006;66(3):246-50.
44. Brooks WD, Fletcher AP, Wilson RR. Spinal cord complications of tuberculous meningitis; a clinical and pathological study. Q J Med. 1954;23(91):275-90.
45. Kumar A, Montanera W, Willinsky R, et al. MR features of tuberculous arachnoiditis. J Comput Assist Tomogr. 1993;17(1):127-30.
46. Gupta RK, Gupta S, Kumar S, et al. MRI in intraspinal tuberculosis. Neuroradiology. 1994;36(1):39-43.
47. Murphy KJ, Brunberg JA, Quint DJ, et al. Spinal cord infection: myelitis and abscess formation. AJNR Am J Neuroradiol. 1998;19(2):341-8.
48. Sharif HS, Aabed MY, Haddad MC. Magnetic resonance imaging and computed tomography of infectious spondylitis. In: Bloem JL, Satoris DJ, editors. MRI and CT of the Musculoskeletal System: A Text Atlas. Baltimore: Williams and Wilkins; 1992. pp. 580-602.
49. Gupta RK, Agarwal P, Rastogi H, et al. Problems in distinguishing spinal tuberculosis from neoplasia on MRI. Neuroradiology. 1996;38 Suppl 1:S97-104.
50. Gupta RK, Jena A, Singh AK, et al. Role of magnetic resonance (MR) in the diagnosis and management of intracranial tuberculomas. Clin Radiol. 1990;41(2):120-7.
51. Awada A, Daif AK, Pirani M, et al. Evolution of brain tuberculomas under standard antituberculous treatment. J Neurol Sci. 1998;156(1):47-52.
52. Bas NS, Güzey FK, Emel E, et al. Paradoxical intracranial tuberculoma requiring surgical treatment. Pediatr Neurosurg. 2005;41(4):201-5.
53. Chen HL, Lu CH, Chang CD, et al. Structural deficits and cognitive impairment in tuberculous meningitis. BMC Infect Dis. 2015;15:279.
54. Ku BD, Yoo SD. Extensive meningeal and prenchymal calcified tuberculoma as long-term residual sequelae of tuberculous meningitis. Neurol India. 2009;57(4):521-2.
55. Marais S, Meintjes G, Pepper DJ, et al. Frequency, severity, and prediction of tuberculous meningitis immune reconstitution inflammatory syndrome. Clin Infect Dis. 2013;56(3):450-60.
56. Post MJ, Thurnher MM, Clifford DB, et al. CNS-immune reconstitution inflammatory syndrome in the setting of HIV infection, part 1: overview and discussion of progressive multifocal leukoencephalopathy-immune reconstitution inflammatory syndrome and cryptococcal-immune reconstitution inflammatory syndrome. AJNR Am J Neuroradiol. 2013;34(7):1297-307.
57. Post MJ, Thurnher MM, Clifford DB, et al. CNS-immune reconstitution inflammatory syndrome in the setting of HIV infection, part 2: discussion of neuro-immune reconstitution inflammatory syndrome with and without other pathogens. AJNR Am J Neuroradiol. 2013;34(7):1308-18.
58. Sun HY, Singh N. Immune reconstitution inflammatory syndrome in non-HIV immunocompromised patients. Curr Opin Infect Dis. 2009;22(4):394-402.

8 CHAPTER

Spinal Tuberculosis

Shivanand Gamanagatti, Jitender Saini

INTRODUCTION

Spinal tuberculosis (TB) is a relatively less common form of TB as compared to pulmonary TB. Overall, osteoarticular TB accounts for 1–2% of all cases of TB, while spinal TB accounts for 0.5–1%. In spinal TB, onset of symptoms is usually insidious and disease progresses slowly.[1,2] Clinical features are largely nonspecific and there is significant delay between the onset of symptoms and establishment of correct diagnosis.[3] Early diagnosis and institution of chemotherapy can prevent significant morbidity and disability in patients with spinal TB. Imaging studies are useful for early diagnosis, initiation of treatment as well as identifying the appropriate site for biopsy when imaging findings are atypical.[3-5]

As mentioned earlier diagnosis of TB infection needs to be established by the microbiological analysis of skeletal lesion for the evidence of tubercle bacilli. However, it may not always be possible, which is supported by the results of many large clinical series.[6-8] In general, the load of *Mycobacterium* in osteoarticular disease is less than that in case of pulmonary TB and rate for positive cultures for acid-fast bacilli (AFB) in osteoarticular tuberculous lesion has been reported by various workers to be between 40% and 88%.[9-13] *Mycobacterium* culture methods are slow and insensitive even in pulmonary TB but these problems get greatly magnified in patients with paucibacillary osteoarticular disease like spinal TB and results in low yield.[14] Histopathological examination of the biopsy specimen is also useful for the diagnosis of spinal TB and is a very useful adjunct to the microbiological examination.

Difficulties discussed earlier make imaging methods as the mainstay for the diagnosis of spinal TB. Plain radiographs are useful in making the diagnosis of spinal TB, however, bony changes can only be detected after significant bony destruction has occurred and the diagnosis is delayed. Magnetic resonance imaging (MRI) and computed tomography (CT) play an important role in early diagnosis of spinal TB.[4,15] Nuclear medicine techniques are also useful for diagnosis of spinal TB, however, they have poor specificity and anatomical details are lacking. In this chapter the pathophysiology of spinal TB is discussed in brief followed by overview of various imaging techniques in spinal TB and relevant imaging findings.

PATHOPHYSIOLOGY

Arterial Anatomy

Vertebral column is supplied by segmental branches arising from the vertebral, subclavian, intercostal, and lumbar arteries. Vertebral body receives blood supply from three types of intraosseous arteries: (i) equatorial, (ii) metaphyseal, and (iii) peripheral. The peripheral arteries supply the outer collar of the vertebral body through short centripetally directed terminal branches. The equatorial arteries supply the central core of the vertebral body subjacent to the nucleus pulposus, and the metaphyseal arteries supply an annular zone between the equatorial arteries and peripheral arteries. Paradiscal regions of the vertebral body are relatively avascular. In children, vertebral bodies are more vascular due to extensive intraosseous anastomosis between various channels of blood supply. With age these anastomotic channels disappear resulting in presence of end arteries. Vascular anatomy is relevant to understanding the pathogenesis of spinal infections.[16,17]

The initial route of entry of *M. tuberculosis* is usually the respiratory tract, followed by hematogenous dissemination. Another mode of *M. tuberculosis* spread to the vertebral bodies is from involved contiguous paraaortic lymph nodes. Vertebral column involvement is most commonly due to hematogenous dissemination via rich arterial arcade is present in the subchondral region of each vertebrae. This vascular plexus allows the hematogenous spread of the infection in the paradiscal region. Batson's plexus, which surrounds the vertebral column, has also been implicated in those cases in which an alternating pattern of vertebral involvement has been described. Batson's paravertebral venous plexus in the vertebra is a valveless system that allows free flow of blood in both directions depending upon the pressure generated by the intra-abdominal and intrathoracic cavities following strenuous activities like coughing. Spread of the infection through intraosseous venous system may be responsible for central vertebral body lesions. In patients with noncontiguous vertebral TB, again it is the vertebral venous system that spreads the infection to multiple vertebrae.[4,18-20]

The tubercle bacillus settles in the vascular cancellous bone and destroys it eventually reaching the cortex. The infection gradually spreads to adjacent vertebra via the disc space. In advanced stages of the disease, progressive vertebral collapse occurs, resulting in kyphosis and gibbus formation. Spinal TB is initially apparent in the anterior-inferior portion of the vertebral body. Later on it spreads into the central part of the body or disc.[1,2,4,18-20]

PATTERNS OF SPINAL TUBERCULOSIS

Paradiscal, anterior, central, and appendiceal lesions are the four common patterns of vertebral involvement in vertebral TB. Paradiscal form is the most common type while anterior, central, and appendiceal types constitute the atypical forms of spinal TB.

Paradiscal disease is characterized by involvement of the contiguous vertebrae. There is involvement of more than one vertebra because segmental arteries supplying the vertebra bifurcate to supply two adjacent vertebrae.

In the central lesion, the disc is not involved, and collapse of the vertebral body produces vertebra plana. Vertebra plana indicates complete compression of the vertebral body. In younger patients, the disc is more often involved because it is more vascularized. In old age, the disc is not primarily involved because of its age-related avascularity.[1,2,4,18-20]

Anterior type of involvement of the vertebral bodies seems to be due to the extension of an abscess beneath the anterior longitudinal ligaments and the periosteum. The infection may spread up and down, stripping the anterior and posterior longitudinal ligaments and involves multiple contiguous vertebrae (subligamentous form). A lack of proteolytic enzymes in mycobacterial infections (in comparison with pyogenic infections) has been suggested as the cause of the subligamentous spread of infection. Intervening disc may preserved early in the course of illness but in later stages it may also get involved. This pattern of disease is usually seen in children and younger individuals.

Appendiceal type involves the posterior arches. Posterior elements are less commonly involved and they may be abnormal along with abnormality of vertebral bodies or rarely isolated involvement of posterior elements may be present.

PATHOLOGY

Following infection, the initial response is accumulation of polymorphonuclear cells, which are rapidly replaced by macrophages and monocytes (mononuclears). The tubercle bacilli are phagocytosed and broken down by mononuclear cells which get transformed into epithelioid cells. Epithelioid cells, which are the hallmark of the tuberculous reaction are large, pale cells with vesicular nucleus, abundant cytoplasm with indistinct margins. Langerhans giant cells are possibly formed by the fusion of a number of epithelioid cells. These are formed only if caseation necrosis has occurred in the lesion, and often they contain tubercle bacilli. After about a week, lymphocytes appear and form a ring around the peripheral part of the lesion. This mass formed by the reactive cells of the reticuloendothelial tissues constitutes a nodule known as the tubercle. During the second week, caseation occurs in the center of the tubercle by coagulation necrosis caused by the protein fraction of the tubercle bacilli. Presence of caseation necrosis is almost diagnostic of tuberculous pathology and such a tubercle is designed as "soft tubercle." A tubercle, however, may not always show central caseation (hard tubercle).[21]

Cold abscess is formed by a collection of products of liquefaction and the reactive exudation. The cold abscess is mostly composed of serum, leucocytes, caseous material, bone debris, and tubercle bacilli.

CLINICAL FEATURES

The clinical course is often indolent, leading to significant delay in diagnosis and treatment resulting in bone or joint destruction. The usual presenting complaints are pain overlying the affected vertebrae, low-grade fever, chills, weight loss, and nonspecific constitutional symptoms. Paraplegia can be the first sign of spinal disease. In addition to weakness, nerve root compression and sensory impairment can also occur. Duration of symptoms ranges from weeks to several years. Historically, this interval was at least 12 months on average, decreasing to between 3 months and 6 months in the recent era.[22] Weight loss has been recorded in 58% of patients and back pain in 90–100% of patients. Neurological involvement has varied in different studies from 32% to 76% with notable differences in severity.[5,23-25] Children may complain of refusal to bear weight, limp and torticollis.

IMAGING MODALITIES

Pathological Basis of the Images

The early tubercular (rich) focus proliferates inside the cancellous or yellow marrow part of the bone leading to group of tubercles. The central part of these tubercles encompasses multinucleated giant and epithelioid cells walled off by lymphocytes. This inflammatory process leads to decalcification and edema inside the vertebral body, which influences the imaging appearance of the bone. As the inflammatory process continues leading to bone destruction and the destroyed bone is replaced by caseous material. This caseous material develops into interosseous abscesses influencing the imaging patterns and is identifiable on cross-sectional imaging. The abscesses (contain necrotic dead tissue material and calcified bone fragments) are surrounded by vascularized wall, which is responsible for rim enhancement following contrast administration.

As the healing phase continues, osteoblastic reaction leads to perceptible osteosclerosis. Finally, new bone formation develops and vertebral bodies may recover their original height, especially if there has been no significant collapse.

Plain Radiographs[26-28]

Plain radiographs may be absolutely normal in early stage of tubercular spondylitis and recognizable changes in vertebrae are seen at a later stage. The typical radiographic appearance is the slowly progressing destruction with only minimal reactive changes in the bone. The radiographic latent period for the spine is 21 days or more, which often delays early diagnosis and treatment. The early Roentgen signs consist of a lytic destructive lesion in the anterior corner of the vertebral endplate, coupled with a recognizable loss of disc space (Fig. 1).

Easily discerned on the anteroposterior (AP) projection is abscess formation, displacing the paraspinal line, particularly well visualized in the thoracic spine, with the adjacent radiolucent lung providing a sharply contrasted peripheral margin (Fig. 2). The lower thoracic-upper lumbar spine is the most common spinal site, with L1 involvement being most prevalent. As an extension of the infectious focus in the lumbar spine, a psoas abscess may form. It can be of varied size and appears as a pear-shaped radiopaque density. Plain radiographs may show erosion and scalloping of the anterior surface

Imaging in Tuberculosis: Clinicopathological Correlation

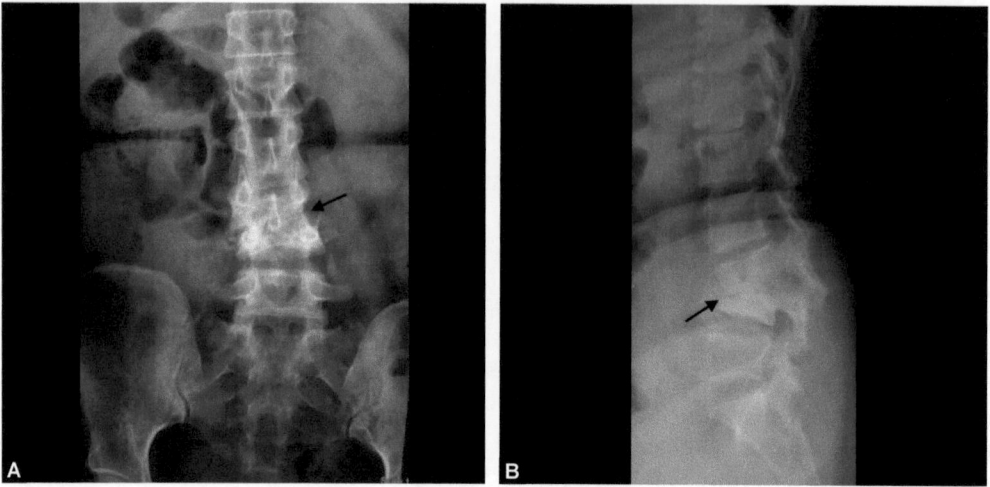

FIG. 1: A, Anteroposterior (AP); and **B,** Lateral radiographs of lumbar spine showing partial collapse of L3 and L4 vertebral bodies with reduced intervening disc space (arrows) associated with right paraspinal soft tissue component

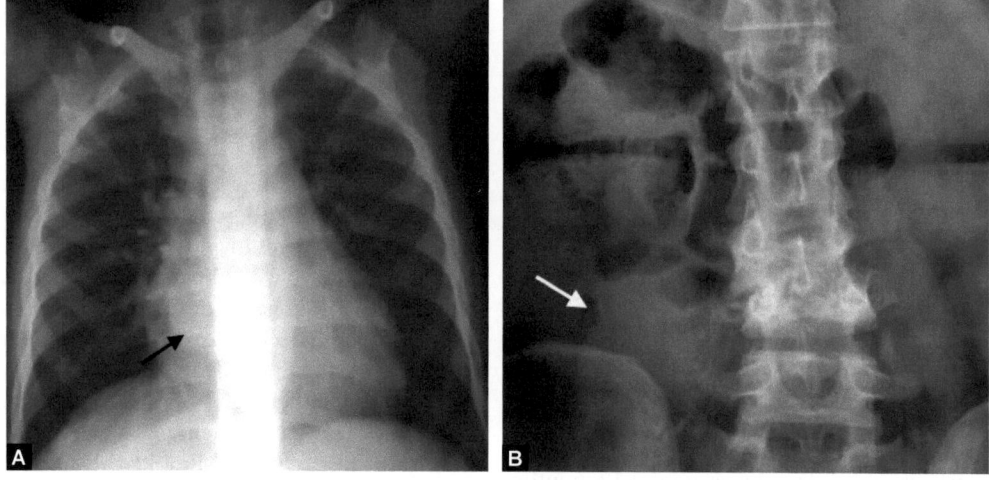

FIG. 2: A Plain radiographs of chest (posteroanterior view); and **B,** Lumbar spine (anteroposterior view) showing displacement of the paraspinal lines (arrows) by paravertebral abscesses

of the vertebral body due to subligamentous extension of a tuberculous abscess (Fig. 3).

Eventually, osteolytic destruction of the vertebral bodies occurs. This process weakens the vertebrae to the extent that pathologic collapse follows. Progressive breakdown of bone, disc disintegration and vertebral collapse finally result in angular kyphosis leading to the development of a gibbus deformity. The degree of angulation varies with the site and extent of vertebral disease. The angulation is often more acute in the thoracic spine than in the cervical or lumbar regions. It is also more severe when only one or two vertebral segments are destroyed.

In long-standing gibbus deformity, tremendous biomechanical stress is placed on the uninvolved vertebral body immediately caudal to the gibbus. This stress may alter the appearance of the vertebra, whereby it becomes taller than it is broad.[28] In chronic healed cases, plain radiographs may show fibrous ankylosis of adjacent vertebrae and sclerosis of the vertebrae (Fig. 4). However bony ankylosis may be seen secondary to superadded bacterial infection.

Spinal Tuberculosis

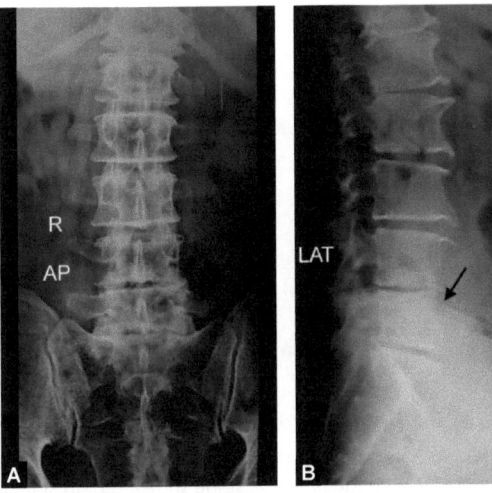

FIG. 3: **A,** Anteroposterior (AP); and **B,** Lateral radiographs of lumbosacral spine showing reduced L4/L5 disc space with scalloping of the anterior surface (arrow) of the L4 and L5 vertebral bodies due to subligamentous extension of abscess

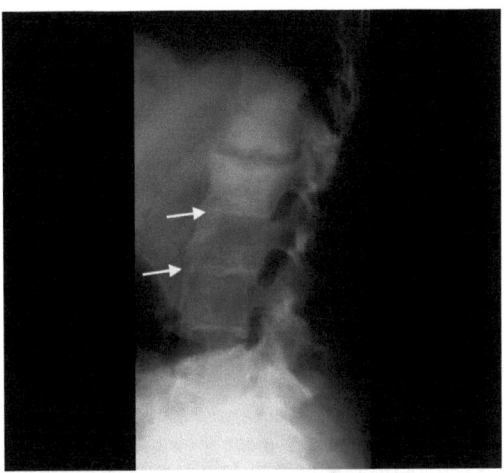

FIG. 4: Lateral radiograph of lumbar spine showing fibrous ankylosis L2–L4 vertebrae (arrows) with sclerosis of L1 and L2 adjacent endplates in a case of chronic healed tuberculous spondylitis

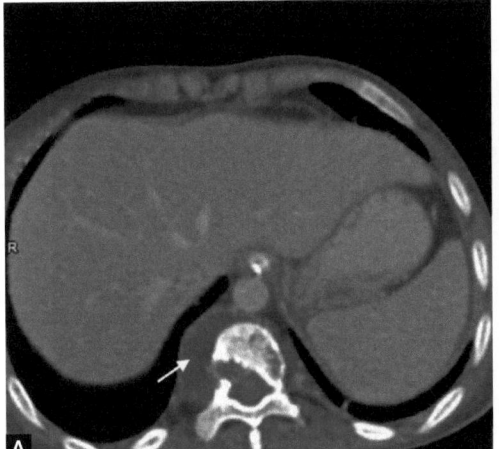
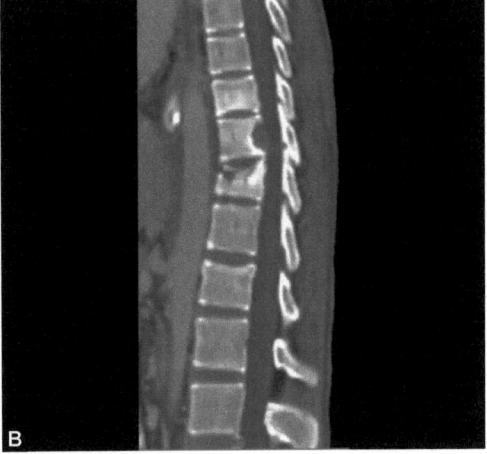

FIG. 5: **A,** Axial; and **B,** Sagittal computed tomography (CT) images showing destruction with sclerosis of D10 vertebra and erosion of the posterior surface of D9 vertebral body with right paravertebral abscess (arrow)

Ultrasound

Ultrasound helps in identifying the accompanied soft tissue abscesses and is also used as guidance for percutaneous drainage of abscesses.

Computed Tomography[29]

Computed tomography is not a routinely used imaging modality in assessing the tuberculous spondylitis but it may be helpful in assessing the cortical breakdown, destruction of cancellous bone as well as spinal distortion in chronic cases (Fig. 5). Multidetector CT (MDCT) using thinnest collimation with multiplanar reconstruction in different planes, can be beneficial to assess the destruction of bone and gibbus/scoliosis deformity of the spine in chronic cases.

One of the major disadvantages of CT as compared to MRI, is difficulty in identifying the early marrow changes of the disease process within the bone. Another disadvantage of CT is its inability to identify subtle epidural soft tissue component due to beam hardening artifact.

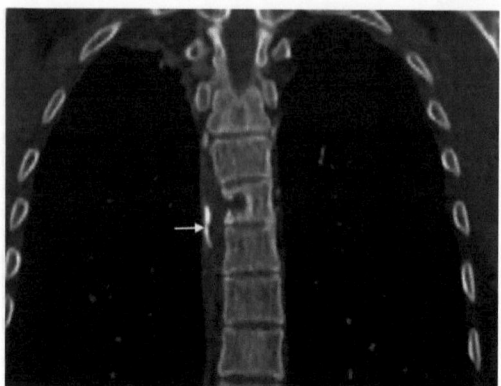

FIG. 6: Coronal three dimensional (3D) reformatted computed tomography image showing erosion of the D4 vertebra associated with right paraspinal soft tissue component with calcification (arrow)

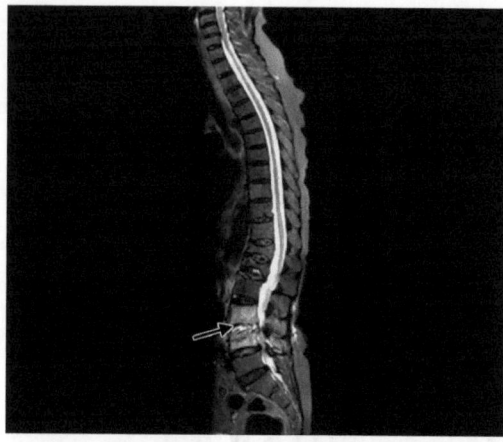

FIG. 7: Sagittal T2W (fat saturated) magnetic resonance (MR) image of whole spine showing high signal intensity within L3–L4 intervertebral disc space (arrow) with hyperintensity of L3 and L4 vertebral bodies suggestive of tuberculous discitis

However, CT is more sensitive in showing subtle soft tissue calcifications as compared to MRI (Fig. 6).

Computed tomography is useful for guiding percutaneous drainage of paravertebral abscesses, which are difficult to access under ultrasound guidance.

Magnetic Resonance Imaging[15,29,30]

Magnetic resonance imaging is the ideal imaging modality for imaging of TB spondylitis because of its ability to identify early marrow changes, its high sensitivity for detecting soft tissue inflammatory changes and to show the relationship of soft tissue component/abscess to spinal cord due to its multiplanar capabilities.

High signal intensity of the intervertebral disc space (higher than adjacent disc spaces) on T2W sequence is an early sign of TB discitis on MRI (Fig. 7). Another, early MRI sign includes enhancement of a vertebral body without height loss, endplate destruction or disc space abnormality (Fig. 8). In early stage, the bone marrow changes of TB spine are nonspecific; consist of a variable high signal intensity on T2W and low signal intensity on T1W images. In advanced stage, very high signal intensity on T2W images centrally and typical rim enhancement following gadolinium administration in the vertebral body suggests intraosseous abscess. Postcontrast T1W images with fat suppression are helpful in showing the paravertebral soft tissue abscesses and epidural extension (Fig. 9). The subligamentous spread of soft tissue up to three or more vertebral body levels within the ligamentous border is another hallmark of tuberculous spondylitis (Fig. 10). This pattern of tuberculous spondylitis with preservation of the intervertebral disc till late and destruction of vertebral body, is usually described in adults and is referred to as a "Floating disc".

Epidural extension of abscess is seen as soft tissue mass with typical peripheral rim enhancement and well-demarcated by the posterior longitudinal ligament. Magnetic resonance imaging helps in demonstrating the thecal sac and spinal cord compression, by the epidural abscess (Fig. 10). Magnetic resonance imaging also helps in demonstrating, the kyphotic/scoliotic deformity in long-standing chronic cases.

Bone and Gallium Scan[31]

Bone scan is not usually performed as a part of routine workup of tuberculous spondylitis, because of very high false-negative rate of 35%. This rate is much higher with gallium scan and is up to 70%.

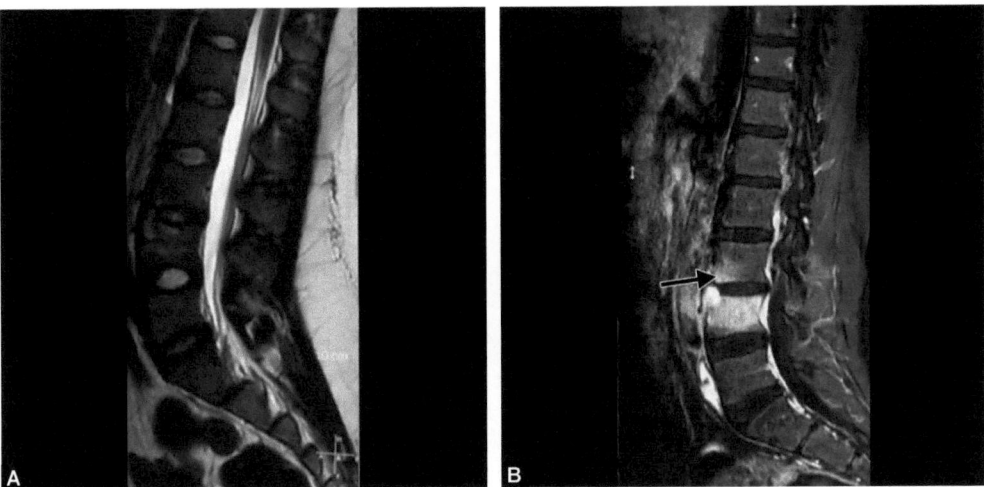

FIG. 8: A, Sagittal T2W; and **B,** Postgadolinium T1W fat-saturated magnetic resonance (MR) images showing patchy hyperintensity and diffuse enhancement following gadolinium administration involving only L4 vertebral body without involvement of intervertebral disc space and no loss vertebral height.
Note: Subtle area of enhancement involving anteroinferior part of L3 vertebra as well (arrow)

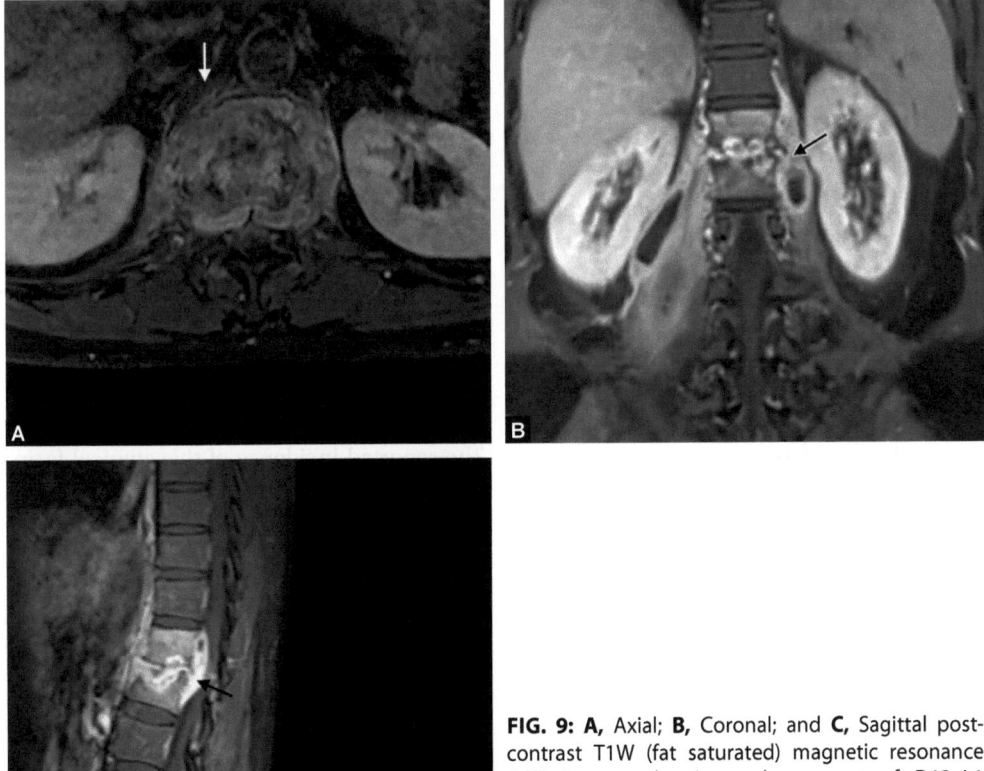

FIG. 9: A, Axial; **B,** Coronal; and **C,** Sagittal post-contrast T1W (fat saturated) magnetic resonance (MR) images showing enhancement of D12–L1 vertebrae with involvement of intervening disc space associated with enhancing soft tissue in prevertebral, paravertebral and epidural spaces (arrows)

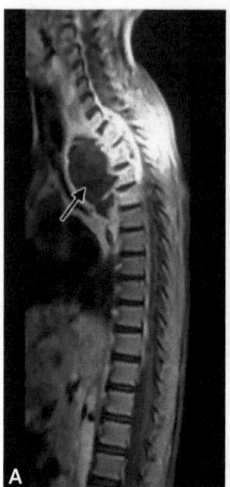 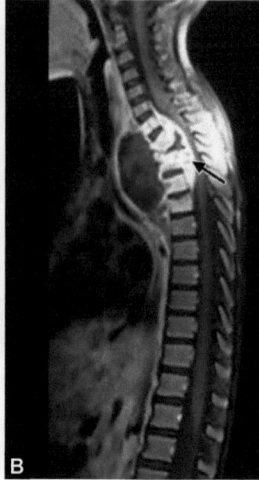

FIG. 10: Sagittal postgadolinium T1W fat-saturated magnetic resonance (MR) images showing enhancement of multiple vertebral dorsal bodies with sparing of intervening disc spaces associated with large prevertebral abscess (arrow), in an example of subligamentous type of tuberculous spondylitis

Note: Large epidural abscess compressing the thecal sac and dorsal cord (arrow)

Cytological and Microbiological Confirmation[32]

Etiological confirmation is usually not required, if the imaging features are typical of tuberculous spondylitis. Microbiological confirmation is made either by demonstration of AFB or tubercle containing epithelioid cells on pathological sample. Imaging helps in obtaining appropriate sample, especially CT-guided biopsy yields adequate material either from the spine itself or from an adjacent soft tissue.

ATYPICAL RADIOGRAPHIC PRESENTATION[33-35]

Concentric Collapse of Vertebral Body

Tubercular infection starting in the center of the vertebral body may lead to concentric collapse of the body. The radiologic feature in these patients is of vertebra plana with preservation of the adjoining disc spaces. It is important to evaluate the patient thoroughly to rule out other pathologic processes such as metastatic deposits, solitary myeloma, and eosinophilic granuloma.

Tuli proposed that the central type of tubercular lesion arises as a result of infection reaching the vertebral body through Batson's venous plexus or the branches of the posterior vertebral artery. The diseased vertebral body, with loss of normal architecture, collapses under axial loading.

Ivory Vertebra

The typical vertebral tuberculous lesion is usually destructive. Occasionally, superadded secondary bacterial (pyogenic) infection may lead to mixed lytic and blastic appearance or a purely sclerotic vertebral body mimicking ivory vertebrae.[5]

Neural Arch Tuberculosis[36,37]

Isolated infection of the posterior elements by TB is rare with an estimated incidence of 2–10% of all cases of spinal TB. The disease may involve the spinous process, lamina, pedicle, apophyseal joint, or the transverse process in isolation or combination (Figs 11 and 12).

Circumferential (Pan) Vertebral Involvement

Simultaneous infection of the anterior and posterior elements of one vertebra is rare and causes significant instability. These patients also are prone to have neurologic complications as a result of instability.

Multiple Vertebral Disease[33]

The reported incidence of this atypical form of spinal TB is approximately 7%. It is estimated that the incidence would be higher if MRI of the entire spine is done. The lesions may be in continuity, affecting from two to four contiguous vertebrae or may affect different levels in different regions of the spine (Figs 12 and 13).

Tuberculous Abscess with no Identifiable Osseous Lesion

A patient with subligamentous tuberculous lesion of the vertebral body starting under the anterior longitudinal ligament may present with a cold abscess in the thigh, abdominal wall/

Spinal Tuberculosis

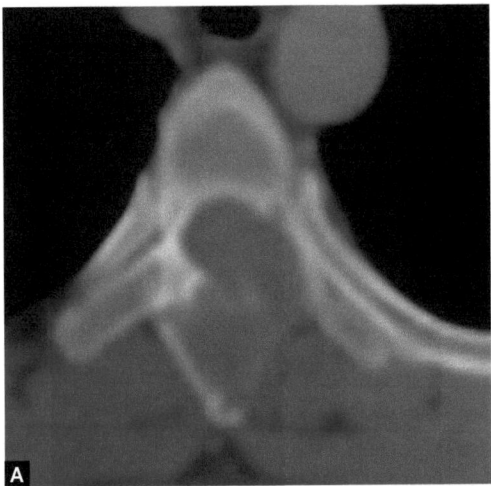
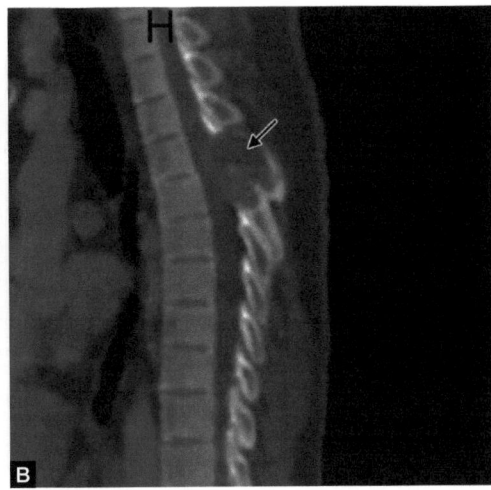

FIG. 11: A, Axial; and **B,** Sagittal reformatted computed tomography (CT) images showing destructive lesion involving posterior elements of dorsal vertebrae (arrow), in a biopsy proven case of tuberculous spondylitis

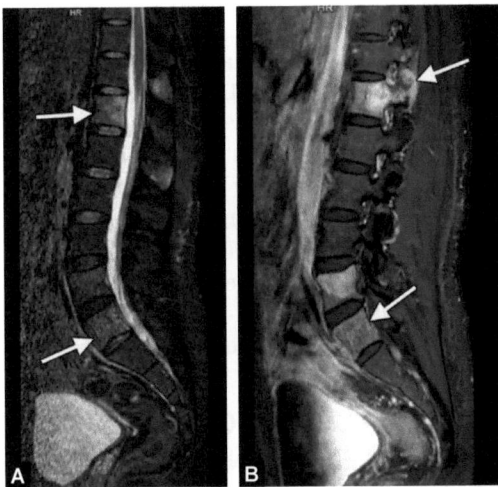

FIG. 12: A, Sagittal fat-saturated T2W; and **B,** Post-gadolinium fat-saturated T1W magnetic resonance images showing T2 hyperintense areas and enhancement following gadolinium administration involving L4 and L5 vertebral bodies (central type of tuberculosis) and body along with posterior elements of D12 vertebra (arrows)

chest wall. The osseous changes in these patients are very minimal or appear late.

Spinal Tumor Syndrome[38]

Spinal tumor syndrome is a condition where patients with spinal TB, who present with compressive myelopathy, radiculopathy or both without any apparent spinal deformity or lesions on plain radiographs. The diagnosis usually is confirmed after surgery and histopathologic evaluation.

RESPONSE ASSESSMENT AND FOLLOW-UP[39]

There is an increasing move away from surgical intervention towards conservative therapy, percutaneous drainage of abscesses, or both. It is therefore critical to monitor treatment response. Magnetic resonance imaging is a valuable diagnostic tool not only for early diagnosis but is also used to effectively monitor treatment response. Particular emphasis should be placed on soft tissue appearance in the early stages. Progressive reduction in gadolinium enhancement and the eventual loss of all enhancement are useful signs. Later on, fat deposition is a useful sign of healing. Gadolinium enhancement patterns vary and a reduction in gadolinium enhancement is a reliable sign, but an increase does not necessarily denote treatment failure.

Follow-up of patients with tuberculous spondylitis has to be based upon both clinical and radiological findings. Usually there is lag of 2 months for radiological improvement of a

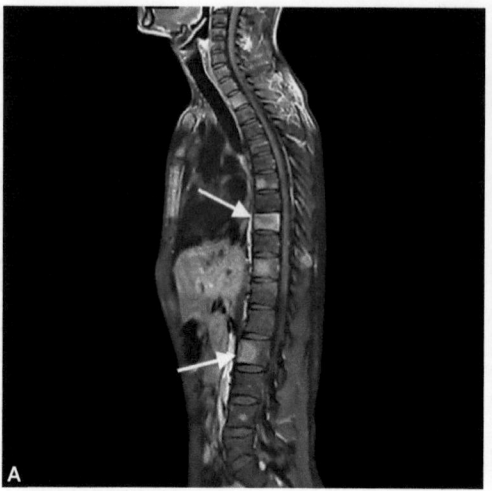
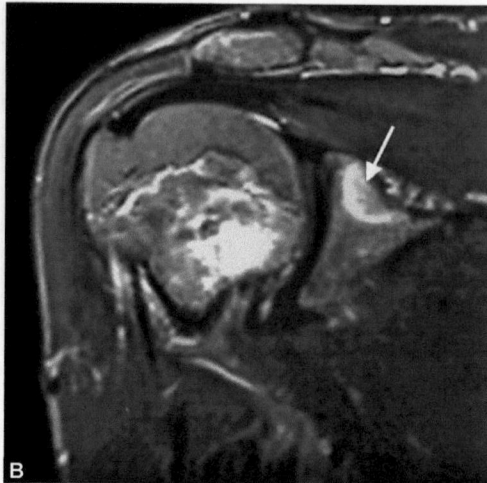

FIG. 13: Multifocal tuberculosis. **A,** Sagittal spine; and **B,** Coronal shoulder short T1 inversion recovery magnetic resonance images showing multiple hyperintense lesions involving vertebral bodies, proximal humerus and glenoid part of scapula (arrows).

lesion to be seen on imaging, as compared to clinical improvement. It takes about 2–3 months to show a radiologically perceptible sclerosis (remineralization), following drug treatment.

Magnetic resonance imaging done at 2–3 months even in a responsive tuberculous spondylitis may show increased inflammatory response giving false impression of progression of disease. Thus, early MRI following the start of drug treatment may be unreliable. However, if MRI findings worsen at 5–6 months of treatment, one should suspect a therapeutically refractory case.

Also, if there is no clinical improvement or there is worsening of spinal abnormality or appearance of a new lesion or failure of healing of ulcer/sinus or dehiscence of wound after 4–5 months of surgery, one should think of either refractory or drug-resistant TB. To label a case as multidrug-resistant TB, drug resistance has to be demonstrated on tissue sample.

Early Healing

Reduction in amount or degree of gadolinium enhancement of soft tissue# (#these findings are the best indicators of early healing).

However, progression of bone or disc changes, either an alteration in signal intensity or increasing destruction, during early course of treatment do not indicate failed treatment.

Late Healing

Signs of healed tubercular lesions on follow-up contrast-enhanced MRI include complete disappearance of marrow edema, resolution of paravertebral collections and replacement of vertebral body marrow by fat, seen as increased signal on T1-weighted images.

These patients should be monitored for at least 2 years, following the completion of treatment regimen and follow-up MRI is performed to show complete resolution of the lesion.

ROLE OF FLUORODEOXYGLUCOSE-POSITRON EMISSION TOMOGRAPHY SCAN[40]

Active TB shows increased uptake on fluorodeoxyglucose-positron emission tomography (FDG-PET) scan, but this increased uptake is nonspecific. It is also seen in neoplastic as well as other granulomatous diseases like brucellosis. Fluorodeoxyglucose-positron emission tomography may be requested in patients with equivocal MRI findings or for response evaluation when there are enhancing areas on MRI, after full clinical resolution of the symptoms and completion of antitubercular treatment (ATT). In such situations, increased uptake on FDG-PET supports presence of active infection. FDG-PET also provides a quantitative measurement of the absolute fraction of the injected dose reaching a tissue called the standard uptake value (SUV). Standard uptake values are raised in cases of active TB.[40]

DIFFERENTIAL DIAGNOSIS[41-45]

The differential diagnosis of tubercular spondylitis includes a wide variety of other infectious and noninfectious disorders. Pyogenic infectious lesions often cannot be differentiated radiographically, and the clinical data is important in the initial diagnosis, whereas aspiration is definitive. An insidious and slow onset of back pain (often of several months' duration), a pulmonary infiltrate (active pulmonary disease is present in 50% of patients with skeletal TB), previous history, a well-defined paraspinal signal abnormality, subligamentous spread up to three or more vertebral body levels, and multiple vertebral involvement or involvement of the entire vertebral body favor the diagnosis of TB of the spine.

Scalloping of the anterior surface of the vertebral bodies, which can occur in subligamentous dissection spread of TB, may also be caused by paravertebral lymphadenopathy owing to metastasis, lymphoma, or myeloma. Occasionally, eosinophilic granuloma involving the spine creating a vertebra plana can mimic early TB. Sometimes it is difficult to distinguish an infection of the spine from a metastasis. Radiologically, the hallmark of spinal infection is erosion of adjacent vertebral endplates and narrowing of the disc space with or without a paravertebral shadow. Metastasis typically does not involve the disc space with erosion of the adjacent vertebral endplates. It usually presents as a lytic/sclerotic lesion in the vertebral body or "winking owl" sign. In problematic cases, CT-guided needle biopsy may be required to differentiate between these entities to ensure prompt diagnosis and treatment.

The presence of pre/paravertebral abscess and the involvement of contiguous vertebrae and intervening discs make the diagnosis of spine TB quite obvious. In cases where these classical features of spine TB are not present, there may be some difficulty in differentiating tuberculous lesions from malignant infiltration. In such cases, diffusion-weighted MRI (DW-MRI) can prove to be a useful tool to arrive at the correct diagnosis. False-negative results can be obtained when there is dense solid caseation within the vertebrae, and in this situation overlap with apparent diffusion coefficient (ADC) values of malignant lesions may be noted. Therefore, diffusion MRI and ADC coefficient values are always best interpreted along with routine MRI sequences and a detailed clinical history and examination.

Other infectious processes (such as brucellosis, fungal infections), sarcoidosis, degenerative, and parasitic diseases can show imaging features similar to tuberculous spondylodiskitis.

One of the most common diagnostic dilemmas is between spinal TB and spinal brucellosis (Figs 14A and B). Some of the salient features which favor the diagnosis of brucellosis include involvement of lumbar spine rather than dorsal spine, sclerosis prior to the start of treatment, absence of gibbus deformity, absence of large soft tissue component or abscesses and presence of typical anterior osteophytes (Parrot's beak) on plain radiographs.

In degenerative disc disease, the affected disc space is narrowed, shows low signal intensity on both T1W and T2W images and does not enhance following contrast administration. However, Modic type 1 degenerative signal changes (hypointense on T1W and high signal on T2W endplate changes attributed to vascularized bone marrow and edema) on conventional MRI sequences can mimic or suggest infection, leading to additional costly and sometimes invasive investigations. Note that in these patients, there is no clinical suspicion of infection, including absent symptoms, and lack of any laboratory data to support infection. If infection could not be definitively excluded on a clinical basis, follow-up imaging is advised which may show minimal change, resolution, or evolution to Modic type 2 changes suggesting degenerative changes rather than infection. Whereas in tuberculous discitis, the affected disc is usually hyperintense on T2W images and enhances strongly following contrast administration. In problematic cases, diffusion-weighted imaging (DWI) may be performed

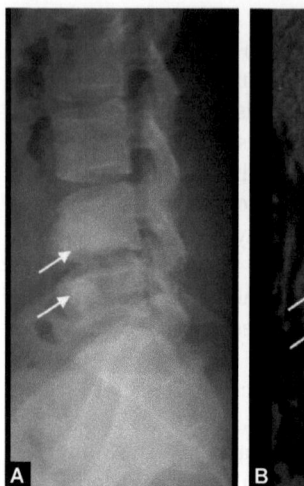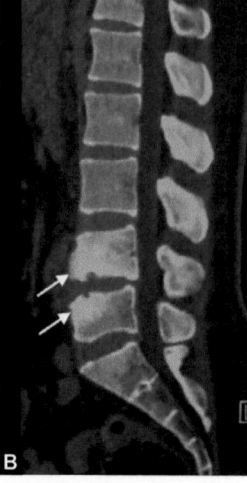

FIG. 14: Chronic granulomatous infection (brucellosis). **A,** Lateral radiograph of lumbar spine; and **B,** Sagittal three-dimensional reformatted computed tomography image of lumbar spine showing sclerosis of anterior parts of L4 and L5 adjacent endplates (arrows) with relatively preserved intervening disc space

to demonstrate claw sign, an indicator of degenerative changes.[44]

In rare instances, CT-guided needle biopsy may be required to differentiate between these entities to ensure prompt diagnosis and treatment.

CONCLUSION

In conclusion, MRI is the imaging modality of choice for early detection of tuberculous spondylitis. Advantages of MRI include, no ionizing radiation, high spatial resolution, allows screening of the whole spine and the demonstration of disease process in multiple planes. Thorough evaluation of the imaging features, such as anterior corner destruction, subligamentous spread, the presence of large paravertebral abscesses and multilevel involvement, will increase the specificity of MRI in the diagnosis of tuberculous spondylitis.

Nevertheless, entities such as pyogenic spondylitis, fungal infections, brucellosis and other granulomatous diseases may pose a diagnostic dilemma and final diagnosis may need histopathological examination.

REFERENCES

1. Tuli SM. Tuberculosis of the Skeletal System: Bones, Joints, Spine and Bursal Sheaths, 3rd edition. New Delhi: Jaypee Brothers Medical Publishers (P) Ltd; 2004.
2. Gardam M, Lim S. Mycobacterial osteomyelitis and arthritis. Infect Dis Clin North Am. 2005;19(4):819-30.
3. Duarte RM, Vaccaro AR. Spinal infection: state of the art and management algorithm. Eur Spine J. 2013;22(12):2787-99.
4. Kilborn T, Janse van Rensburg P, Candy S. Pediatric and adult spinal tuberculosis: imaging and pathophysiology. Neuroimaging Clin N Am. 2015;25(2):209-31.
5. Jain R, Sawhney S, Berry M. Computed tomography of vertebral tuberculosis: patterns of bone destruction. Clin Radiol. 1993;47(3):196-9.
6. Grange JM. The rapid diagnosis of paucibacillary tuberculosis. Tubercle. 1989;70(1):1-4.
7. Martin T, Cheke D, Natyshak I. Broth culture: the modern "guinea-pig" for isolation of mycobacteria. Tubercle. 1989;70(1):53-6.
8. Moon MS, Moon YW, Moon JL, et al. Conservative treatment of tuberculosis of the lumbar and lumbosacral spine. Clin Orthop Relat Res. 2002;(398):40-9.
9. Dobson J. Tuberculosis of the spine; an analysis of the results of conservative treatment and of the factors influencing the prognosis. J Bone Joint Surg Br. 1951;33-B(4):517-31.
10. Weinberg JA. The surgical excision of psoas abscesses resulting from spinal tuberculosis. J Bone Joint Surg Am. 1957;39-A(1):17-27.
11. Hald J. The value of histological and bacteriological examination in tuberculosis of bones and joints. Acta Orthop Scand. 1964;35:91-7.
12. Kemp HB, Jackson JW, Jeremiah JD, et al. Anterior fusion of the spine for infective lesions in adults. J Bone Joint Surg Br. 1973;55(4):715-34.
13. Masood S. Diagnosis of tuberculosis of bone and soft tissue by fine-needle aspiration biopsy. Diagn Cytopathol. 1992;8(5):451-5.
14. Delogu G, Zumbo A, Fadda G. Microbiological and immunological diagnosis of tuberculous spondylodiscitis. Eur Rev Med Pharmacol Sci. 2012;16 Suppl 2:73-8.
15. Desai SS. Early diagnosis of spinal tuberculosis by MRI. J Bone Joint Surg Br. 1994;76(6):863-9.
16. Ratcliffe JF. The arterial anatomy of the developing human dorsal and lumbar vertebral body. A microarteriographic study. J Anat. 1981;133(Pt 4):625-38.
17. Ratcliffe JF The anatomy of the fourth and fifth lumbar arteries in humans: an arteriographic study in one hundred live subjects. J Anat. 1982;135(Pt 4):753-61.
18. Moore SL, Rafii M. Imaging of musculoskeletal and spinal tuberculosis. Radiol Clin North Am. 2001;39(2):329-42.
19. De Vuyst D, Vanhoenacker F, Gielen J, et al. Imaging features of musculoskeletal tuberculosis. Eur Radiol. 2003;13(8):1809-19.
20. Yao DC, Sartoris DJ. Musculoskeletal tuberculosis. Radiol Clin North Am. 1995;33(4):679-89.

21. Williams GT, Williams WJ. Granulomatous inflammation—a review. J Clin Pathol. 1983;36(7):723-33.
22. Janssens JP, de Haller R. Spinal tuberculosis in a developed country. A review of 26 cases with special emphasis on abscesses and neurologic complications. Clin Orthop Relat Res. 1990;(257):67-75.
23. Perronne C, Saba J, Behloul Z, et al. Pyogenic and tuberculosis spondylodiskitis (vertebral osteomyelitis) in 80 adult patients. Clin Infect Dis. 1994;19(4):746-50.
24. Nussbaum ES, Rockswold GL, Bergman TA, et al. Spinal tuberculosis: a diagnostic and management challenge. J Neurosurg. 1995;83(2):243-7.
25. Hodgson SP, Ormerod LP. Ten-year experience of bone and joint tuberculosis in Blackburn 1978-1987. J R Coll Surg Edinb. 1990;35(4):259-62.
26. Stäbler A, Reiser MF. Imaging of spinal infection. Radiol Clin North Am. 2001;39(1):115-35.
27. Hetem SF, Schils JP. Imaging of infections and inflammatory conditions of the spine. Semin Musculoskelet Radiol. 2000;4(3):329-47.
28. Rowe LJ, Yochum TR. Infection (nonsuppurative osteomyelitis-tuberculosis). In: Yochum TR, Rowe LJ (Eds). Yochum and Rowe's Essentials of Skeletal Radiology, 3rd edition. Lippincott: Williams & Wilkins; 2004. pp. 1398-412.
29. Sharif HS, Morgan JL, al Shahed MS, al Thagafi MY. Role of CT and MR imaging in the management of tuberculous spondylitis. Radiol Clin North Am. 1995;33(4):787-804.
30. Joseffer SS, Cooper PR. Modern imaging of spinal tuberculosis. J Neurosurg Spine. 2005;2(2):145-50.
31. Pandit HG, Sonsale PD, Shikare SS, Bhojraj SY. Bone scintigraphy in tuberculous spondylodiscitis. Eur Spine J. 1999;8(3):205-9.
32. Mondal A. Cytological diagnosis of vertebral tuberculosis with fine-needle aspiration biopsy. J Bone Joint Surg. 1994;76(2):181-4.
33. Naim-ur-Rahman. Atypical forms of spinal tuberculosis. J Bone Joint Surg Br. 1980;62-B(2):162-5.
34. Pande KC, Pande SK, Babhulkar SS. An atypical presentation of tuberculosis of the spine. Spinal Cord. 1996;34(12):716-9.
35. Pande KC, Pande SK, Babhulkar SS. Concentric collapse of the vertebral body: an atypical form of spinal tuberculosis. Neurol Inf Epidemiol. 1997;2(1):225-7.
36. Ragland RL, Abdelwahab IF, Braffman B, et al. Posterior spinal tuberculosis: a case report. AJNR Am J Neuroradiol. 1990;11(3):612-3.
37. Solomon A, Sacks AJ, Goldschmidt RP. Neural arch tuberculosis: a morbid disease. Radiographic and computed tomographic findings. Int Orthop. 1995;19(2):110-5.
38. Parmar H, Shah J, Patkar D, et al. Intramedullary tuberculomas: MR findings in seven patients. Acta Radiol. 2000;41(6):572-7.
39. Gillams AR1, Chaddha B, Carter AP. MR appearances of the temporal evolution and resolution of infectious spondylitis. AJR Am J Roentgenol. 1996;166(4):903-7.
40. Jain AK, Dhammi IK, Modi P, Kumar J, Sreenivasan R, Saini NS. Tuberculosis spine: Therapeutically refractory disease. Indian J Orthop. 2012;46(2):171-8.
41. Smith AS, Weinstein MA, Mizushima A, et al. MR imaging characteristics of tuberculous spondylitis vs vertebral osteomyelitis. AJR Am J Roentgenol. 1989;153(2):399-405.
42. Güler N, Palanduz A, Ones U, et al. Progressive vertebral blastomycosis mimicking tuberculosis. Pediatr Infect Dis J. 1995;14(9):816-8.
43. Paus B. Tumour, tuberculosis and osteomyelitis of the spine. Differential diagnostic aspects. Acta Orthop Scand. 1973;44(4):372-82.
44. Palle L, Reddy MB, Reddy KJ. Role of magnetic resonance diffusion imaging and apparent diffusion coefficient values in the evaluation of spinal tuberculosis in Indian patients. Indian J Radiol Imaging. 2010;20(4):279-83.
45. Patel KB, Poplawski MM, Pawha PS, et al. Diffusion-weighted MRI "claw sign" improves differentiation of infectious from degenerative modic type 1 signal changes of the spine. AJNR Am J Neuroradiol. 2014;35(8):1647-52.

9

CHAPTER

Head and Neck Tuberculosis

Jeffrey Hawk, Ashu S Bhalla, Ashok Srinivasan

INTRODUCTION

Tuberculosis (TB) continues to be a prevalent disease in the developing world; and while the disease is typically seen in the chest, abdomen, and brain, involvement of different anatomic locations in the head and neck is not unusual. This chapter is focused on the different clinical manifestations and imaging appearance of TB presenting in the head and neck.

CERVICAL SPINE AND COMPLICATIONS

Clinical Presentation

The clinical presentation in patients with cervical spine TB often consists of neck pain, dysphagia, fever, night sweats, weight loss and progressive respiratory symptoms including dyspnea or stridor.[1,2] Symptoms can be insidious with a slow onset. A chronic course with progressive worsening is commonly seen when treatment is delayed. Airway compromise and vascular involvement marks an extreme in the spectrum of this disease, and has been reported as a cause of death in rare cases.[2] Neurologic symptoms can ensue when the disease tracks beneath the posterior longitudinal ligament along the anterior epidural space leading to mass effect on the cord. This includes paresthesias, paraparesis, quadriparesis, bowel and bladder dysfunction.

Cervical spine TB with complicating prevertebral abscess is managed with conservative measures initially with antituberculous antibiotics when appropriate. Often, however, it requires percutaneous or surgical drainage, sometimes requiring placement of fusion hardware. Treatment approaches to cervical spine TB have been evaluated, comparing conservative measures to surgical approaches.[3]

Imaging Appearance

The cervical spine is the least common site to be affected by TB, with lower thoracic and lumbar involvement being much more common. Typically, multiple levels are affected, primarily involving the vertebrae and sparing the intervertebral disks until later in the course of disease. Spread can be seen in a craniocaudal fashion deep to the anterior (paraspinal disease) and posterior (epidural disease) longitudinal ligaments over several levels. In tuberculous spondylitis there may be skip lesions, with intervening segments of relatively normal spine. Involvement of the posterior elements is also seen.

The predilection for vertebral involvement with relative disk sparing in TB is contrary to pyogenic spondylodiskitis, in which the disks are involved in a destructive fashion early in the disease. In pyogenic spondylodiskitis, this occurs secondary to extension from an adjacent vertebral body. The disks can be the primary site of involvement in pyogenic spondylodiskitis in young children.

Initially, cervical spine and prevertebral involvement may be detected on plain radiographs of the neck. On lateral radiographs, thickening of the retropharyngeal/prevertebral soft tissues, vertebral body destruction, straightening or reversal of cervical lordosis can be seen.

If spinal involvement is suspected, cross-sectional imaging including computed tomography (CT) [or preferably magnetic resonance imaging (MRI)] is indicated. This provides information on the levels of involvement, vertebral body disease not apparent on radiographs, soft tissue extension into the prevertebral or epidural space, potential airway or vascular compromise, spinal cord compromise, and nodal disease. Cross-sectional imaging also assists with treatment planning and approach. Dedicated MR and CT cross-sectional imaging of the neck will often include some of the lung apices and the lower intracranial structures and basal cisterns, allowing assessment of these areas for tuberculous involvement as well.

Computed tomography should be performed with contrast if possible, with multiplanar reconstructions and bone and soft tissue algorithms. Computed tomography is best for evaluating osseous destructive changes in the vertebral bodies. It also performs fairly well in assessment of anterior soft tissue extension. It can identify developing tuberculous abscesses as prevertebral or retropharyngeal low attenuation fluid collections with an irregular, enhancing peripheral rim. Adjacent soft tissue fat stranding can be identified as retropharyngeal effusions. Computed tomography is not ideal for assessment of epidural disease and meningeal involvement, and often significant disease in these areas can be underappreciated or frankly overlooked on CT. Computed tomography is not adequate for assessment of the spinal cord, though it may be able to give some idea of the degree of mass effect on the cord if present.

If available and not contraindicated, MRI should be performed in all cases of suspected tuberculous spondylitis. Magnetic resonance imaging should be performed with and without gadolinium contrast, if possible. The most useful sequences include axial and sagittal fluid-sensitive sequences (short T1 inversion recovery or fat-saturated fast spin-echo), precontrast T1 without fat saturation, and postcontrast fat-saturated T1 sequences in the axial and sagittal planes. Magnetic resonance imaging is best for evaluating soft tissue involvement extending from the vertebral bodies including prevertebral and most importantly, epidural disease. Epidural and prevertebral/retropharyngeal collections will often be heterogeneous on T1WI and T2WI, with expected heterogeneously high signal on T2WI and heterogeneous low to intermediate T1WI signal. Peripheral, irregular enhancement is seen along these collections if a well-defined abscess has developed. Otherwise, diffuse enhancement in these areas represents phlegmon, with its associated risks of progression to abscess. Cervical spine MR can demonstrate enhancement of the cervical spinal dura and show involvement of the basal cisterns. Magnetic resonance imaging is also suited for assessment of spinal cord involvement and/or mass effect and associated secondary changes in the cord. Figure 1 depicts the imaging features in a patient with retropharyngeal abscess likely related to dens involvement.

Differential Diagnosis

The primary differential diagnosis to consider in tuberculous spondylitis is pyogenic (bacterial) spondylodiskitis. As discussed earlier, pyogenic spondylodiskitis involves the disks early and often does not have an extensive craniocaudal extent, usually involving two vertebral body levels. Other granulomatous processes, fungal infections and *Actinomyces* may also be in the differential diagnosis when TB is being considered. Involvement limited to a single vertebra with osseous destruction may overlap with the appearance of neoplastic processes, either primary or metastatic. If there is primary retropharyngeal or prevertebral involvement with minimal to no diskovertebral disease, consider tuberculous adenitis of the retropharyngeal nodes, with or without superimposed abscess.

Imaging in Tuberculosis: Clinicopathological Correlation

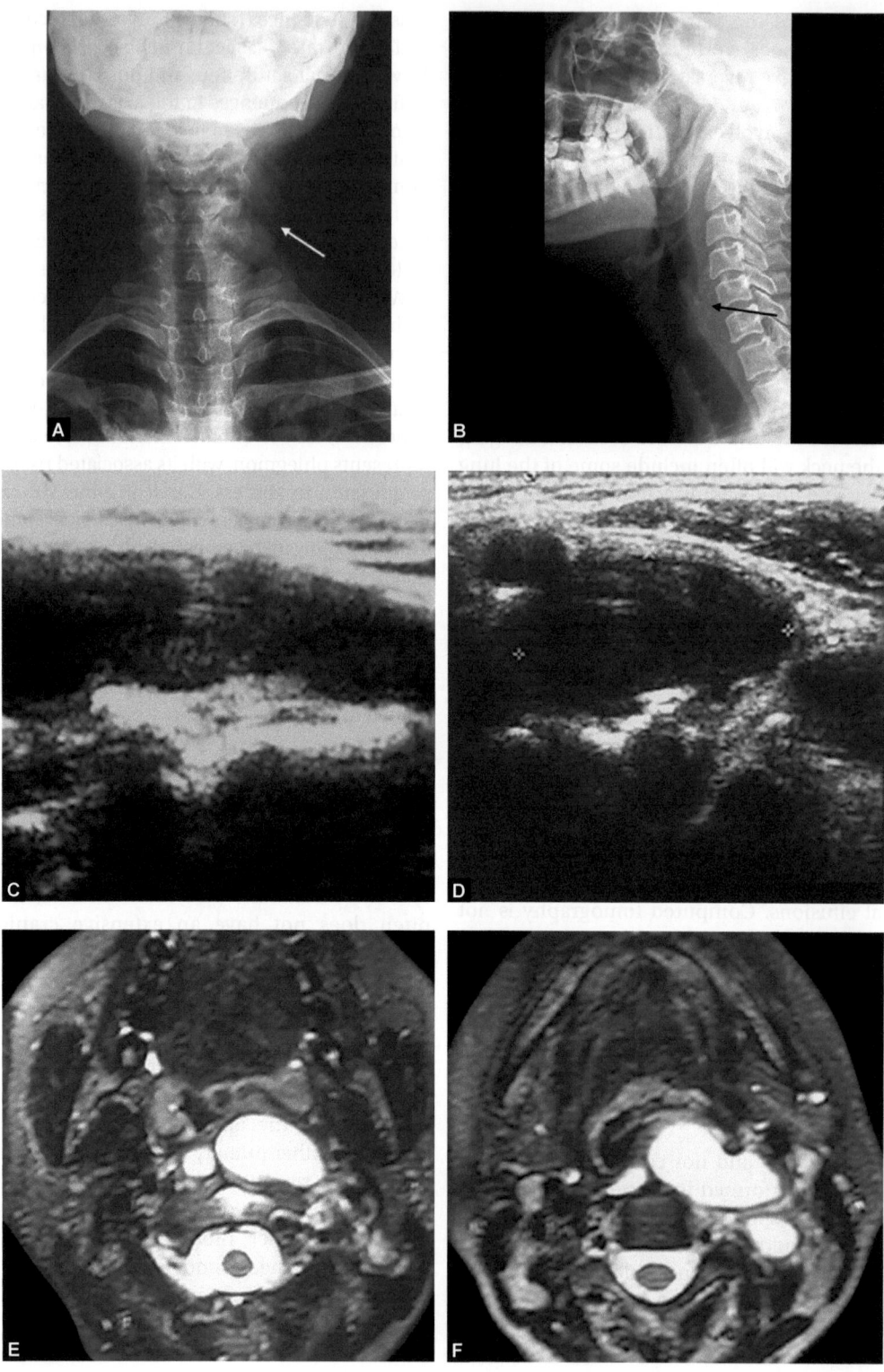

Continued

Continued

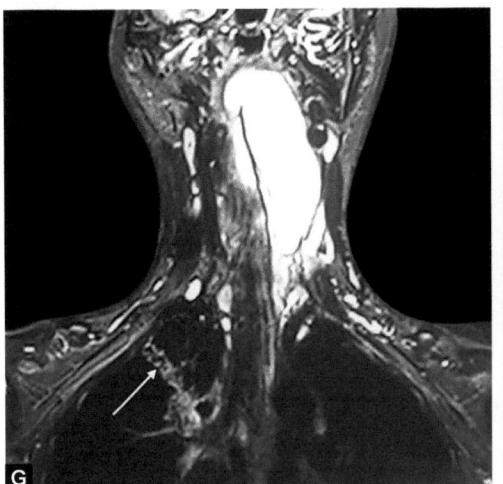
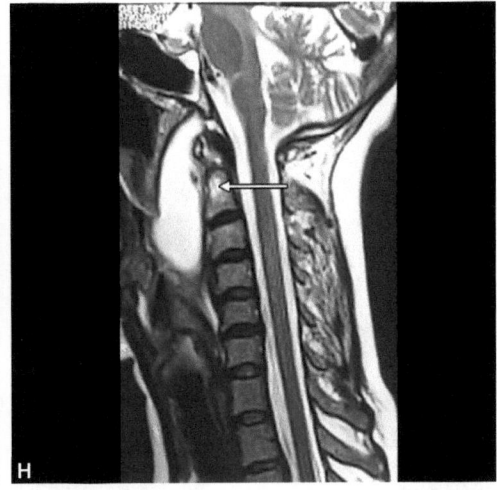

FIG. 1: Retropharyngeal abscess. A 32-year-old lady reported to the emergency room with left-sided neck pain and swelling of 1 week duration. **A,** Frontal and **B,** lateral radiographs of soft tissue neck reveal a swelling on left side neck (long arrow in A), widened retropharyngeal space (arrow in B) with a normal cervical spine. Note also made of right upper zone lung abnormality; **C,** ultrasonography neck sagittal and **D,** axial reveal an anechoic collection in the retropharyngeal and posterior cervical space. Patient underwent magnetic resonance imaging subsequently. **E and F,** T2W fat suppressed axial cranial to caudal and **G,** coronal images confirm the location of abscess in retropharyngeal and left posterior cervical space; and **H,** the sagittal T2W sequence reveals subtle hyperintensity in the base of odontoid (black arrow) suggesting a possible origin for the abscess. Fibrotic lesion is noted in right upper zone lung (arrow in G)

LYMPH NODES

Clinical Presentation

Perhaps one of the most common manifestations of TB in the head and neck is lymphadenopathy. Tuberculous adenitis commonly presents with palpable, nontender, enlarged lymph nodes. They typically involve level 5 (posterior cervical, spinal accessory chain) and less commonly the internal jugular chain (levels 2, 3, and 4). Concomitant pulmonary TB may or may not be present. Reactive cervical lymphadenopathy can also be seen with other tuberculous processes in the head and neck, such as spondylodiskitis, retropharyngeal abscesses and so forth. As with TB elsewhere in the body, immunosuppression [human immunodeficiency virus (HIV), organ transplant, lymphoproliferative diseases, chemotherapy] is a contributing factor.

Imaging Appearance

Tuberculous adenitis is best assessed with contrast-enhanced neck CT. Tuberculous nodes may be partially calcified and may show central necrosis, with peripheral enhancement. Adjacent soft tissue inflammatory changes and fat stranding may also be present. The nodes are most commonly found in the posterior cervical chain, and may be unilateral.

On MRI, nodes can demonstrate high intensity on T2WI, with central nonenhancing areas of necrosis on gadolinium contrast-enhanced sequences. Magnetic resonance imaging is not well-suited for detection of calcifications, but signal voids may be seen on all sequences if larger calcifications are present. Adjacent fat stranding and inflammatory changes are best detected on T1WI without fat saturation, seen as low signal infiltration of the adjacent high signal fat, and T2WI with fat saturation, seen as high signal infiltration of the adjacent low signal saturated fat. Figure 2 depicts the imaging features in a patient with tuberculous lymphadenitis.

Nodes are easily visualized with ultrasound due to their superficial location. As expected, central necrosis is fluid like and more hypo-

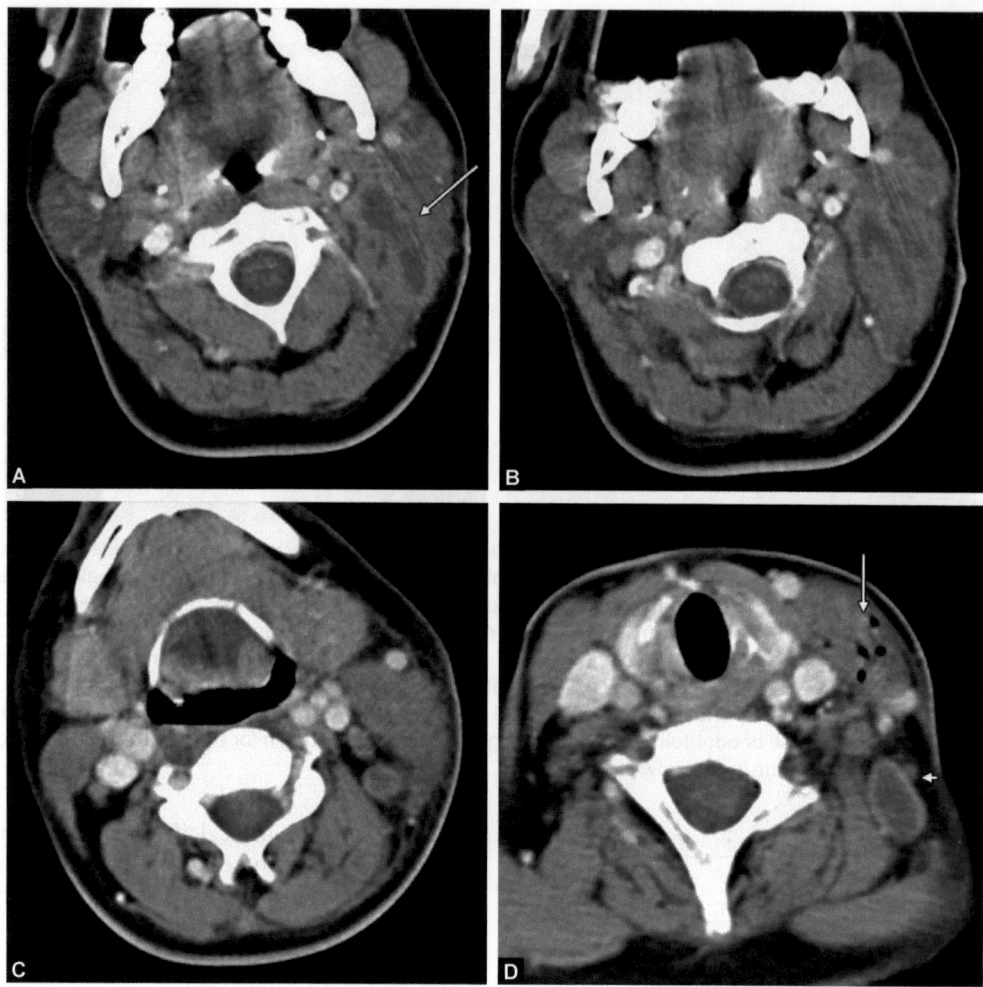

FIG. 2: Nodal tuberculosis. Contrast-enhanced computed tomography images (cranial to caudal) of a 22-year-old male reveal a heterogeneous, conglomerate nodal mass showing areas of necrosis within (arrow) located in the left posterior cervical space. Few discrete lymph nodes showing central necrosis and rim enhancement are also seen (arrow head). Air specks in the sternocleidomastoid muscle (arrow) are consequent to a previous fine-needle aspiration cytology. The aspirate was acid-fast bacilli positive (arrow in D)

echoic than the surrounding node without demonstrable blood flow. Calcifications may shadow.

Differential Diagnosis

The differential diagnosis of tuberculous adenitis is broad, and often the diagnosis is guided by ancillary clinical information. In the case of necrotic nodes in an adult, one must always consider metastatic disease from head and neck squamous cell carcinoma, especially those associated with human papillomavirus. In children, necrotizing lymphadenitis is a relatively common reaction to routine upper aerodigestive bacterial infections like pharyngitis and tonsillitis. Other entities that may mimic necrotic lymph nodes in the head and neck include complicated or uncomplicated branchial cleft cysts, thyroglossal duct cysts, thymic cysts, laryngoceles, ranulas, various upper aerodigestive diverticula, and lymphoceles/cystic hygromas. Except for lymphoceles/cystic hygromas and perhaps type 3 basal cell carcinomas, many of these other cystic entities are commonly located in spaces other than the posterior triangle of the neck, helping differentiate them from necrotic tuberculous adenitis.

Calcified lymph nodes may be seen after treatment for lymphoma and in various granulomatous processes such as fungal infection, sarcoidosis, or silicosis. Metastatic papillary thyroid carcinoma may also present with lymph node calcifications. Also in the differential diagnosis of tuberculous lymphadenitis are nodes from cat-scratch disease, Castleman disease, and HIV.

MUCOSAL SPACE AND ACCESSORY ORGANS

Clinical Presentation

In the mucosal space of the head and neck, many sites of involvement by TB have been described. These include the oral cavity, larynx, tonsils, nasopharynx, and accessory organs such as submandibular and parotid glands.

In the larynx, all levels may be involved, including the supraglottis (particularly the epiglottis and aryepiglottic folds), glottis and subglottis. When the glottis is involved, laryngeal TB presents with cough, dysphagia, hoarseness or a change voice quality. This is due to inflammatory and ultimately fibrotic changes that develop. The fibrosis often leads to voice changes that persist even after treatment.[4] In advanced cases, laryngeal involvement can present with dyspnea. It is frequently associated with pulmonary TB.

Tuberculosis has been reported as a cause of tonsillitis and peritonsillar abscess. It may involve the oral cavity including the tongue manifesting as glossitis. Tuberculosis of the nasopharynx can clinically present with nasal obstruction, rhinorrhea and obstructive symptoms of the eustachian tube, including otitis, and conductive hearing loss.[5]

Though relatively rare, TB can infect the salivary glands. The parotid is the most common of the salivary glands to be involved and can have an acute or chronic presentation.[6] It can present as an acute painful swelling or as an indolent, chronic, and progressive enlargement. Involvement of the submandibular glands is even rarer than parotid involvement. Submandibular TB can also present in an acute fashion or as a more indolent, progressive enlargement.

Imaging Appearance

The appearance of tuberculous laryngitis is relatively nonspecific on imaging. Truncation of the free edge of the epiglottis has been described as a finding in tuberculous epiglottis.[7] Mucosal thickening/asymmetry and submucosal fat stranding can be observed at involved laryngeal sites. Cervical lymphadenopathy can accompany tuberculous laryngitis.

Mucosal space asymmetry, swelling, and submucosal edema with blurring of fat planes can be part of the imaging presentation of tuberculous involvement of the nasopharynx. It can also present as a mass-like extension into the nasopharyngeal cavity. Nasopharyngeal TB usually does not invade adjacent structures in the aggressive way that carcinoma often does.

Subacute or chronic tuberculous parotitis often appears as single or multifocal intraparotid lesions which may demonstrate some component of cystic/necrotic change. On CT, this manifests as areas of enhancing abnormality with central nonenhancing hypodensity if necrosis is present. On ultrasound, these necrotic areas appear hypoechoic or anechoic with surrounding hyperemia. As would be expected on MR, acute and subacute parotitis appears as high signal on T2WI, particularly in the areas of cystic change/necrosis, with lack of enhancement of the necrosis. Acute parotitis and submandibular sialadenitis may present as diffuse heterogeneous enlargement of the respective gland with adjacent periglandular fat stranding.

Differential Diagnosis

A primary consideration with tuberculous involvement of the mucosal space is head and neck mucosal space carcinoma. In the larynx, the main consideration is squamous cell carcinoma. The presence of associated lymphadenopathy, sometimes with associated necrosis, can further confuse the picture. Often additional clinical information, tissue diagnosis, and microbiologic studies are required to make the distinction.

With nasopharyngeal involvement, nasopharyngeal carcinoma, lymphoma, and, in children, rhabdomyosarcoma should all be considered. As mentioned, TB does not typically demonstrate the invasive appearance that can be seen with entities such as nasopharyngeal carcinoma and rhabdomyosarcoma. Other causes of nasopharyngeal asymmetry or adenoidal enlargement including HIV (which can often coexist with TB), amyloidosis and reactive lymphoid hyperplasia must be considered, as should other granulomatous processes such as sarcoidosis and granulomatosis with polyangiitis.

In the case of chronic tuberculous parotitis or submandibular sialadenitis, it may be confused with other, more common salivary gland maladies, such as benign mixed tumors, Kuttner tumors in the case of the submandibular glands or malignant primary parotid and submandibular neoplasms. As in other sites in the head and neck, diagnosis often requires histologic and microbiologic confirmation. Acute tuberculous parotitis may be confused with bacterial or viral causes of parotitis. Acute tuberculous sialadenitis should be distinguished from postobstructive sialadenitis from stones or tumors, and bacterial, viral and autoimmune etiologies. Figures 3 and 4 demonstrate the imaging features in two patients with TB of the thyroid gland and parotid gland, respectively.

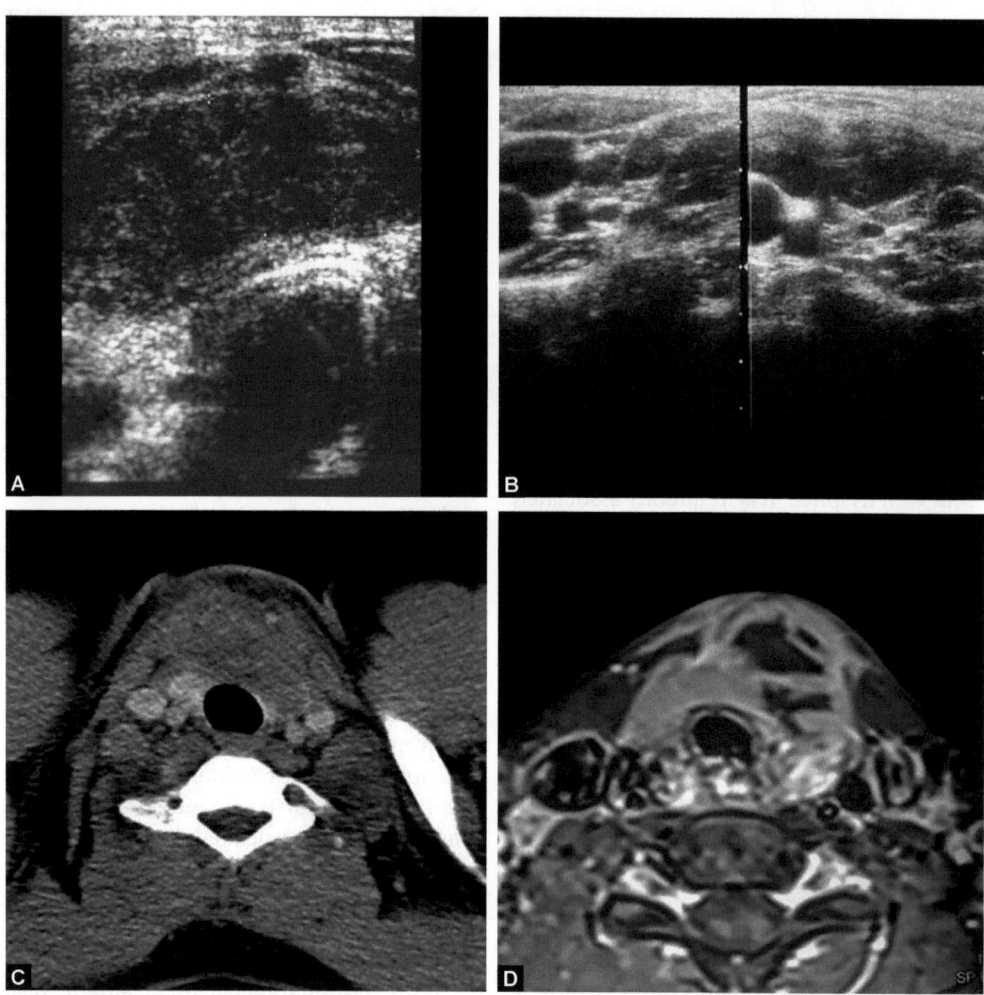

FIG. 3: Thyroid tuberculosis. **A** and **B,** ultrasonography of an 11-year-old boy shows enlarged, heterogeneous isthmus and left lobe of thyroid with hypoechoic areas within. Enlarged lymph nodes are also noted; **C,** contrast-enhanced computed tomography shows the lesion is hypodense; **D,** contrast-enhanced T1W axial magnetic resonance image reveals rim enhancement and central necrosis in the thyroid lesion

Head and Neck Tuberculosis

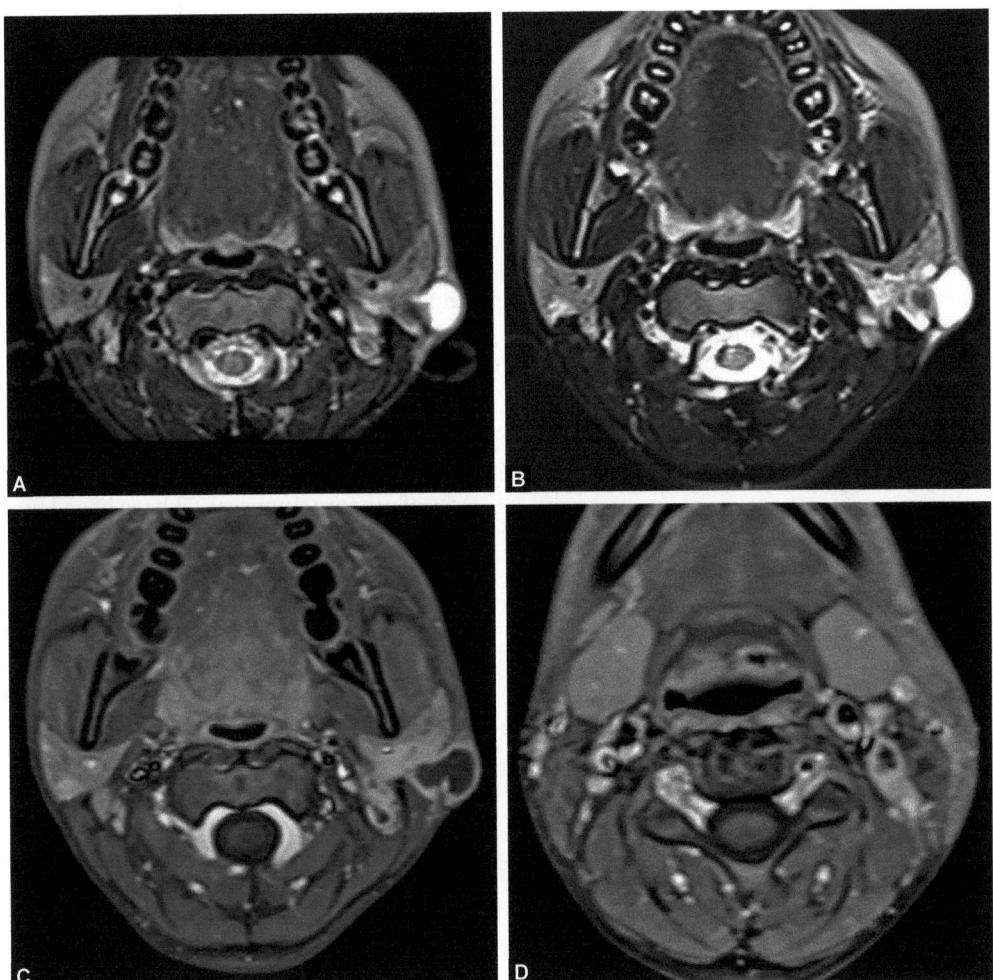

FIG. 4: A 30-year-old male patient with swelling in left preauricular region. **A** and **B,** T2W axial images show a hyperintense lesion in superficial lobe of the left parotid gland; **C** and **D,** gadolinium-enhanced T1W axial images show a rim enhancing lesion suggestive of abscess. Enlarged draining lymph nodes are also noted

ORBIT

Clinical Presentation

Though orbital TB is rare, TB can reach the orbit via direct spread from an adjacent head and neck site such as the paranasal sinuses, or via hematogenous spread typically from the lungs. Even with the rarity of orbital TB, the extreme prevalence of TB infection worldwide inevitably leads to cases of orbital disease. Often symptoms can be nonspecific and high clinical suspicion must be held to avoid delays in diagnosis. Cases of orbital TB leading to orbital apex syndrome have been described.[8] In a review of the literature on orbital TB, Madge and colleagues[9] discuss multiple patterns of orbital involvement by TB; periostitis, tuberculoma/cold abscess with or without osseous involvement, lacrimal gland adenitis and direct spread from sinonasal TB.[9] Tuberculosis can present as chorioretinal lesions and lesions over the sclera and cornea on clinical examination.[10]

Imaging Appearance

Tuberculosis can involve multiple orbital structures including the globe, extraocular muscles, lacrimal gland, lacrimal duct and sac, orbital fat, and optic nerve.

Involvement of the lacrimal gland can lead to diffuse enlargement of the gland and enhancement. Tuberculomas can present as focal areas of mass like abnormality, which can calcify, especially when treated. Defined fluid collections with relatively little surrounding edema (compared to pyogenic orbital cellulitis/abscess) can be seen. Linear enhancement along the meningeal covering of the optic nerves and extraocular muscle edema can be observed with optic nerve and extraocular myositis, respectively.

Contrast-enhanced CT of the orbit will suffice for evaluation of most cases of orbital TB, particularly in the anterior two-thirds of the orbit or for disease extending from the paranasal sinuses. Disease involving the optic nerve, globe, orbital apex or if there is suspicion of intracranial extension of orbital TB or orbital extension of intracranial TB, multisequence MRI is indicated. This should include coronal precontrast T1 without fat saturation, coronal postcontrast fat-saturated T1 and coronal T2 sequences. The orbital apices, orbital fissures, cavernous sinus, and anterior and middle cranial fossae should be closely evaluated.

Differential Diagnosis

Differential diagnostic considerations in orbital tuberculosis are myriad given the variety of imaging findings in orbital TB. Fluid collections can mimic pyogenic abscess or subperiosteal abscess though often with less adjacent fat stranding, hematic cysts when internal contents are complex, lymphangiomas, dermoids, epidermoids, and the rare orbital meningocele. Tuberculomas and presentations with orbital disease demonstrating soft tissue involvement can appear similar to hemangiomas, pseudotumor, metastasis, primary orbital malignancies such as rhabdomyosarcoma in children, and lymphoma. Optic nerve involvement can mimic optic neuritis, metastasis, lymphoma, leukemia, sarcoidosis, optic nerve glioma, and potentially meningioma. Lacrimal gland involvement can appear similar to bacterial or viral adenitis, lymphoma, epithelial malignancies of the lacrimal gland, and sarcoidosis. Involvement of the globe should be distinguished from chorioretinitis, scleritis and episcleritis of other causes, choroidal tumors, choroidal and retinal detachments, hemorrhages, and effusions.

Clearly, clinical, microbiological, and laboratory information and the temporal course of disease is indispensable in adding specificity and narrowing the differential diagnosis.

SINONASAL CAVITIES

Clinical Presentation[11-14]

Sinonasal TB is most often secondary, however, cases of primary sinonasal TB have been known to occur. The presentation of TB of the paranasal sinuses and nasal cavity can include obstructive symptoms, persistent nasal discharge, reduced sense of smell, and alteration in the quality of phonation. These symptoms are often chronic and can masquerade as more typical forms of rhinosinusitis. Sinonasal TB can extend into the orbit or the intracranial compartment.

Imaging Appearance

On CT, paranasal sinus involvement often appears as mucosal thickening of the affected sinus with various degrees of sinus opacification, particularly if the tuberculous process obstructs normal sinus egresses. At times, this opacification may demonstrate increased attenuation, and may be mass-like, particularly if a sinonasal tuberculoma is present. These can enhance. Destructive osseous changes can occur and can involve ethmoid air cell septae and the nasal septum. Chronic osteitis can be seen in the walls of the involved sinus and destruction of the walls of the paranasal sinuses can be seen. Occasionally, calcification within the sinonasal opacities is present.

When sinonasal disease is detected, close evaluation of the orbit, anterior and middle cranial fossae, skull base, and cavernous sinuses is prudent to fully appreciate the extent of disease. The effects on osseous sinonasal structures and bones of the skull base are best assessed with multiplanar CT. Magnetic resonance imaging should be performed whenever intracranial or posterior/apical orbital involvement is suspected.

Differential Diagnosis

The differential diagnosis includes more common forms of chronic sinusitis and sarcoidosis. Tuberculomas may mimic sinonasal polyposis or allergic fungal sinusitis. Granulomatosis with polyangiitis and other aggressive processes such as sinonasal neoplasms (squamous cell carcinoma, melanoma, lymphoma, adenocarcinoma, etc.) can have a similar appearance when osseous destruction and/or enhancement is seen.

MISCELLANEOUS

Tuberculosis can also affect other anatomical structures in the head and neck. Figures 5 and 6 show the imaging features in two patients with tuberculous involvement of the mandible and masticator space muscles, respectively.

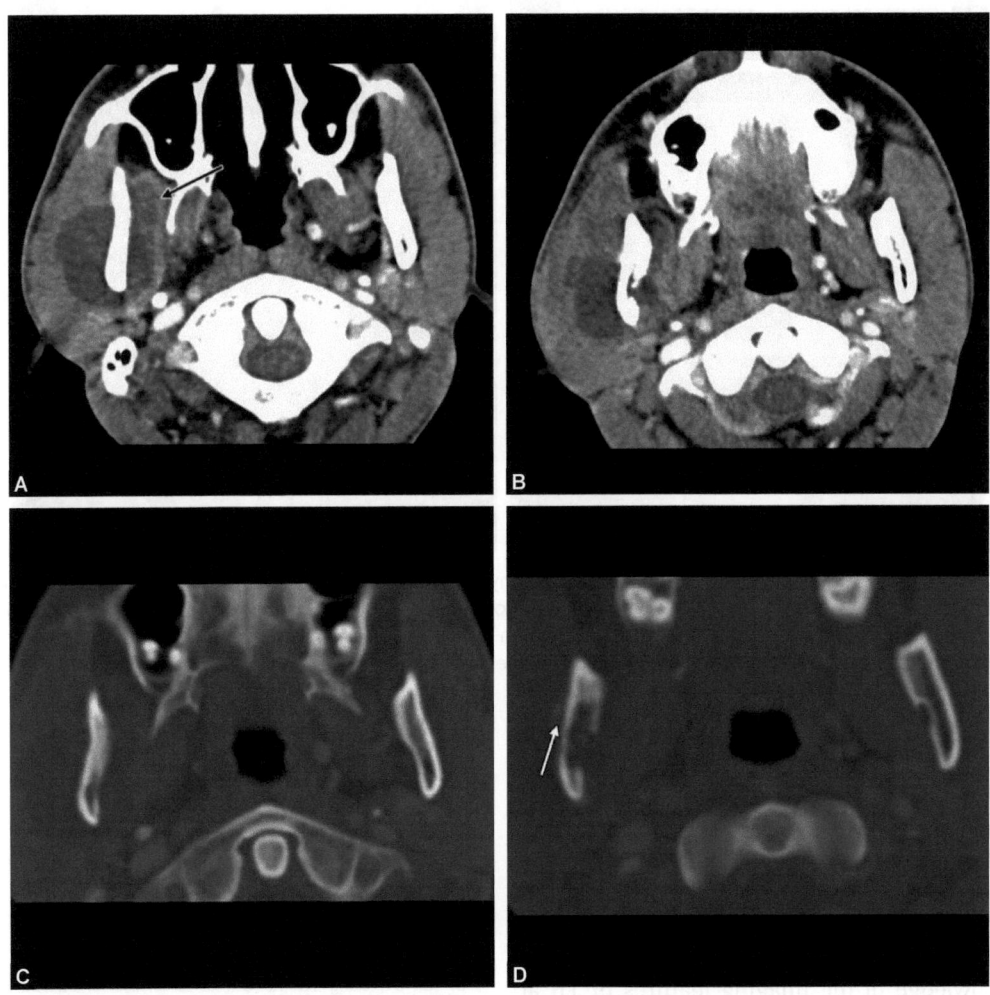

FIG. 5: Tuberculous osteomyelitis. Contrast-enhanced computed tomography images of a 21-year-old male presenting with pain and fullness of right side of the face. **A** and **B,** There is a fluid collection with rim enhancement seen in the right masseteric space (black arrow). The abscess is centered around the ramus of the mandible; **C** and **D,** bone window reveals irregular, ill-defined areas of lysis and sclerosis in the underlying mandibular ramus, along with periosteal reaction (white arrow).

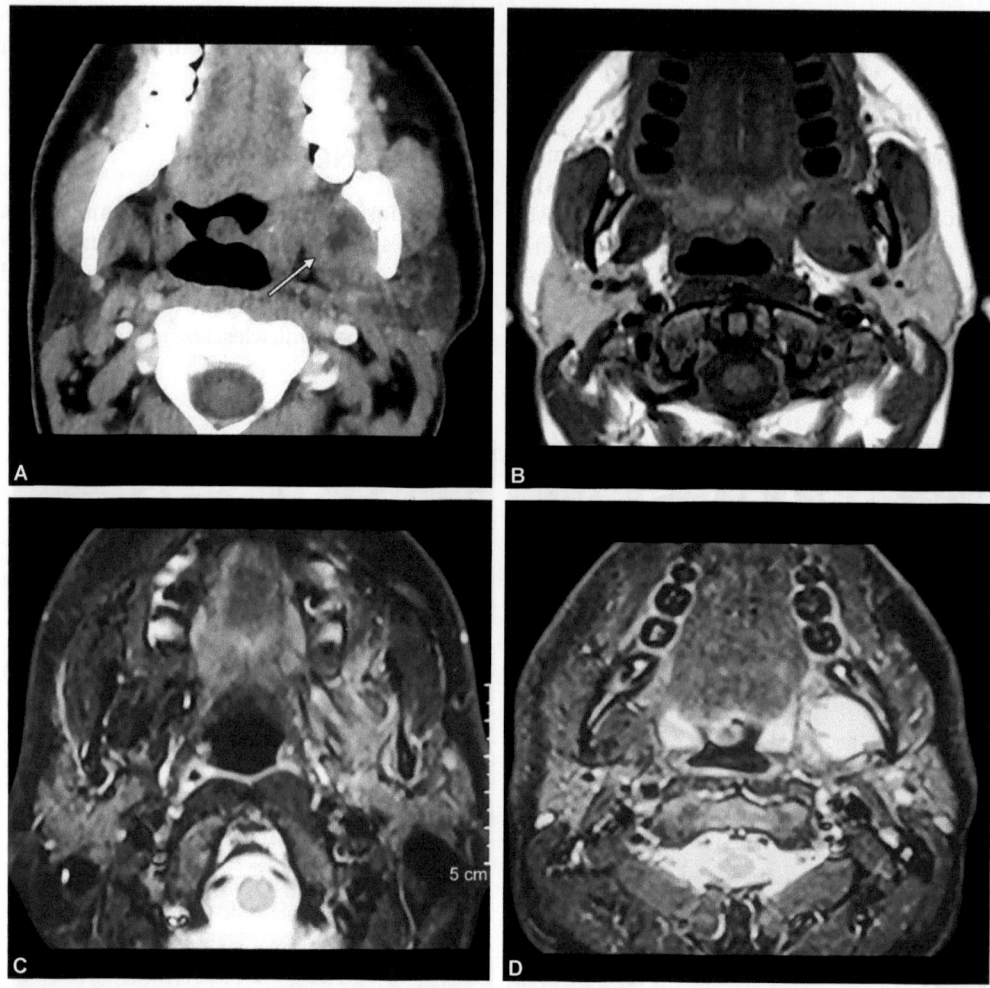

FIG. 6: Tuberculous myositis. **A,** Computed tomography; **B,** T1W magnetic resonance (MR); **C** and **D,** T2W fat suppressed images of a 21-year-old man with history of being treated for pulmonary TB a year back. Medial pterygoid muscle on the left side has an abscess within (arrow). More cranial MR section reveals edema of the lateral pterygoid and masseter also. Bone window images (not shown) did not reveal any bone erosion

CONCLUSION

While the involvement of the head and neck by TB may not be common, it is important to be aware of the different sites of potential affliction so that a comprehensive imaging evaluation can be performed for the benefit of the patient. Knowledge of the imaging features of TB at different anatomical sites in the head and neck is crucial for achieving this goal, and where appropriate, providing a differential diagnosis.

REFERENCES

1. Alawad AA, Khalifa AF. A Rare Cause of Retropharyngeal Abscess: Cervical Pott's Disease. Am J Trop Med Hyg. 2015;92(5):884.
2. Hugar BS, Chandra YP, Babu PR, et al. Fatal case of retropharyngeal abscess associated with Pott's disease. J Forensic Leg Med. 2013;20(6):567-9.
3. Qu JT, Jiang YQ, Xu GH, et al. Clinical characteristics and neurologic recovery of patients with cervical spinal tuberculosis: should conservative treatment be preferred? A retrospective follow-up study of 115 cases. World Neurosurg. 2015;83(5):700-7.

4. Lucena MM, da Silva FS, da Costa AD, et al. Evaluation of voice disorders in patients with active laryngeal tuberculosis. PLoS One. 2015;10(5):e0126876.
5. Darouassi Y, Chihani M, Elktaibi A, et al. Association of laryngeal and nasopharyngeal tuberculosis: a case report. J Med Case Rep. 2015;9:2.
6. Vyas S, Kaur N, Yadav TD, et al. Tuberculosis of parotid gland masquerading parotid neoplasm. Natl J Maxillofac Surg. 2012;3(2):199-201.
7. El Ayoubi F, Chariba I, El Ayoubi A, et al. Primary tuberculosis of the larynx. Eur Ann Otorhinolaryngol Head Neck Dis. 2014;131(6):361-4.
8. Tanawade RG, Thampy RS, Wilson S, et al. Tuberculous Orbital Apex Syndrome with Severe Irreversible Visual Loss. Orbit. 2015;34(3):172-4.
9. Madge SN, Prabhakaran VC, Shome D, et al. Orbital tuberculosis: a review of the literature. Orbit. 2008;27(4):267-77.
10. Cameron JA, Nasr AM, Chavis P. Epibulbar and ocular tuberculosis. Arch Ophthalmol. 1996;114(6):770-1.
11. Kim KY, Bae JH, Park JS, et al. Primary sinonasal tuberculosis confined to the unilateral maxillary sinus. Int J Clin Exp Pathol. 2014;7(2):815-8.
12. Budu VA, Bulescu IA, Schnaider A, et al. A rare case of concomitant tuberculosis of the nose, paranasal sinuses and larynx: clinical, histological and immunohistochemical aspects. A case report. Rom J Morphol Embryol. 2015;56(2 Suppl):833-6.
13. Moon WK, Han MH, Chang KH, et al. CT and MR imaging of head and neck tuberculosis. Radiographics. 1997;17(2):391-402.
14. Kar IB, Panda SN, Mishra N, et al. Resurgence of tuberculosis: a rare case of primary orbitomaxillary tuberculoma. Oral Surg Oral Med Oral Pathol Oral Radiol. 2013;116(1):e27-31.

10
CHAPTER

Imaging in Chest Tuberculosis

Ashu S Bhalla, Ankur Goyal

INTRODUCTION

Tuberculosis (TB) can affect any organ, and can have protean clinical and imaging manifestations. Lungs are the most commonly affected and frequently the first site of involvement due to airborne exposure [pulmonary TB (PTB)]. All other sites of involvement are clubbed under extrapulmonary TB (EPTB). Chest TB (CTB) manifests in the form of involvement of lungs, lymph nodes (LNs), pleura, and chest wall, in descending order of frequency. Cardiac involvement is rare and involvement of dorsal spine has been covered elsewhere in the book.

ROLE OF IMAGING

- *Detection of disease:* Chest X-ray (CXR) is usually the preliminary imaging investigation, followed by contrast-enhanced computed tomography (CECT) (if required) in a case of suspected TB. Ultrasonography may be done in case of chest wall abscess
- *Qualification of disease activity:* Whether there is active infection or only sequelae is an important question to be answered by imaging and laboratory parameters
- *Evaluating treatment response in follow-up:* Patients are usually followed-up using CXR for lung parenchymal lesions, ultrasonography for pleural effusion and chest wall abscess, and CECT for mediastinal LNs
- *Detect complications:* Imaging helps in detection of complications like bronchial artery hypertrophy, aneurysms, aspergillomas, and bronchopleural fistula so as to guide appropriate management
- *Diagnose healed tuberculosis with confidence:* Patients with healed TB may continue to be symptomatic. It is important to confidently diagnose such cases so as to avoid unnecessary institution of antitubercular therapy (ATT), because these patients require only symptomatic treatment.

IMAGING MODALITIES

Chest-X ray

Chest-X ray posteroanterior projection is usually performed as an initial investigation along with sputum microscopy. It is the most frequently employed investigation for diagnosis and follow-up and may be the only radiological investigation required in sputum-positive cases. It is widely available, easy to perform, cheap, and involves low radiation exposure. Other conventional views (lateral and lordotic views) are seldom used nowadays. Table 1 enlists the indications of doing a CXR.

Ultrasonography

Ultrasonography is employed to detect pleural effusion, characterize the nature of effusion, guide thoracocentesis and follow-up. It is definitive for distinguishing pleural thickening from mild effusion. It is also useful in evaluation of chest wall cold abscess. Ultrasonography may also give information regarding concomitant involvement of liver, spleen, abdominal LNs, and ascites. Ultrasonography is free from ionizing radiation, widely available, easy to perform and can be done at the bedside.

Table 1: Indications of doing a chest radiograph and computed tomography	
Indications of chest X-ray	**Indications of computed tomography**
• Evaluation of patients suspected to have CTB • In a patient suspected/diagnosed to have extrathoracic TB, as a baseline workup • For assessing treatment response in a diagnosed case of CTB • After any thoracic intervention (thoracocentesis, etc.) • In evaluation of symptomatic patients with past history of TB	• For diagnosis of CTB in patients with equivocal CXR or/and equivocal clinical profile • For diagnosis in patients with high index of suspicion (like immunocompromised) and those likely to have atypical imaging features (retrovirus infected patients) • Initial CECT for complete disease assessment in patients suspected to have additional extrapulmonary involvement • To assess disease activity in case of equivocal CXR/persistent radiographic lesions • In evaluation of symptomatic patients with past history of antitubercular therapy: When no prior radiographs available for comparison or if there is appearance of new findings • Imaging of suspected complications of TB

CECT, contrast-enhanced computed tomography; CTB, chest tuberculosis; CXR, chest X-ray; TB, tuberculosis.

Computed Tomography

Multidetector CT is the investigation of choice in case of nondiagnostic CXR.[1] It is an important tool in detecting radiographically occult disease as well as has higher specificity than CXR.[2] Computed tomography is more accurate than CXR in evaluation of LNs in primary TB and early detection of bronchogenic spread of infection in reactivation TB. Contrast-enhanced computed tomography (CECT) is the modality of choice for evaluation of mediastinal and hilar lymphadenopathy and for demonstration of necrosis within. It also helps in the evaluation of pleural effusions by demonstrating thickening and enhancement of the pleural layers in empyema. Computed tomography is better at assessment of disease activity in case of equivocal CXR and in evaluation of complications. It enables earlier detection of lesions and can also be used to classify the etiology of parenchymal involvement.[1] Computed tomography enables comprehensive evaluation of lung lesions, airways, mediastinum, pleural effusions, diaphragm, axillae, supraclavicular regions, soft tissues, and bones of the chest wall. Table 1 enumerates the indications of doing a chest CT.

The initial CT evaluation should thus be a contrast-enhanced examination so as to have optimal characterization of LNs, effusion and soft tissues of the chest wall. High-resolution CT (HRCT) reconstructions using high spatial resolution algorithm and narrow collimation, enable accurate detection and characterization of pulmonary nodules. A noncontrast CT is sufficient in the follow-up of parenchymal lesions but contrast administration is required for following patients with lymph nodal disease. Computed tomography findings enable accurate diagnosis of active CTB noninvasively, which is especially relevant in sputum-negative patients and permits early institution of ATT. Exposure to ionizing radiation and intravenous contrast-related issues are the limitations.

Magnetic Resonance Imaging

Conventional sequences (T1 and T2-weighted), subtracted postcontrast imaging and newer sequences like diffusion-weighted imaging serve as problem-solving investigations. One particular indication where they are employed is evaluation of mediastinum, to assess disease activity in persistent lymphadenopathy (where CECT may be equivocal), and in case of mediastinal fibrosis. Peripheral ring enhancement and central diffusion restriction are hallmarks of active disease. Magnetic resonance imaging (MRI) is useful in follow-up of mediastinal disease in children and young adults because it is free from ionizing radiation. Magnetic resonance imaging can also be employed to characterize effusions and is a reasonable alternative to CT for evaluation of lung findings in pregnant patients.[3] High cost, limited availability, and long acquisition times are the drawbacks.

Positron Emission Tomography-Computed Tomography

Fluorodeoxyglucose-positron emission tomography integrated with computed tomography (^{18}F-FDG-PET/CT) is employed in the workup of pyrexia of unknown origin, to localize the site of infection, inflammation, or malignancy. It may also be used in assessing disease activity and therapeutic response, however, high radiation exposure is a problem. Also FDG uptake is nonspecific and neoplasms may mimic TB.

PATHOPHYSIOLOGY AND IMAGING FINDINGS

The conventional classification of CTB into primary and postprimary (or reactivation) forms is helpful because it helps to understand the disease process and corresponding imaging manifestations. Age of the patient, underlying immune status, and prior exposure are the important determinants of the type of TB infection. Radiological patterns have been described for both primary and postprimary TB (PPT), but there is considerable overlap and recent studies question this categorization.

Primary TB occurs in patients not previously exposed to the bacilli and is usually airborne. Since it is the first exposure to the bacilli, it affects children, especially in the endemic areas. However it is now increasingly seen in adults as well, more so in the nonendemic regions. The primary parenchymal consolidation is known as the Ghon focus, which together with draining lymphatics and regional LNs constitutes the primary Ghon's complex.[4] This gangliopulmonary involvement is characteristic of primary TB. Other manifestations which can occur in primary TB are pleural TB, tracheobronchial involvement, and miliary dissemination; however these may be seen in reactivation disease as well. Isolated hilar and/or paratracheal adenopathy is the most common disease manifestation in children.[5]

Parenchymal involvement is usually evident as dense homogenous consolidation on imaging related to caseous exudates.[6] It is usually unilateral, commonly located in the middle and lower zones (Fig. 1A). Chest X-ray may show air space consolidation in 70% and evidence of lymphadenopathy in 95% of children with primary infection. Chest X-ray evidence of lymphadenopathy is less common in adults (43%).[7] On the contrary, radiographically evident lung involvement is more common in adults.[7] Computed tomography better demonstrates the consolidation which is commonly seen in middle lobe, basal segments of lower lobes, and anterior segment of upper lobes. Lymphadenopathy is also unilateral (on the same side as consolidation) and commonly involves hilar, paratracheal and subcarinal regions, in decreasing order of frequency (Fig. 1B). Bilateral lymph node enlargement can be seen in one-third of the cases. Computed tomography is more accurate than CXR in detecting mediastinal and hilar lymphadenopathy and a contrast-enhanced study helps in demonstrating central necrosis, thus increasing the diagnostic confidence (Figs 1C and D). The central low attenuation represents caseous necrosis while peripheral enhancement represents the vascular granulomatous tissue.[8] Homogenous enhancement is commonly seen in children, and heterogeneous enhancement may also be seen. Surrounding perinodal fat shows streakiness and suggests active disease. The necrotic LNs may coalesce to form abscesses in the mediastinum or neck (Fig. 1E). It may be noted here that isolated consolidation is nonspecific. However when it occurs in predisposed locations along with ipsilateral mediastinal adenopathy, a diagnosis of TB can be made. Similarly necrotic LNs may also be seen in metastases and histoplasmosis.

In majority of cases, the parenchyma lesion resolves without sequelae, while in rest there may be small calcified foci and tuberculomas. Together with calcified hilar LN, this is suggestive of a previous infection. In majority of the cases, the primary infection remains confined to chest; however in up to 10%, there is hematogenous dissemination, leading to progressive primary TB. This disseminated disease often occurs in very young and immunocompromised children. Local complications include bronchial

Imaging in Chest Tuberculosis

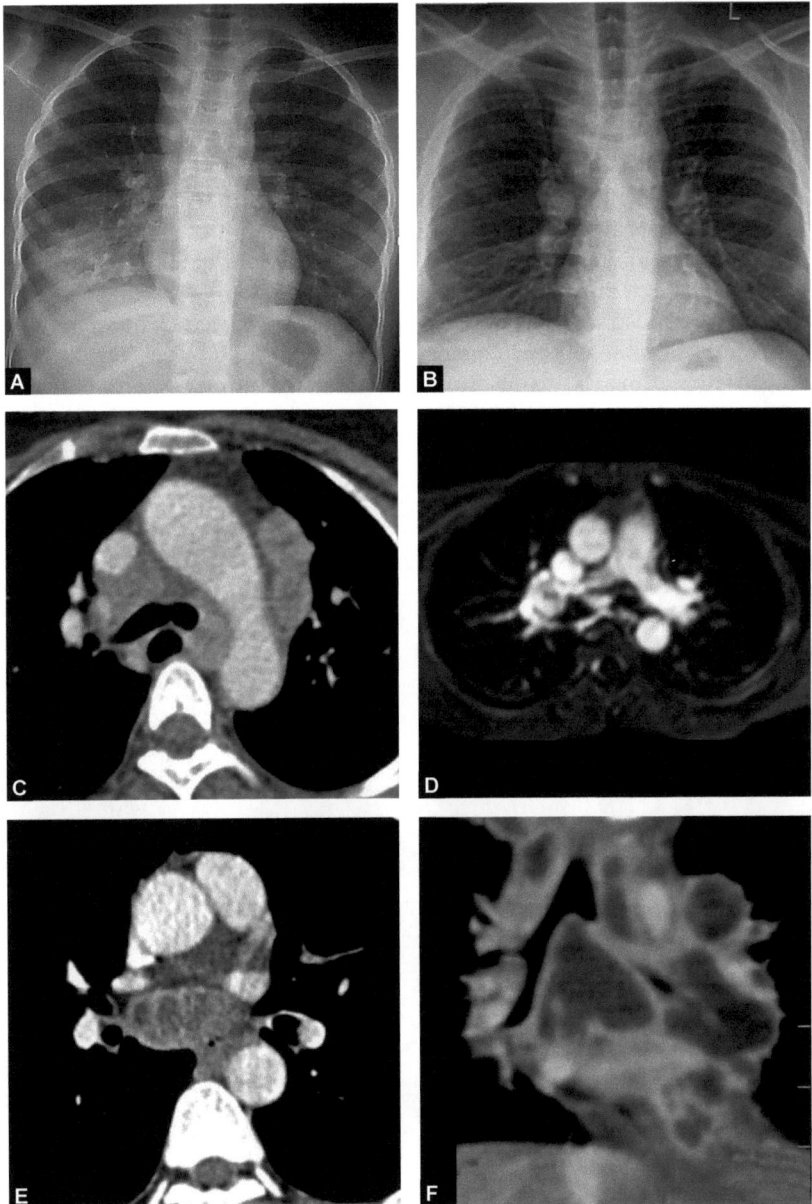

FIG. 1: Imaging in active tuberculosis. **A,** Chest radiograph in an adolescent patient shows right lower zone consolidation and lymph node enlargement in right hilar and paratracheal locations; **B,** a 14-year-old male shows enlarged lymph nodes in right paratracheal and hilar regions on chest X-ray; without any lung parenchymal findings; **C,** axial contrast-enhanced computed tomography (CECT) section (mediastinal window) in a 40-year-old female patient shows enlarged lymph nodes in precarinal, prevascular and paraesophageal regions with central necrosis and perinodal fat stranding; **D,** axial postcontrast fat-suppressed T1W magnetic resonance image of a different patient shows central hypointense focus of necrosis in persistent right hilar lymph node, suggesting residual active disease; **E,** axial CECT scan (mediastinal window) in an 18-year-old female patient demonstrates conglomerate rim-enhancing lymph nodes in retrocardiac location; and **F,** coronal CECT image in a 4-year-old child shows extensive necrotic conglomerate mediastinal and hilar lymphadenopathy with compression of left main and left lower lobe bronchus. There is resultant collapse of left lower lobe

compression (due to lymphadenopathy) (Fig. 1F) leading to distal pneumonia/atelectasis and perforation into the bronchus leading to spread of the infection.

Reactivation TB (or PPT) occurs in persons previously sensitized to TB infection and thus classically described to occur in adults.[4] It usually occurs due to endogenous causes (reactivation of dormant bacilli due to immunosuppression, malnutrition, or debilitation) but may occur due to exogenous repeat exposure. The hallmark of PPT is formation of cavities, bronchogenic spread, progressive fibrosis, and lung destruction. Postprimary TB commonly involves the apical and posterior segments of upper lobes and superior segment of lower lobes. Multiple segments are usually involved and bilateral involvement is common.[9] Recent studies[10] have found that children and adolescents also show similar destructive lung changes, questioning the traditional distinction of primary and reactivation TB. Also adolescents have been found to develop adult-type disease within 2 years of primary infection, suggesting that incomplete control of recent primary infection may be responsible rather than reactivation of healed infection.[11]

Cavities have thick irregular walls and may develop air-fluid levels (Fig. 2A). A significant amount of fluid content however suggests superimposed pyogenic infection.[6] Surrounding consolidation or clustered nodules are frequently seen (Figs 2B and C). With healing, the wall of the cavity becomes less thick. Endobronchial

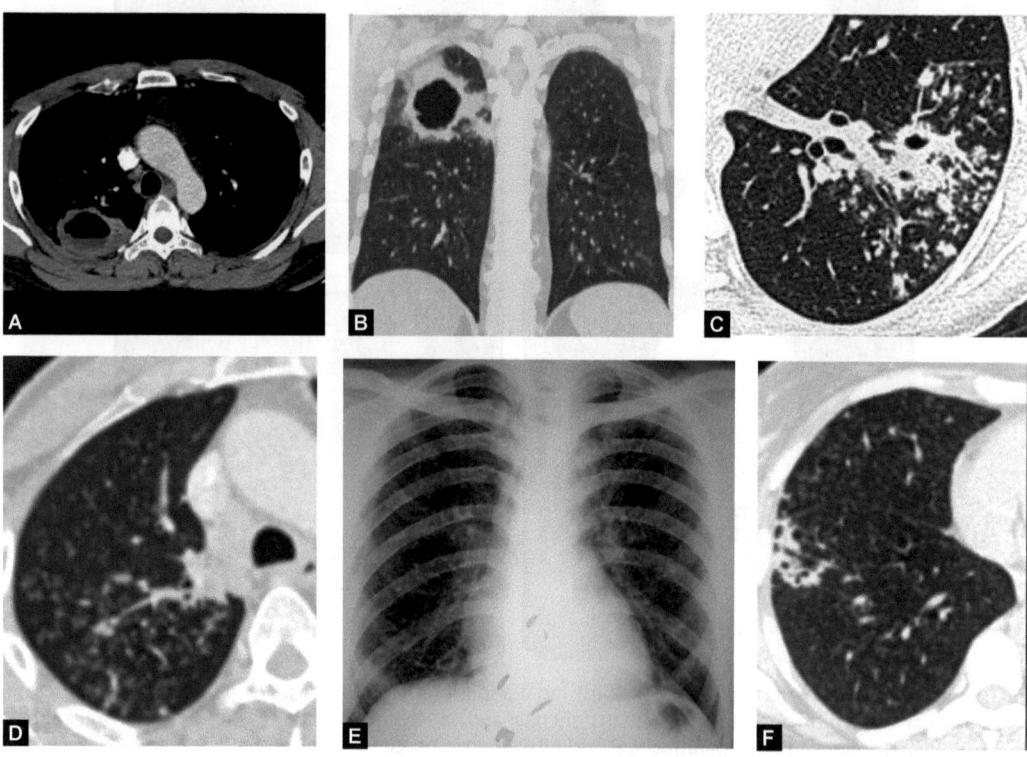

FIG. 2: Imaging in active TB (continued). **A,** Axial contrast-enhanced computed tomography section (mediastinal window) in a 34-year-old male patient shows thick-walled cavity in the posterior segment of right upper lobe with air-fluid level within; **B,** coronal reformat (lung window) demonstrates the cavity better, with surrounding consolidation, suggesting reactivation TB; **C,** different patient with reactivation TB depicts small thick-walled cavities with surrounding centrilobular nodules in left lower lobe; **D,** a 53-year-old female patient shows ill-defined centrilobular nodules with branching tree-in-bud lesions in right lower and middle lobes; **E,** chest X-ray of a different patient shows multiple ill-defined nodules randomly distributed in both lungs suggestive of miliary TB; and **F,** axial CT scan (lung window) shows innumerable randomly distributed lung nodules with patchy areas of pneumonitis

spread results from liquefaction of an area of caseous necrosis and bronchial communication. Chest X-ray reveals multiple ill-defined air space nodules (5-10 mm) in a segmental or lobar distribution. Computed tomography demonstrates endobronchial active infection in 95% cases, usually in the form of well-defined 2-4 mm nodules in centrilobular distribution with branching "tree-in-bud" pattern (Fig. 2D).[12] Latter are not specific for TB and can occur in any endobronchial infection, small airway disease, aspiration or inhalation of foreign substances, connective tissue diseases, and even neoplasms. Mediastinal/hilar lymphadenopathy is uncommon in PPT.[13] Complications include rupture of cavities into pleural space, leading to empyema. A bronchopleural fistula may also develop. Erosion into adjacent vessel may lead to life-threatening hemoptysis (erosion into pulmonary arterial branch known as Rasmussen pseudoaneurysm). Erosion into vessels also leads to hematogenous dissemination.

Fibroatelectasis and destructive lung changes commonly occur with chronic infection and healing. Upper lobes commonly show volume loss with hilar retraction, mediastinal shift, fissural displacement, and compensatory hyperinflation in remaining lung. Associated apical pleural thickening with extrapleural fat proliferation and fibrocalcific parenchymal lesions are also seen. Combined with bronchiectasis and cavitation, there is distortion of the involved parenchyma. The healed tubercular cavities may harbor aspergilloma, and such patients commonly present with hemoptysis. Hemoptysis may also occur due to hypertrophy of bronchial arteries and nonbronchial systemic collaterals due to chronic inflammation involving bronchi and lungs.

OTHER PATTERNS OF INVOLVEMENT

Following patterns may be seen both in primary as well as reactivation forms.

Miliary Tuberculosis

It results from hematogenous dissemination of the bacilli, leading to the development of multiple small granulomatous lesions in various organs such as lungs, liver, spleen, and brain. In the early stages, CXR may be normal and CT (HRCT) is more sensitive in detecting radiographically occult disease. Computed tomography classically shows 1-3 mm well-defined nodules randomly distributed in lungs, often associated with interstitial septal thickening and/or ground glass (Figs 2E and F). These nodules are actually located in pulmonary interstitium and there may be basal predominance of findings due to gravity-linked increased blood flow. If untreated, the nodules coalesce, become evident on radiographs, and may present as "snowstorm" appearance. Miliary involvement of the lungs usually heals without any sequelae and calcification is distinctly unusual. Miliary distribution of nodules may also be seen in metastases (e.g., thyroid carcinoma), pneumoconiosis, other infections (like fungal), hypersensitivity pneumonitis, and tropical pulmonary eosinophilia.

Tuberculomas

These are well-defined round lesions ranging from 0.5-5 cm and may be solitary or multiple. They are seen in both primary TB and PPT and usually indicate healed infection. Smaller satellite nodules may be seen in the vicinity. Majority remain stable in size and calcification is often seen. These nodules may cavitate and sometimes have irregular margins.

Pleural Involvement

Pleura is involved more commonly in primary TB wherein it presents as unilateral large free effusion, usually without loculations (Fig. 3A). It occurs as a delayed hypersensitivity response to mycobacterial antigens and thus microbiological analyses are frequently negative.

In PPT, effusions are smaller, loculated, and microbiologically positive because they result from rupture of a cavity into the pleural space. Three phases may be seen in pleural involvement of PPT. One is the exudative phase where there is smooth enhancement and thickening of visceral and parietal pleura (split pleura sign) on CECT. Second is fibrinopurulent phase where the effusion consists of pus (empyema).

Internal echogenic debris and septations are better demonstrated on ultrasonography. There is usually associated rib crowding and volume loss of ipsilateral hemithorax (Fig. 3B). Pleural empyema may track into the chest wall to form subcutaneous abscess (empyema necessitans). Final stage is the organizing phase where there is chronic empyema and fibrothorax. These present as persistent pleural collections with extensive pleural thickening and calcification with extrapleural fat proliferation. In fibrothorax, there is diffuse pleural thickening and little effusion (that too organized).

Spontaneous appearance of air-fluid level in effusion or hydropneumothorax refractory to thoracocentesis should lead one to search for bronchopleural fistula. Computed tomography is the investigation of choice to demonstrate the site of communication between bronchial tree and pleural space.

Healing occurs by resolution of effusion, which often requires percutaneous drainage. Residual pleural thickening and calcification suggest sequelae to old infection.

Tracheobronchial Tuberculosis

Involvement of the tracheobronchial tree occurs by perforation of an involved LN into the bronchial tree (usually in primary TB) or by endobronchial spread (in PPT). Acute involvement manifests as wall thickening, enhancement, and circumferential narrowing of the involved segment (Fig. 3C). Adjacent LN enlargement or peribronchial soft tissue thickening may also be seen. Uncommonly, there may be irregular intraluminal polypoid mass as well. Small airway involvement is seen as "tree-in-bud" nodules in centrilobular distribution. Healing can produce fibrotic bronchial stenosis and postobstructive bronchiectasis/atelectasis. Calcified peribronchial LNs can erode into adjacent bronchus, producing broncholiths. Latter may also occur due to inspissated secretions. Secondary amyloidosis may develop in the background of chronic inflammation. However the most common type of bronchial involvement is cicatricial bronchiectasis secondary to destructive fibrosis of lung parenchyma.

Extranodal Mediastinal Tuberculosis

Tuberculosis can also involve the esophagus, resulting from spread of infection from adjacent lymphadenitis. In acute phase, there may be wall thickening and later on strictures may result. Traction diverticulae can result due to adjacent periadenitis. Rarely tracheoesophageal fistulas may develop.

Tuberculosis pericarditis manifest as pericardial thickening and effusion with calcification developing in late stages (Fig. 3D). Constrictive pericarditis is a common complication with fibrous or calcified pericardial thickening.

Fibrosing mediastinitis/mediastinal fibrosis can be focal or diffuse. Focal type is more common and seen as localized mass in the right paratracheal, subcarinal, or hilar regions. Diffuse form manifests as plaque-like or ill-defined hypodense soft tissue thickening (Fig. 3D) which may cause narrowing of tracheobronchial tree, pulmonary vessels or superior vena cava obstruction. Hyperintensity on T2W MR images suggests active inflammation while diffuse hypointensity indicates fibrous tissue. Calcification may also be seen, however is more common in focal form.[14] Nontubercular causes of mediastinal fibrosis include histoplasmosis, autoimmune diseases, and radiation therapy.

Chest Wall Tuberculosis

Involvement of the thoracic cage is relatively uncommon in TB; when affected, it can involve the bones (ribs, sternum), joints (sternoclavicular and costochondral joints) as well as soft tissues (breast) (Fig. 3E). Rib involvement presents as lytic bone destruction and cold abscess. Joint involvement is seen as widening of the joint space, articular surface irregularity, and mixed lytic-sclerotic involvement of the subchondral regions. Breast involvement usually occurs in the form of abscess which may develop skin ulceration and discharging sinus. Ultrasonography depicts ill-defined hypoechoic lesion with internal mobile debris.

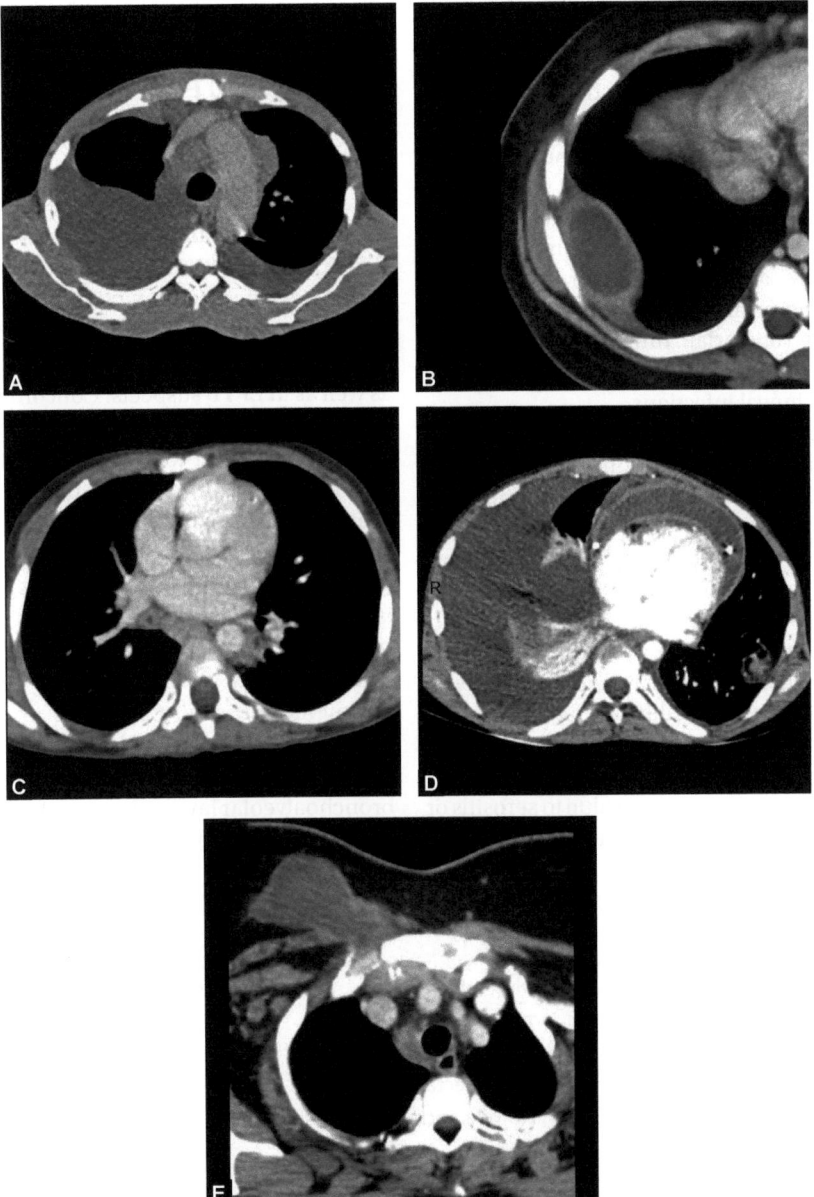

FIG. 3: Imaging in active tuberculosis (continued). **A,** Axial contrast-enhanced computed tomography (CECT) image (mediastinal window) shows bilateral pleural effusion (right > left) along with hypodense mediastinal lymphadenopathy; **B,** axial CECT image (mediastinal window) of a 13-year-old child shows loculated right effusion with enhancing pleural layers and rib crowding, suggestive of empyema; **C,** axial CECT image (mediastinal window) of a 35-year-old male patient reveals circumferential wall thickening and luminal narrowing of right lower lobe bronchus; **D,** axial CECT image (mediastinal window) of an 18-year-old male patient shows pericardial effusion and thickening with drainage catheter *in situ*. Also, note is made of free right-sided effusion and a cavity in left lower lobe; and **E,** axial CECT image (mediastinal window) of a 39-year-old female patient shows an abscess in the right breast with involvement of sternum, costal cartilage and also sternoclavicular joint (seen in a cranial section). Necrotic lymph nodes are seen in right paratracheal and axillary locations

DIFFERENTIAL DIAGNOSES

Imaging findings are often nonspecific and unless there is concordance between clinical profile, laboratory investigations, and radiology, other diseases must also be considered as differentials.

- Findings of active endobronchial infection (such as consolidation, acinar nodules on CXR, and centrilobular nodules on CT) may occur in nontubercular etiology as well (bacterial, fungal). Nodules with surrounding ground glass halo are typically seen in fungal infections
- Presence of consolidation (without thoracic lymphadenopathy) is nonspecific and can occur due to both infective and noninfective causes
- Bilateral hilar lymphadenopathy is commonly seen in sarcoidosis and may occur in lymphoma and metastases
- Thick-walled cavity may be seen in malignancy where irregularity and nodularity of the wall may help in differentiation
- Semi-invasive fungal infections commonly mimic chest TB
- Bilateral effusion is usually due to serositis or underlying liver/heart/renal disease.

IMAGING FEATURES OF ACTIVE AND HEALED CHEST TUBERCULOSIS (TABLE 2 AND FIGS 1 TO 4)

Conventionally sputum microscopy ± culture has been used to detect active TB infection. Recent studies suggest that more sensitive polymerase chain reaction-based techniques like GeneXpert MTB/RIF are also useful and have an added advantage of detecting drug resistance. Chest X-ray is a good screening modality and a baseline CXR is usually advocated both in CTB as well as in EPTB suspects. Concordant clinical and CXR findings obviate the need of doing a CT, especially if microbiological analysis is positive. Also, a normal CXR has high negative predictive value for active TB. However, if the clinical suspicion is high or in special situations (like immunocompromised status) or if CXR is equivocal/indeterminate, CT is indicated. If even the CT features are indeterminate for disease activity, then blood tests (erythrocyte sedimentation rate, C-reactive protein, total leukocyte counts, and differential leukocyte counts, respectively), Mantoux test, and bronchoalveolar lavage (in case of parenchymal involvement) are used to resolve the ambiguity.

Table 2: Indicators of chest tuberculosis disease activity on chest X-ray and computed tomography

Active tuberculosis	Healed tuberculosis	Indeterminate for disease activity
• Air space nodules/clustered/centrilobular nodules in predisposed regions • Consolidation in predisposed regions with ipsilateral LN enlargement • Miliary nodules • Thick-walled cavity • Cavity with surrounding consolidation • Unilateral hilar/paratracheal LN enlargement with central necrosis or heterogeneous enhancement • Conglomeration of LNs or obscuration of perinodal fat • Unilateral effusion/empyema with split pleura sign	• Thin-walled cavity ± aspergilloma • Bronchiectasis • Fibroparenchymal/reticular opacities • Atelectasis/collapse • Well-defined small nodules ± calcification (tuberculomas) • Subcentimetric calcified/homogeneously enhancing mediastinal LNs • Pleural thickening/calcification without effusion	• Consolidation/centrilobular nodules in other segments—nonspecific • Ground glass opacities: It may suggest superimposed secondary infections or aspiration related • Cavity with air-fluid level: It usually indicates secondary infection • Equivocal nodules on CXR (miliary/air space) • Equivocal hilar prominence on CXR/widening of paratracheal stripe • Borderline enlarged discrete LNs with homogeneous enhancement and preserved perinodal fat

CXR, chest X-ray; LNs, lymph nodes.

Tissue sampling (from LNs, lung lesion or thoracocentesis for effusion) is also frequently done for microbiological/pathological evidence of TB. Nevertheless, there may still be cases where ATT is presumptively started and monitoring of clinical response on follow-up is the only way to confirm the diagnosis. Following imaging features suggest active TB (Figs 1 to 3):

- Air space (acinar) nodules/clustered/centrilobular nodules in predisposed regions: Presence of ill-defined fluffy coalescent air space nodules on CXR suggests active infection. Large nodules (1–4 cm) clustered in a peribronchial distribution suggest active infection and may be surrounded by tiny satellite nodules. Similarly centrilobular nodules on CT with sharply marginated linear branching opacities suggest bronchogenic spread of infection in clinically suspected patients
- Consolidation in predisposed regions with ipsilateral LN enlargement points towards the diagnosis of active TB
- Miliary nodules indicate hematogenous spread of infection
- Thick-walled cavities represent necrotizing consolidation and are surrounded by centrilobular nodules
- Unilateral hilar/paratracheal LN enlargement (with central necrosis or heterogeneous enhancement, conglomeration of nodes and/or obscuration of perinodal fat)
- Unilateral effusion/empyema with split pleura sign
- Pericardial effusion ± thickening
- Chest wall abscess with/without involvement of underlying bones and/or joints.

Radiological features in patients with healed TB (Fig. 4) include pulmonary sequelae (fibroparenchymal lesions, calcific foci, and atelectasis), tuberculomas, thin-walled cavities (may be colonized with mycetoma), traction bronchiectasis, small calcified LNs, and pleural thickening/calcification without effusion (Table 2).

Table 2 enumerates the imaging features which are definitive of active TB (Figs 1 to 3), definitive for healed TB (sequelae) (Fig. 4), and features indeterminate for disease activity.

Figures 5 demonstrates examples of complications in CTB, as enumerated earlier.

TUBERCULOSIS IN IMMUNOCOMPROMISED PATIENTS

Immune-suppressed individuals like those who are retrovirus positive, diabetics and elderly debilitated patients show atypical radiological features. There is increased prevalence of miliary dissemination, lymphadenopathy, effusion, and extrapulmonary involvement; but cavitation is rare.[13] Middle lobe and basal involvement may be seen. Nodules are commonly seen and associated ground-glass opacities (GGOs) may also be seen. This is especially seen in case CD4 T-lymphocyte count is less than 200 cells/mm^3.

Another phenomenon which is unique to retrovirus infected patients is immune reconstitution inflammatory syndrome; it occurs as a result of recovery of the patient's immune status [due to antiretroviral therapy (ART)] evidenced by rising CD4 T-lymphocyte count. This leads to mounting of a robust inflammatory response to an opportunistic infection (subclinical or currently/previously treated infection).[15] Immune reconstitution inflammatory syndrome is associated with both TB and atypical mycobacteria and occurs within 2–3 months after initiation of ART. Imaging manifestations include worsening necrotic lymphadenopathy and lung infiltrates. Less common manifestations include nervous system involvement and hepatosplenomegaly. Diagnosis is challenging and resistance to ATT may need to be ruled out. The management includes continuation of ATT as well as ART and additionally steroids may be started. Drug-related hypersensitivity may also confound the scenario by causing fever and LN enlargement.

IMAGING IN NONTUBERCULOUS MYCOBACTERIAL INFECTION

Nontuberculous mycobacteria infections may present similar to the PPT, when it is called "classic" or cavitary disease, and nonclassic or bronchiectatic disease.[16] Predisposing factors include underlying lung disease, occupational

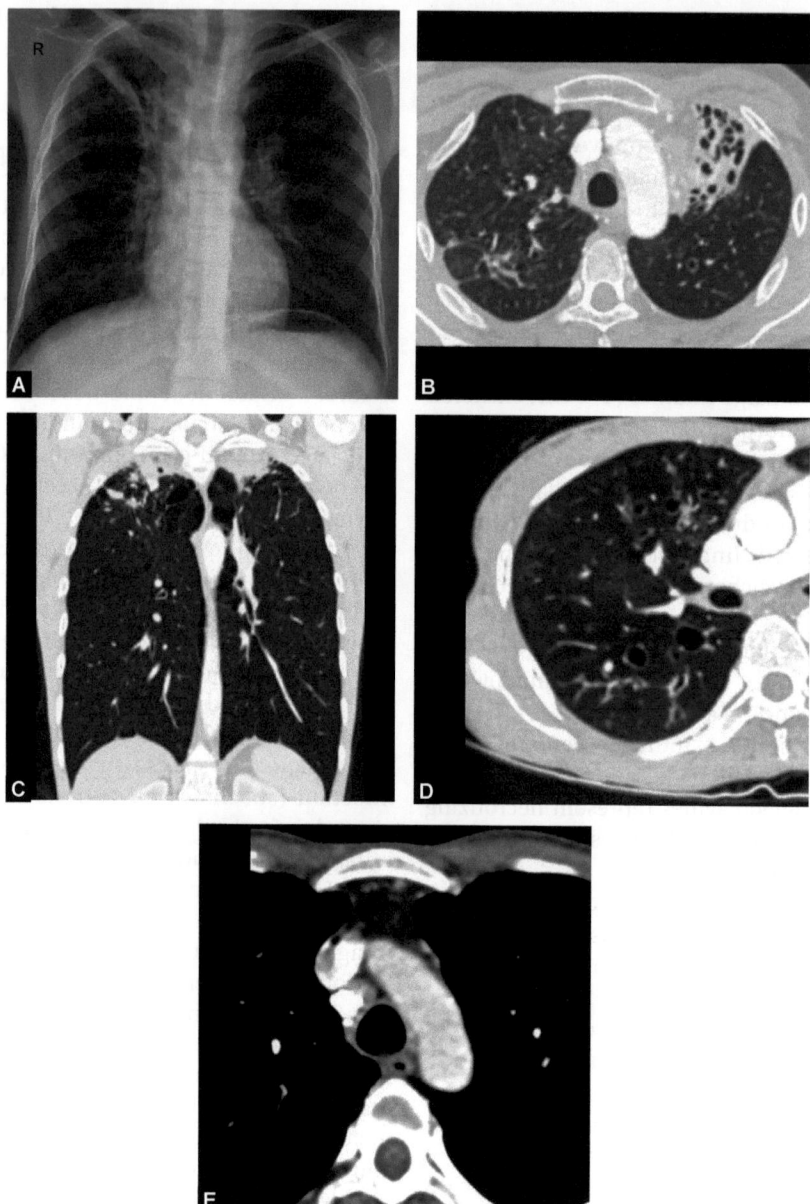

FIG. 4: Imaging features of healed tuberculosis (sequelae). **A,** chest X-ray in a 38-year-old male patient shows fibrobronchiectasis and atelectasis involving right upper zone; **B,** axial contrast-enhanced computed tomography (CECT) image (lung window) in a different patient shows fibrobronchiectasis involving left upper lobe along with volume loss. Few fibroparenchymal lesions are also seen in posterior segment of right upper lobe; **C,** coronal CT image (lung window) in a different patient depicts volume loss in both lung apices along with apical pleural thickening; **D,** axial CECT image (mediastinal window) in a 26-year-old male shows multiple small thin-walled cavities and bronchiectasis involving right lower (superior segment) and middle lobes. A subcentimetric calcified tuberculomas is also seen in right lower lobe; and **E,** axial CECT image (mediastinal window) in a different patient shows a densely calcified pretracheal lymph node

Imaging in Chest Tuberculosis

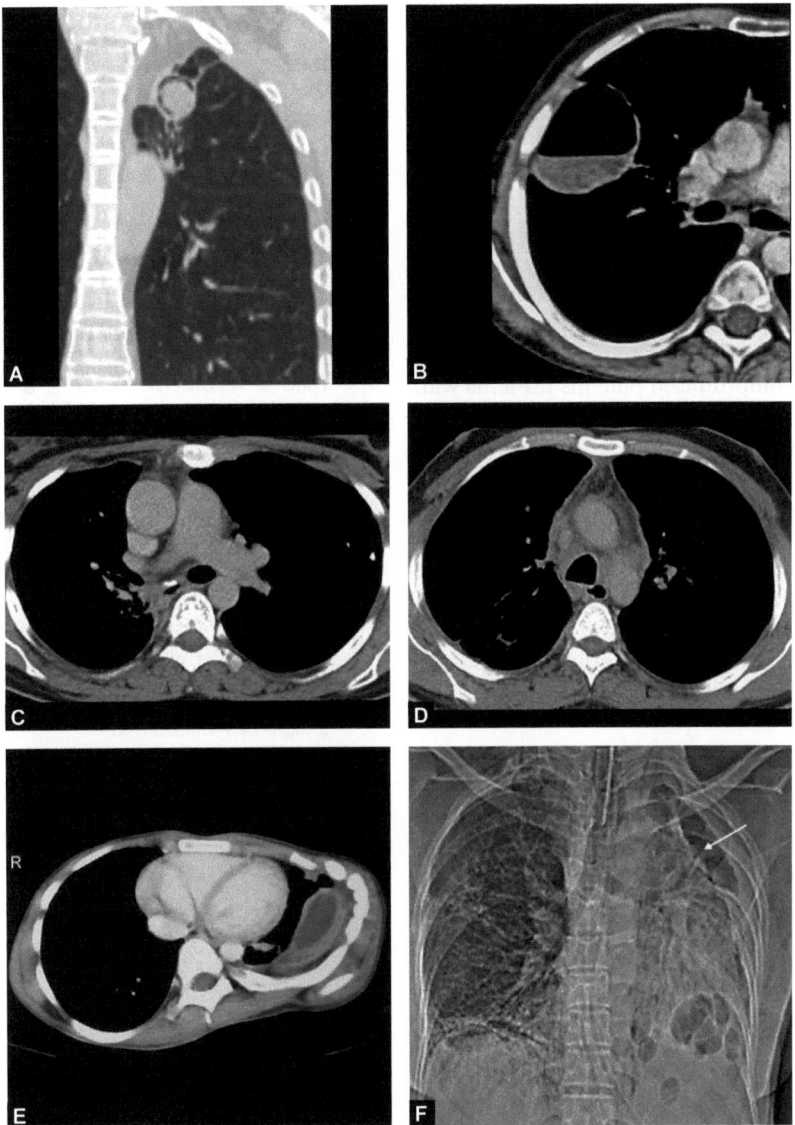

FIG. 5: Complications of tuberculosis (TB). **A,** Coronal CT image (lung window) of a 59-year-old male patient shows a thin-walled cavity in left upper lobe with mobile soft tissue content within, indicative of aspergilloma. Surrounding fibrobronchiectatic changes and atelectasis are seen; **B,** axial contrast-enhanced computed tomography (CECT) image (mediastinal window) in a 14-year-old male patient (treated case of pulmonary TB, now presenting with fever and cough) shows a thin-walled cavity with air-fluid level within, suggesting superimposed infection; **C,** axial CECT image (mediastinal window) in a 46-year-old female patient shows a calcified peribronchial lymph node with narrowing of right lower lobe bronchus. Note is also made of fibrobronchiectasis right lower lobe and tiny calcified granulomas bilaterally; **D,** axial CECT image (mediastinal window) in a 32-year-old male patient shows ill-defined soft tissue thickening in the mediastinum, surrounding the aorta, superior vena cava and trachea, indicative of diffuse mediastinal fibrosis; **E,** axial CECT image (mediastinal window) in a 42-year-old male patient with chronic empyema shows loculated left-sided pleural effusion with marked pleural thickening and enhancement. There is severe volume loss in left hemithorax with rib crowding; and **F,** CT topogram image of a 49-year-old female patient with persistent dyspnea and recurrent left pneumothorax, shows an abnormal communication between bronchus and pleural space, indicating a bronchopleural fistula (arrow)

factors, immune-suppression connective tissue disease, and debility. Imaging in classic disease reveals upper lobe cavities (which are small and thin-walled), bronchogenic spread, cicatrization, atelectasis, and pleural thickening. As in PPT, LN enlargement and pleural involvement is less common. Nonclassic form manifests with bronchiectasis and bronchiolitis (mosaic attenuation and centrilobular nodules).[17] Right middle lobe and lingula are most commonly involved. Consolidation and GGO may also be seen. Nontuberculous mycobacteria infection in immunocompromised patients presents with disseminated disease and mediastinal adenopathy is common.

CONCLUSION

Chest radiograph and CT are the workhorse in diagnostic evaluation and follow-up of suspected TB patients. However imaging should be used judiciously to limit radiation exposure and for optimal utilization of resources.

REFERENCES

1. Bhalla AS, Goyal A, Guleria R, et al. Chest tuberculosis: Radiological review and imaging recommendations. Indian J Radiol Imaging. 2015;25(3):213-25.
2. Feng F, Shi YX, Xia GL, et al. Computed tomography in predicting smear-negative pulmonary tuberculosis in AIDS patients. Chin Med J (Engl). 2013;126(17): 3228-33.
3. Rizzi EB, Schinina' V, Cristofaro M, et al. Detection of Pulmonary tuberculosis: comparing MR imaging with HRCT. BMC Infect Dis. 2011;11(1):243.
4. Van Dyck P, Vanhoenacker FM, Van den Brande P, et al. Imaging of pulmonary tuberculosis. Eur Radiol. 2003;13(8): 1771-85.
5. Marais BJ, Gie RP, Schaaf HS, et al. A proposed radiological classification of childhood intra-thoracic tuberculosis. Pediatr Radiol. 2004;34(11):886-94.
6. Cardinale L, Parlatano D, Boccuzzi F, et al. The imaging spectrum of pulmonary tuberculosis. Acta Radiol. 2015; 56(5):557-64.
7. Leung AN, Müller NL, Pineda PR, et al. Primary tuberculosis in childhood: radiographic manifestations. Radiology. 1992;182(1):87-91.
8. Pombo F, Rodríguez E, Mato J, et al. Patterns of contrast enhancement of tuberculous lymph nodes demonstrated by computed tomography. Clin Radiol. 1992;46(1):13-7.
9. Burrill J, Williams CJ, Bain G, et al. Tuberculosis: a radiologic review. Radiographics. 2007;27(5):1255-73.
10. Veedu PT, Bhalla AS, Vishnubhatla S, et al. Pediatric vs adult pulmonary tuberculosis: A retrospective computed tomography study. World J Clin Pediatr. 2013;2(4):70-6.
11. Marais BJ, Gie RP, Schaaf HS, et al. The natural history of childhood intra-thoracic tuberculosis: a critical review of literature from the pre-chemotherapy era. Int J Tuberc Lung Dis. 2004;8(4):392-402.
12. Hatipoğlu ON, Osma E, Manisali M, et al. High resolution computed tomographic findings in pulmonary tuberculosis. Thorax. 1996;51(4):397-402.
13. Skoura E, Zumla A, Bomanji J. Imaging in tuberculosis. Int J Infect Dis. 2015;32:87-93.
14. Rossi SE, McAdams HP, Rosado-de-Christenson ML, et al. Fibrosing mediastinitis. Radiographics. 2001;21(3):737-57.
15. Venkatanarasimha N. HIV, HAART, and IRIS: tuberculosis versus malignancy. AJR Am J Roentgenol. 2010;195(5): W376.
16. Martinez S, McAdams HP, Batchu CS. The many faces of pulmonary nontuberculous mycobacterial infection. AJR Am J Roentgenol. 2007;189(1):177-86.
17. Koh WJ, Lee KS, Kwon OJ, et al. Bilateral bronchiectasis and bronchiolitis at thin-section CT: diagnostic implications in nontuberculous mycobacterial pulmonary infection. Radiology. 2005;235(1):282-8.

CHAPTER 11

Lymph Node Tuberculosis

Naveen Kalra, Chirag K Ahuja, Niranjan Khandelwal

INTRODUCTION

Lymph nodes are the most common site of extrapulmonary tuberculosis (TB). Tubercular lymphadenitis is the leading form of tubercular infection in the developing countries including the Indian subcontinent accounting for close to 35% of cases.[1] Isolated cervical lymphadenopathy is the most common presentation in immunocompetent patients. Multifocal involvement is more common, often with intrathoracic and intra-abdominal lymphadenopathy and associated pulmonary disease in immunocompromised patients, especially human immunodeficiency virus (HIV) seropositive cases.[1] The diagnosis of TB involves a combination of positive biochemical markers and suggestive imaging findings in an appropriate clinical setting.

LOCATION

In the general population, tuberculous lymphadenitis most frequently involves the cervical lymph nodes followed in frequency by mediastinal, axillary, mesenteric, hepatoportal, perihepatic and inguinal group of lymph nodes, many a times in conjunction with lung and other local solid organ involvement.[2,3] The common presenting complaint is presence of a supraclavicular or posterior cervical region swelling or multiple painless slow growing masses developing over weeks to months.[4,5] The lymphadenopathy is more often bilateral. The lymphadenopathy in abdominal TB falls along the lymphatic drainage sites of the small bowel and liver which may be seeded hematogenously and characteristically occurs in mesenteric, peripancreatic, periportal and para-aortic groups of lymph nodes. The nodes may be scattered singly or are seen as conglomerate masses with central necrosis.

CLINICAL FEATURES

The common systemic complaints of these patients are fever, weight loss, fatigue, and night sweats. Mediastinal lymphadenitis may present with distressing cough as a prominent symptom while abdominal complaints may be heaviness, pain, constipation or loose stools. Initially the nodes are firm, discrete, and mobile with an intact and free overlying skin. Subsequently these may become matted with inflammation of the overlying skin. In more advanced stage, the nodes may soften leading to formation of abscesses and sinus tracts which may be difficult to heal.[1]

Paradoxical reaction during antituberculosis treatment is a well-known phenomenon first described in 1955 by Chloremis et al.[6] It is defined as the clinical or radiological worsening of pre-existing tuberculous lesions or development of new lesions in a patient who initially improves with antituberculosis therapy[7] in the absence of disease relapse. Its incidence ranges from 11–15% of patients with TB, more commonly seen in HIV-positive patients.[8] It is seen frequently in those with extrapulmonary TB involving the central nervous system, cervical and mediastinal lymph nodes, and in cases of disseminated TB.[8,9] The mechanism is immune restoration which mounts a response on various body systems.[10]

PATHOLOGY AND PATHOGENESIS

Tuberculous lymphadenitis is a local manifestation of the systemic disease caused by *Mycobacterium tuberculosis*.[11] It may occur during primary tuberculous infection or as a result of reactivation of dormant focus of infection or at times direct extension from a contiguous active focus. The initial sites of spread of infection from the lung parenchyma are hilar, mediastinal and paratracheal lymph nodes followed by supraclavicular lymph nodes reflecting the lymphatic drainage routes for the lung parenchyma. Cervical lymphadenitis may represent a spread from the primary focus of infection in the tonsils or adenoids or at times, paranasal sinuses disease.[12] The initial stage of superficial lymph node involvement leads to progressive multiplication of tubercular bacilli, resulting in the onset of delayed hypersensitivity, which is accompanied by hyperemia, swelling, necrosis, and caseation of the center of the nodes. This may, if untreated, lead to inflammation and matting with the adjoining nodes. Asymptomatic intestinal or hepatic TB may spread through their respective lymphatic drainage sites to the mesenteric, hepatic or peripancreatic lymph nodes, resulting in essentially the same phenomenon as elsewhere.

Pathologically, tuberculous lymphadenitis is a chronic specific granulomatous inflammation with caseation necrosis. The characteristic morphological element is the tuberculous granuloma (caseating tubercle), which consists of giant multinucleated cells (Langhans cells), surrounded by epithelioid cells aggregates, T-cell lymphocytes and few fibroblasts. Granulomatous tubercles evolve to central caseous necrosis and tend to become confluent, replacing the lymphoid tissue.

Jones and Campbell[13] classified peripheral tuberculous lymph nodes into following five stages:
- Stage 1: Enlarged, firm, mobile, and discrete nodes showing nonspecific reactive hyperplasia
- Stage 2: Large rubbery nodes fixed to surrounding tissue owing to periadenitis
- Stage 3: Central softening due to abscess formation
- Stage 4: Collar-stud abscess formation
- Stage 5: Sinus tract formation.

DIFFERENTIAL DIAGNOSIS

Tuberculous lymphadenopathy should be differentiated from lymphadenitis due to other causes, the most common of which is reactive hyperplasia, followed by disease states, like lymphoma, sarcoidosis, metastases, and less frequently generalized lymphadenopathy of HIV,[14] lymphadenitis caused by atypical mycobacteria other than TB and fungi. In general, multiplicity, matting, and caseation favor TB while rubbery consistency of lymph nodes favors lymphoma. Metastatic lymph nodes are usually hard and fixed to the underlying structures or the overlying skin.

DIAGNOSIS OF TUBERCULOUS LYMPHADENITIS

Tuberculin skin test is positive in majority of patients of tuberculous lymphadenitis, the probability of false-negative test being less than 10%.[15,16] A chest radiograph should be obtained in all such patients. It not only excludes any coexisting intrathoracic disease but the presence of an active or healed pulmonary lesion acts as a supportive evidence for tuberculous lymphadenitis in cases where the diagnosis remains in doubt, e.g., biopsy suggesting granulomatous pathology but a negative culture. Polymerase chain reaction amplification of *M. tuberculosis* deoxyribonucleic acid is an accurate method for diagnosis of TB and has proven to be sensitive and specific for the rapid detection of the disease especially in various fluid samples.[17]

IMAGING

Imaging currently forms the primary investigative noninvasive modality in the diagnostic algorithm of TB. The affected lymph nodes can be imaged by plain radiographs, ultrasound (US), computed tomography (CT), and magnetic resonance imaging (MRI), with most of the recent emphasis being on CT imaging. In early cases, however, US, CT, and MRI allow just the detection of enlarged lymph nodes and may not be successful in identifying the etiology.[18,19] Additional parameters apart from size are shape, internal architecture, extranodal extension, and vascularity that may improve diagnostic rate.[20] US-guided fine-needle aspiration cytology of lymph nodes has been shown to be an accurate method of diagnosis but is an invasive and operator-dependent examination.[21,22]

Plain Radiography

Chest radiograph forms the initial screening imaging modality for suspected nodal or extranodal TB. The various findings that may be seen are mediastinal, hilar or axillary lymphadenopathy. Lymphadenopathy is typically unilateral and right sided, involving the hilum and right paratracheal region although it is bilateral in about one-third of cases. Although lymphadenopathy is usually associated with other manifestations of TB, it can be the sole radiographic abnormality especially in infants. There may be combination of calcified hilar nodes along with a parenchymal Ghon focus (Ranke complex) which is suggestive of previous TB. Chest radiography may be useful in longitudinal follow-up of patients undergoing antitubercular treatment to look for resolution or worsening of the disease.

Plain radiography is not very useful in assessing lymph node TB other than in the chest. Elsewhere, it may be helpful in associated osseous involvement in bone TB.

Ultrasound

Ultrasound is a widely available, noninvasive, easy-to-perform, and radiation free imaging modality for evaluation of lymph nodes. The various parameters that can be assessed by an US examination are number, size, and location of the enlarged lymph nodes. The pattern of central and peripheral echogenicity, presence of calcification, and conglomeration are other variables which can assist in the diagnosis of TB (Fig. 1). Adding a duplex mode with color Doppler imaging aids in the assessment of vascularity of the lymph nodes further assisting in arriving at a diagnosis. In a few US studies, it has been shown that tuberculous nodes are rounded, hypoechoic with no visible hilum, have blurred margins or show matting and perinodal edema.[23] Cystic necrosis and internal echoes are often encountered. The Doppler appearance may sometimes mimic malignancy due to vessel

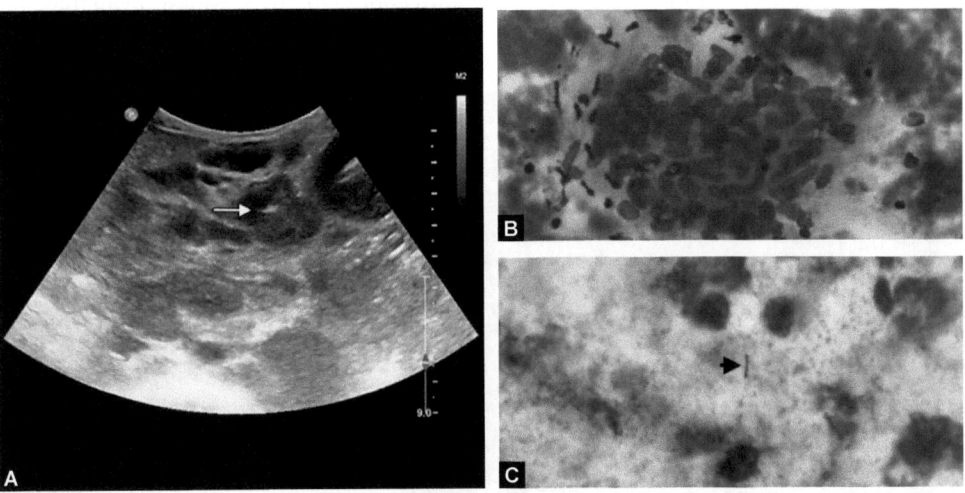

FIG. 1: Axial transabdominal ultrasound **A,** shows presence of multiple large mesenteric and retroperitoneal lymph nodes showing hypoechoic centres suggestive of necrosis. Needle-in-situ noted in one of the mesenteric lymph node (arrow). **B,** cytopathology smear shows an epitheloid cell granuloma (May Grünwald-Giemsa x 40X); and **B,** presence of an acid-fast bacillus (Ziehl–Neelsen stain x 100X) *(For color version, see Plate 10)*
Courtesy: Images B and C: Dr Nalini Gupta, Professor, Department of Cytology, PGIMER, Chandigarh, India.

dislocation by necrosis.[24] Thick capsule and microcalcifications may also be observed.[25]

Real-time elastography is an advanced sonographic technique based on the differential stiffness of organs. This modality has shown reasonable results in differentiating tumors of the breast, thyroid, prostate, pancreas, and lymph nodes.[26] Most research in lymph node evaluation has focused on the differentiation of benign and malignant superficial lymph nodes.[27] The concept of stiffness evolved over time when it was realized on clinical palpation that metastatic lymph nodes are hard and lymph nodes of TB are of tough texture.[28] The hardness was highest for metastasis followed by lymphoma and TB in that order according to a study by Fu et al.[29]

Contrast-enhanced US (CEUS) is another improvisation of US which involves the application of US contrast agents to standard sonography. It does not entail the risk of radiation and nephrotoxicity as is seen with contrast-enhanced CT (CECT), especially in seriously ill and chronic kidney disease patients who have to undergo repeated examinations. The contrast agents used are microbubbles stabilized by a shell having a high degree of echogenicity. The size of microbubble particle is smaller than that of a red blood cell. Contrast-enhanced US provides information on both macro- and microvasculature and perfusion patterns of a lesion (Fig. 2). It exploits the differences in blood flow characteristics between normal and pathological tissue.[30] As of now, CEUS has been described for the evaluation of liver lesions[30] as well as few nonliver lesions, especially involving superficially located lymph nodes.[31] Yang et al.[32] studied the enhancement pattern of tubercular lymphadenitis in affected patients. They identified rim enhancement in 46.8% patients, inhomogeneous enhancement in 33.9% patients, and nonenhancement in 19.3% cases. Rim enhancement was more common in nodes less than or equal to 20 mm in diameter while inhomogeneous enhancement was more common in the lymph nodes more than 20 mm in diameter. Contrast-enhanced US can also be used to direct the needle in a tubercular lymph node to a non-necrotic area which is likely to yield the best results in a suspected tubercular lymph node.[33] Though it is a promising tool, it has yet to find a place in the diagnostic algorithm of TB.

Computed Tomography

Computed tomography is currently the workhorse for diagnosing pathologies of the chest and abdomen. It is widely available, quick to perform, and has high resolution. The

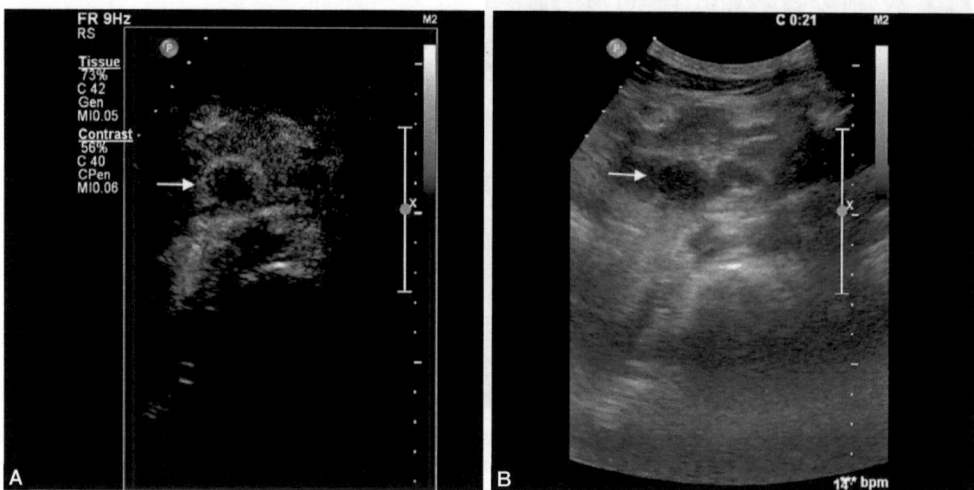

FIG. 2: Contrast enhanced **A**, and corresponding gray scale **B**, ultrasound images demonstrate presence of central necrosis and peripheral enhancement (arrow) in a patient of tubercular lymphadenitis at the porta hepatis *(For color version, see Plate 10)*

main disadvantages are radiation exposure and administration of iodine-based contrast medium which may have an adverse effect on the patient's renal parameters especially in renal failure and diabetics. Computed tomography is more sensitive than chest radiography for assessing lymphadenopathy. The features of tubercular lymphadenitis that are characteristically seen on CECT are lymph node enlargement, loss of normal reniform shape, homogenous or peripheral enhancement, central necrosis, conglomeration (Fig. 3), dermal and subcutaneous manifestations of inflammation in the form of thickening of the overlying skin, engorgement of the lymphatics, and thickening of the adjacent muscles. Lymph nodes greater than 2 cm in diameter generally develop low attenuation centers secondary to necrosis because of the outgrowth of the vascular supply towards the center of the lesion.[34]

Apart from the classical peripheral enhancement typical of TB, the other patterns of enhancement are nonhomogenous enhancement, homogenous enhancement, and homogenous nonenhancement. Moreover, the same nodal group may show different patterns of contrast enhancement, possibly related to the different stages of the pathological process. The presence of calcification (peripheral or sometimes amorphous or nodular) favors a tubercular etiology over other diagnoses, especially in endemic areas. Thus, the suggestive features of TB on CECT are the presence of conglomerate nodal mass with central necrosis, thick irregular rim of contrast enhancement, variable degree of enhancement in smaller nodes, and presence of calcification. Malignant and other inflammatory lymph nodes, on the other hand, generally demonstrate homogeneous enhancement.

Magnetic Resonance Imaging

Magnetic resonance imaging gives a much better soft tissue contrast than CT scan; however, it is highly sensitive to motion due to its long sequence durations. The other advantage includes radiation free nature and disadvantages include high cost and requirement of expertise. The sequences often employed include T1, T2, and gadolinium-enhanced T1 along with diffusion-weighted imaging (DWI) which analyzes intercellular water motion.[35] Tubercular lymph nodes have increased central T2 hyperintensity which corresponds to T1 hypointensity indicative of central necrosis and presence of peripheral enhancement (Fig. 4). Lymph nodes appearing hypointense on T2-weighted images either show

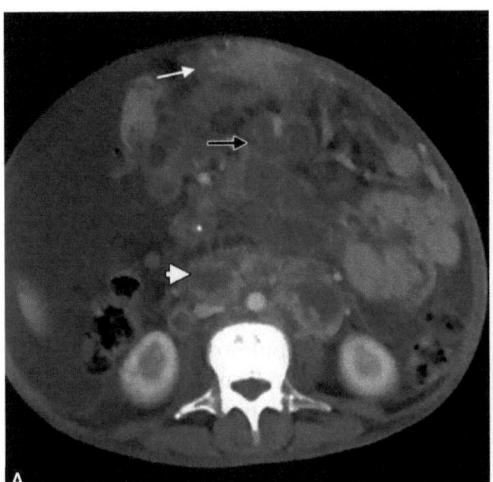 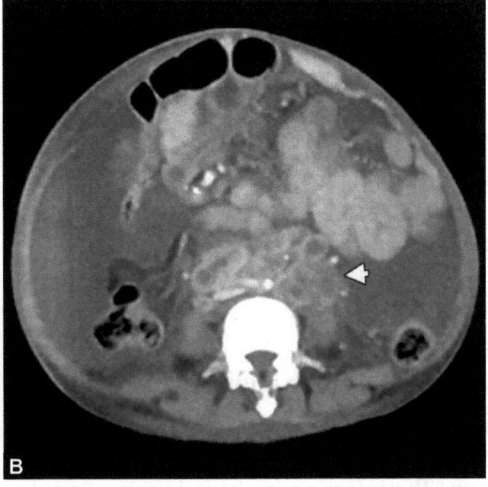

FIG. 3: Axial contrast enhanced computed tomography sections **A,** and **B,** show presence of enlarged conglomerate necrotic retroperitoneal (arrowhead) and mesenteric (black arrow) lymph nodes. Note the typical peripheral enhancement with hypoenhancing centres. Also noted is massive ascites and omental thickening (straight white arrow).

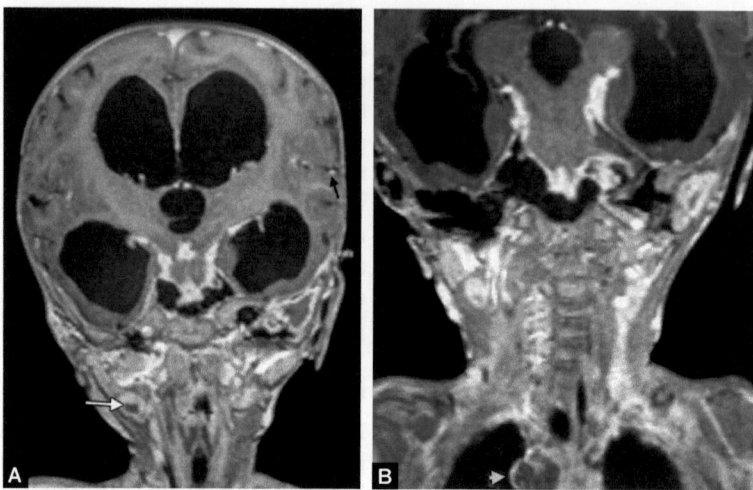

FIG. 4: Coronal gadolinium enhanced T1 weighted images show classical basal meningitis with associated hydrocephalus in a patient of disseminated tuberculosis. Also noted are presence of typical peripherally enhancing necrotic lymph nodes in the neck (arrow) and mediastinum (arrowhead).

solid caseation or calcification and the latter can be confirmed with susceptibility-weighted imaging. Diffusion-weighted imaging may show diffusion restriction which may be secondary to the presence of inflammatory cells in the pus that impede the motion of water molecules. Few studies have shown that low apparent diffusion coefficient (ADC) values favor malignancy while a higher ADC value favor an infective etiology of lymph node enlargement.[36] However, this is not well applicable to tubercular lymph nodes which may behave more like malignancy on DWI images. Magnetic resonance imaging is particularly helpful in TB of the brain and spine which may clinch the diagnosis when associated lymph nodes are difficult to be classified into one pathology or the other.

REGION SPECIFIC TUBERCULAR LYMPHADENOPATHY

Peripheral Tubercular Lymphadenopathy

The peripheral lymph nodes comprise the cervical, axillary, inguinal, popliteal, and cubital group. The infection in these is secondary to involvement of the structures drained by the respective lymph node group, e.g., inguinal nodes in lower limb involvement, cervical nodes in tonsillar/head and neck involvement. Typical inflammatory enhancement occurs to variable degree ranging from diffuse homogenous pattern to classical peripheral pattern. Conglomeration and adjoining inflammation may ensue leading to development of discharging sinuses in untreated patients. Imaging features, as on other sites, are typical of TB if there is presence of coalescence, peripheral enhancement, and central necrosis.

Central Tubercular Lymphadenopathy

Thoracic Tuberculosis

Initially tubercular bacilli lodge in the lung parenchyma, commonly in the apical segment. There may be subsequent involvement of the draining lymphatics and then of the lymph node group. The lymph nodes involved are the mediastinal group (pretracheal, paratracheal, tracheobronchial, precarinal, subcarinal, and aortopulmonary groups) and the hilar group. Apart from enlargement, there may be central cavitation (necrosis), peripheral enhancement along with foci of calcification. Sometimes, the lymph nodes may rupture into the bronchi leading to endobronchial spread of the disease and scattering of the bacilli to other pulmonary sites. Uncommon manifestations observed in patients with mediastinal lymph node involvement include dysphagia,[37,38] esophagomediastinal fistula,[39,40] and tracheoesophageal fistula.[41] Rarely there may be erosion of the adjoining vasculature leading to varying severity of hemoptysis. Chronic involvement may lead to cicatrization and distortion of the adjoining anatomy. Lymphadenopathy secondary to lymphomatous involvement is usually homogeneous and encases the major vessels (Fig. 5). The other common etiology is sarcoidosis wherein the nodes are seen in paratracheal, subcarinal, and hilar locations. Lung parenchymal involvement typically clinches the diagnosis (Fig. 6).

Abdominal Tuberculosis

Abdominal TB is a great mimicker as it may involve a variety of organs and tissues, e.g., gastrointestinal tract, peritoneum, lymph nodes, and solid viscera, and may mimic diseases like inflammatory bowel disease, colonic malignancy and other gastrointestinal infections. Lymphadenopathy is the most common manifestation of abdominal TB.[42] The presenting symptoms are abdominal pain or signs of compression of adjoining structures like intestinal obstruction and obstructive jaundice. Tuberculous abdominal lymphadenopathy can develop via oral, hematogenous, and loco-

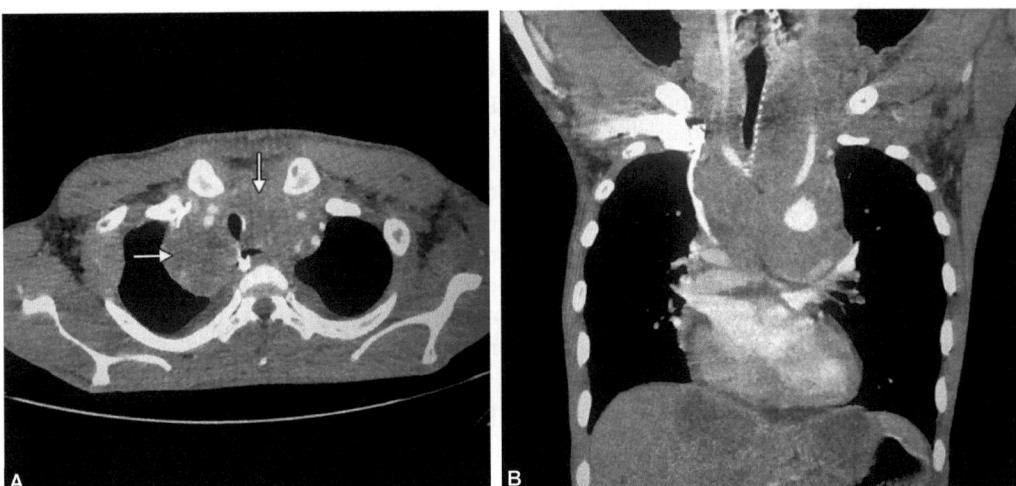

FIG. 5: Lymphoma: **A,** Axial CECT of chest showing a large homogeneous anterior and middle mediastinal mass (arrows) encasing blood vessels and causing tracheal compression and deviation to right; **B,** Coronal reformat.

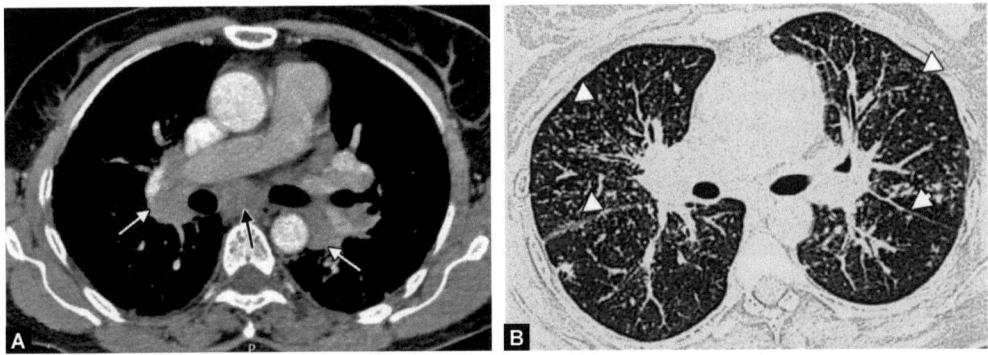

FIG. 6: Sarcoidosis: Mediastinal **A,** and lung **B,** window settings of a contrast enhanced CT scan showing relatively homogeneous mediastinal (subcarinal) and hilar lymph nodes (arrows) along with interstitial lung disease (arrowheads).

regional routes.[43] From the oral route, the bacilli lodge in the lymphoid tissue of the intestinal submucosal layer to form epithelioid tubercles. These tubercles drain into the peripancreatic and superior mesenteric lymph nodes through lymphatics of the ileocecum, jejunum, ileum, and the right side of the colon and subsequently into the cisterna chyli.[44,45] The left side of the colon is rarely involved and so does its drainage into the inferior mesenteric lymph nodes and lower para-aortic lymph nodes. In a study by Zhang et al.,[46] the predominant anatomic distribution of TB lymphadenitis was in the lesser omentum (60.0%), the mesentery (65.5%), the anterior pararenal space (63.6%), and the upper paraaortic regions (60.0%). This finding was consistent with the known lymphatic drainage routes.

Tubercular lymphadenitis has been described to evolve through different stages with different enhancement patterns at variable junctures.[47] In early stage, the lymphoid tissues proliferate and form non-necrotic tubercles and caseating granulomas. In this stage, CT shows homogenous enhancement of the affected lymph nodes. In the next stage, the lymph node undergoes central caseation necrosis with an intact peripheral capsule. This gives typical peripheral enhancement of the peripheral inflammatory lymphatic tissues with nonenhancing central necrotic core. Subsequently, capsular destruction takes place resulting in periadenitis and fusion of adjacent lymph nodes. At this stage, there is multilocular enhancement of the coalesced lymph nodes. The last stage is the healing stage wherein the lymph nodes undergo fibrosis and calcification, the latter is easily picked up on CT scan.[43,45] The typical pattern of peripheral enhancement and central nonenhancing necrosis is seen in up to 80% of cases.[48,49]

Other differentials of necrotic lymph nodes that need to be excluded are Whipple disease[50] and the cavitating mesenteric lymph node syndrome of celiac disease.[44,51] Lymph nodes affected in Whipple disease have high fat content which is responsible for the low CT attenuation value [10–20 Hounsfield unit (HU)]. This lymphadenopathy responds to antibiotic therapy. The lymphadenopathy associated with the cavitating mesenteric lymph node syndrome of celiac disease also has a low CT attenuation value. However, these lymph nodes are truly cavitating nodes.

Lymphoma is also a close differential in many such patients. Tuberculosis predominantly involves lesser omental, mesenteric and upper paraaortic lymph nodes, whereas lower para-aortic lymph nodes are involved more often in lymphoma. Tuberculous lymphadenopathy commonly shows peripheral rim enhancement, often with a multilocular appearance, whereas lymphomatous adenopathy characteristically shows homogenous attenuation.

CONCLUSION

Imaging in lymph node TB has evolved from plain radiography to MRI, yet the mainstay of identification of tuberculous etiology still remains the typical peripheral enhancement, central necrosis and conglomeration. Many times, antitubercular treatment is started on the basis of these typical findings in patients in endemic zones. However tissue diagnosis is still essential in atypical cases and to ascertain drug resistance.

REFERENCES

1. Sharma SK, Mohan A. Extrapulmonary tuberculosis. Indian J Med Res. 2004;120(4):316-53.
2. Brizi MG, Celi G, Scaldazza AV, et al. Diagnostic imaging of abdominal tuberculosis: gastrointestinal tract, peritoneum, lymph nodes. Rays. 1998;23(1):115-25.
3. Thompson MM, Underwood MJ, Sayers RD, et al. Peripheral tuberculous lymphadenopathy: a review of 67 cases. Br J Surg. 1992;79(8):763-4.
4. Kanlikama M, Mumbuç S, Bayazit Y, et al. Management strategy of mycobacterial cervical lymphadenitis. J Laryngol Otol. 2000;114(4):274-8.
5. Penfold CN, Revington PJ. A review of 23 patients with tuberculosis of the head and neck. Br J Oral Maxillofac Surg. 1996;34(6):508-10.
6. Choremis CB, Padiatellis C, Zoumboulakis D, et al. Transitory exacerbation of fever and roentgenographic findings during treatment of tuberculosis in children. Am Rev Tuberc. 1955;72(4):527-36.
7. Cheng VC, Ho PL, Lee RA, et al. Clinical spectrum of paradoxical deterioration during antituberculosis therapy in non-HIV-infected patients. Eur J Clin Microbiol Infect Dis. 2002;21(11):803-9.
8. Cheng VC, Yam WC, Woo PC, et al. Risk factors for development of paradoxical response during anti-

tuberculosis therapy in HIV-negative patients. Eur J Clin Microbiol Infect Dis. 2003;22(10):597-602.
9. Breen RA, Smith CJ, Bettinson H, et al. Paradoxical reactions during tuberculosis treatment in patients with and without HIV co-infection. Thorax. 2004;59(8):704-7.
10. Singh A, Rahman H, Kumar V, et al. An unusual case of paradoxical enlargement of lymph nodes during treatment of tuberculous lymphadenitis in immunocompetent patient and literature review. Am J Case Rep. 2013;14:201-4.
11. Dheda K, Barry CE, Maartens G. Tuberculosis. Lancet. 2016;387(10024):1211-26.
12. Fogel N. Tuberculosis: a disease without boundaries. Tuberculosis (Edinb). 2015;95(5):527-31.
13. Jones PG, Campbell PE. Tuberculous lymphadenitis in childhood: the significance of anonymous mycobacteria. Br J Surg. 1962;50(221):302-14.
14. Bem C. Human immunodeficiency virus-positive tuberculous lymphadenitis in Central Africa: clinical presentation of 157 cases. Int J Tuberc Lung Dis. 1997;1(3):215-9.
15. Artenstein AW, Kim JH, Williams WJ, et al. Isolated peripheral tuberculous lymphadenitis in adults: current clinical and diagnostic issues. Clin Infect Dis. 1995;20(4):876-82.
16. Cantrell RW, Jensen JH, Reid D. Diagnosis and management of tuberculous cervical adenitis. Arch Otolaryngol. 1975;101(1):53-7.
17. Schluger NW, Kinney D, Harkin TJ, et al. Clinical utility of the polymerase chain reaction in the diagnosis of infections due to Mycobacterium tuberculosis. Chest. 1994;105(4):1116-21.
18. Curtin HD, Ishwaran H, Mancuso AA, et al. Comparison of CT and MR imaging in staging of neck metastases. Radiology. 1998;207(1):123-30.
19. Esen G. Ultrasound of superficial lymph nodes. Eur J Radiol. 2006;58(3):345-59.
20. van den Brekel MW, Castelijns JA, Snow GB. The size of lymph nodes in the neck on sonograms as a radiologic criterion for metastasis: how reliable is it? AJNR Am J Neuroradiol. 1998;19(4):695-700.
21. van den Brekel MW, Castelijns JA, Stel HV, et al. Occult metastatic neck disease: detection with US and US-guided fine-needle aspiration cytology. Radiology. 1991;180(2):457-61.
22. van den Brekel MW, Castelijns JA, Stel HV, et al. Modern imaging techniques and ultrasound-guided aspiration cytology for the assessment of neck node metastases: a prospective comparative study. Eur Arch Otorhinolaryngol. 1993;250(1):11-7.
23. Khanna R, Sharma AD, Khanna S, et al. Usefulness of ultrasonography for the evaluation of cervical lymphadenopathy. World J Surg Oncol. 2011;9:29.
24. Ahuja AT, Ying M. Sonographic evaluation of cervical lymph nodes. Am J Roentgenol. 2005;184(5):1691-9.
25. Butnaru A, Dudea SM, Şerban A, et al. Ultrasound-histopathological correlations in tuberculous adenitis. Rev Rom Ultrason. 2003;5:191-7.
26. Dewall RJ. Ultrasound elastography: principles, techniques, and clinical applications. Crit Rev Biomed Eng. 2013;41(1):1-19.
27. Ying L, Hou Y, Zheng HM, et al. Real-time elastography for the differentiation of benign and malignant superficial lymph nodes: a meta-analysis. Eur J Radiol. 2012;81(10):2576-84.
28. Bhatia KS, Cho CC, Yuen YH, et al. Real-time qualitative ultrasound elastography of cervical lymph nodes in routine clinical practice: interobserver agreement and correlation with malignancy. Ultrasound Med Biol. 2010;36(12):1990-7.
29. Fu Y, Shi YF, Yan K, et al. Clinical value of real time elastography in patients with unexplained cervical lymphadenopathy: quantitative evaluation. Asian Pac J Cancer Prev. 2014;15(13):5487-92.
30. Claudon M, Dietrich CF, Choi BI, et al. Guidelines and good clinical practice recommendations for Contrast Enhanced Ultrasound (CEUS) in the liver - update 2012: A WFUMB-EFSUMB initiative in cooperation with representatives of AFSUMB, AIUM, ASUM, FLAUS and ICUS. Ultrasound Med Biol. 2013;39(2):187-210.
31. Piscaglia F, Nolsøe C, Dietrich CF, et al. The EFSUMB Guidelines and Recommendations on the Clinical Practice of Contrast Enhanced Ultrasound (CEUS): update 2011 on non-hepatic applications. Ultraschall Med. 2012;33(1):33-59.
32. Yang G, Zhang W, Li J, et al. The value of contrast-enhanced ultrasound in the diagnosis of tuberculous mesenteric lymphadenitis. Chinese J Med Ultrasound. 2015;7:531-5.
33. Zhang W, Yang G, Pei Y, et al. Application of contrast-enhanced ultrasound in needle biopsy of tuberculous cervical lymph node. Zhonghua Er Bi Yan Hou Tou Jing Wai Ke Za Zhi. 2014;49(3):240-2.
34. Curvo-Semedo L, Teixeira L, Caseiro-Alves F. Tuberculosis of the chest. Eur J Radiol. 2005;55(2):158-72.
35. Shao H, Yang ZG, Xu GH, et al. Tuberculosis in the abdominal lymph nodes: evaluation with contrast-enhanced magnetic resonance imaging. Int J Tuberc Lung Dis. 2013;17(1):90-5.
36. Perrone A, Guerrisi P, Izzo L, et al. Diffusion-weighted MRI in cervical lymph nodes: differentiation between benign and malignant lesions. Eur J Radiol. 2011;77(2):281-6.
37. Singh B, Moodley M, Goga AD, et al. Dysphagia secondary to tuberculous lymphadenitis. S Afr J Surg. 1996;34(4):197-9.
38. Gupta SP, Arora A, Bhargava DK. An unusual presentation of oesophageal tuberculosis. Tuber Lung Dis. 1992;73(3):174-6.
39. Ohtake M, Saito H, Okuno M, et al. Esophagomediastinal fistula as a complication of tuberculous mediastinal lymphadenitis. Intern Med. 1996;35(12):984-6.
40. Im JG, Kim JH, Han MC, et al. Computed tomography of esophagomediastinal fistula in tuberculous mediastinal lymphadenitis. J Comput Assist Tomogr. 1990;14(1):89-92.
41. Lee JH, Shin DH, Kang KW, et al. The medical treatment of a tuberculous tracheo-oesophageal fistula. Tuber Lung Dis. 1992;73(3):177-9.
42. Mathieu D, Ladeb MF, Guigui B, et al. Periportal tuberculous adenitis: CT features. Radiology. 1986;161(3):713-5.
43. Pereira JM, Madureira AJ, Vieira A, et al. Abdominal tuberculosis: imaging features. Eur J Radiol. 2005;55(2):173-80.

44. Yang ZG, Min PQ, Sone S, et al. Tuberculosis versus lymphomas in the abdominal lymph nodes: evaluation with contrast-enhanced CT. AJR Am J Roentgenol. 1999;172(3):619-23.
45. Vanhoenacker FM, De Backer AI, Op de BB, et al. Imaging of gastrointestinal and abdominal tuberculosis. Eur Radiol. 2004;14 Suppl 3:E103-15.
46. Zhang G, Yang ZG, Yao Z, et al. Differentiation between tuberculosis and leukemia in abdominal and pelvic lymph nodes: evaluation with contrast-enhanced multidetector computed tomography. Clinics. 2015;70(3):162-8.
47. Pombo F, Rodriguez E, Mato J, et al. Patterns of contrast enhancement of tuberculous lymph nodes demonstrated by computed tomography. Clin Radiol. 1992;46(1):13-7.
48. Zhang M, Li M, Xu GP, et al. Neoplasm-like abdominal nonhematogenous disseminated tuberculous lymphadenopathy: CT evaluation of 12 cases and literature review. World J Gastroenterol. 2011;17(35):4038-43.
49. Kim SY, Kim MJ, Chung JJ, et al. Abdominal tuberculous lymphadenopathy: MR imaging findings. Abdom Imaging. 2000;25(6):627-32.
50. Friedman HD, Hadfield TL, Lamy Y, et al. Whipple's disease presenting as chronic wastage and abdominal lymphadenopathy. Diagn Microbiol Infect Dis. 1995;23(3):111-3.
51. Schmitz F, Herzig KH, Stüber E, et al. On the pathogenesis and clinical course of mesenteric lymph node cavitation and hyposplenism in celiac disease. Int J Colorectal Dis. 2002;17(3):192-8.

12
CHAPTER

Imaging in Abdominal Tuberculosis

Raju Sharma, Madhusudhan KS, Devasenathipathy Kandasamy

INTRODUCTION

Tuberculosis (TB) is one of the leading causes of death worldwide, killing 1.5 million people in 2014 and around 6 million new cases were reported in the same year. India has the largest number of cases constituting 23% of all TB patients in the world followed by Indonesia and China. Abdominal TB (ATB) accounts for a significant percentage of the total disease burden in developing countries with reported incidence of 17% of all patients admitted with TB.[1] There has been a resurgence of ATB even in the developed countries in recent years which is mainly attributed to the increased incidence of acquired immunodeficiency syndrome (AIDS), increased use of immuno-suppressive therapy and rise in prevalence of multidrug-resistant TB.

Abdominal TB can develop from (i) reactivation of a dormant focus in the abdomen, (ii) hematogenous or lymphatic spread from an ongoing active TB, (iii) ingestion of the pathogen, or (iv) by direct extension from adjacent tissues.[2] Most of the patients of intestinal TB present with symptoms like abdominal pain, vomiting, diarrhea, abdominal distension, and perianal fistulae.[3] Systemic symptoms like fever, weight loss, loss of appetite, and malaise may be present. Although TB can involve any part of the gastrointestinal (GI) tract, it has a predilection to involve ileocecal region and ascending colon, which accounts for 50–90% cases.[4,5] The sites of involvement in descending order of frequency are the ileocecal junction, followed by the ileum, cecum, ascending colon, jejunum, rest of the colon, rectum, duodenum, ano perineum, esophagus, and stomach.[6,7]

The diagnosis of ATB is challenging because it can mimic various other diseases such as Crohn's disease, amebic infections, carcinoma, sarcoidosis, lymphoma, metastasis, and fungal infections. Sometimes aspirate or biopsy is necessary to confirm the diagnosis although the yield from the specimen is often poor.[8,9] Imaging plays a very important role in diagnosing, evaluating the extent of spread, disease-related complications, and in assessing response to therapy. Imaging can also help in guiding aspiration or biopsy.

IMAGING MODALITIES

Radiography

The wide availability of cross-sectional modalities has relegated the role of radiographs in the evaluation of ATB to a minor one. However, abdominal radiographs can show features of bowel obstruction in the form of dilated bowel loops with multiple air-fluid levels (Fig. 1). Enteroliths and calcified lymph nodes can be seen sometimes on radiograph, which should point towards the diagnosis of TB. Associated active pulmonary TB can be seen in up to 20% of patients with ATB.[10] Evidence of active or old TB on chest radiograph can be a supporting feature for ATB, however a normal chest radiograph does not rule out ATB.

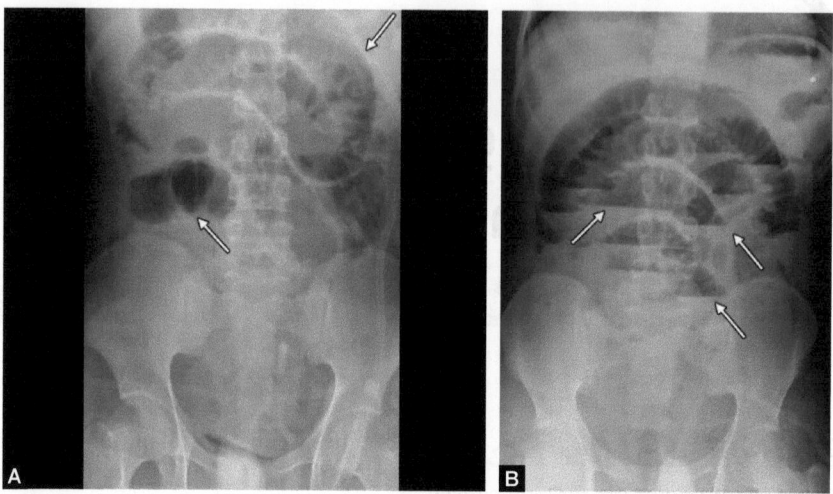

FIG. 1: Small bowel obstruction. **A,** Supine; and **B,** erect plain radiographs of the abdomen of a 30-year-old male with ileal tuberculosis presenting with acute abdomen showing dilated small bowel loops (arrows) with multiple air-fluid levels (arrows in B) suggesting acute small bowel obstruction

Barium Studies

Barium meal follow through (BMFT) is still used in the evaluation of subacute small bowel obstruction and many characteristic findings are described for bowel TB. With the advent of multidetector computed tomography the use of BMFT has decreased. However, BMFT is a good modality to show the mucosal lesions such as ulcerations and hypertrophic changes.[3,11,12] Barium studies may also show abnormally dilated bowel loops, strictures, mucosal nodularity, fistulas, wide separation of loops due to lymphadenopathy, kinking and matted loops due to peritoneal involvement. Barium enema is useful for suspected colonic involvement.[13] Conventional barium enteroclysis, performed after inserting a nasojejunal tube, results in better distension of the bowel and provides double contrast which helps in detection of subtle strictures and in demonstration of early mucosal abnormalities.[14] However, it is becoming obsolete because of the advent of newer techniques such as CT enterography (CTE) and magnetic resonance enterography (MRE). The limitation of barium study is that it does not give information about the extraluminal abnormalities which is often vital to reach a diagnosis.

Ultrasonography

Ultrasound (US) is widely available and inexpensive modality, which is often used as the first-line imaging for patient presenting with abdominal complaints. Ultrasound may be used to demonstrate bowel wall thickening, fistulas, abscess and enlarged mesenteric and retroperitoneal lymph nodes.[3,15] High frequency transducer can better demonstrate bowel wall thickening.[16] Color Doppler ultrasonography (USG) is useful in assessing active inflammatory segments, which show increased vascularity. USG-guided drainage procedures (intra-abdominal collection and psoas abscesses) are increasingly being performed to minimize the risk of injuring vital structures. The major advantage of USG is absence of ionizing radiation especially important in pediatric population. Ultrasound is very sensitive for detection of fluid in the abdomen. Septations and debris within the fluid sometimes can only be demonstrated on US which suggests the exudative nature of the fluid seen in TB.[17,18] Ultrasound can also show the presence of peritoneal thickening, nodularity, and enlarged lymph nodes. Subjective nature of the modality and inability to evaluate all the abdominal structures optimally are its limitations.

Computed Tomography

Computed tomography can show the spectrum of imaging findings of ATB. Intravenous contrast media administration with oral contrast is a must for complete evaluation of abdominal structures. It can show bowel wall as well as extraluminal abnormalities. It is also capable of demonstrating complications such as obstruction, perforation and abscess formation, vascular complications, fistulae, and intussusceptions. Contrast-enhanced CT (CECT) can demonstrate the presence of necrosis or calcification within the lymph node.[19] Ascites, peritoneal thickening and nodularity can also be detected on CECT.[20]

Computed tomography enteroclysis and CTE can evaluate the bowel loops in distended state.[21,22] Computed tomography enteroclysis is invasive as it needs nasojejunal intubation, whereas CTE is a noninvasive technique using water mixed with osmotically active agents such as mannitol. Because of comparable bowel distension and noninvasiveness of the procedure CTE is preferred over CT enteroclysis. Since bowel is distended, wall thickening, mucosal abnormality and subtle strictures are demonstrated much better on CTE than on conventional CECT. Computed tomography enterography allows better anatomical localization of the disease and examination of all bowel loops including the ileal loops.

Magnetic Resonance Imaging

Magnetic resonance imaging (MRI) is not routinely used for the evaluation of ATB but is a problem solving tool in specific clinical situations. Magnetic resonance enterography may be preferred over CTE because of radiation concerns, in children for the evaluation of GI-TB and for follow-up when response to therapy needs to be assessed. Magnetic resonance imaging is also useful and is the imaging modality of choice in anorectal TB and perianal fistula.[23]

ILEOCECAL AND SMALL BOWEL TUBERCULOSIS

Almost 90% cases of GI-TB tend to involve the ileocecal region. Various reasons which are proposed for this preferential involvement are:

- Physiological stasis
- Abundant lymphoid tissue
- Increased rate of absorption
- Closer contact of tubercle bacilli with the mucosa
- Relatively neutral pH environment.[4,5,24]

Ileocecal TB can present in three classic forms:
1. Ulcerative (60%)
2. Hypertrophic (10%)
3. Ulcerohypertrophic (30%) that mimics malignancy.[5,25]

The ulcerative variety occurs in patients with reduced immunity and hypertrophic form is seen in those with a competent immune system.

Barium studies in early stage of the disease may show spasm, mucosal fold edema, and hypermotility of ileocecal valve along with accelerated bowel transit.[5,26,27] In advanced stages, barium studies show stricture at terminal ileum with proximal dilatation, deformed ileocecal valve and contracted and pulled-up cecum (Fig. 2). Ileocecal valve may be fixed, irregular, gaping, and incompetent due to inflammation or fibrosis. Fleischner's sign (inverted umbrella sign), describes narrowed terminal ileum with thickening of the ileocecal valve lips and/or wide gaping of the ileocecal valve (Fig. 2). Stierlin's sign is rapid emptying of barium in cecum due to persistent irritability of mucosa (Fig. 2). String sign is defined as persistent narrow stream of barium in a segment of bowel indicating stenosis (Fig. 2). Goose neck deformity is dilated terminal ileum, which appears hanging from the shrunken, pulled-up cecum. Other signs include conical cecum (contracted and pulled-up cecum) and purse-string stenosis (focal stenosis opposite ileocecal valve with dilated terminal ileum and smooth cecum).

Computed tomography enterography in the early stage of the disease shows circumferential bowel wall thickening of terminal ileum, ileocecal junction, and cecum. Later, the more characteristic appearance of asymmetric thickening of ileocecal valve and medial wall of the cecum appear (Fig. 3). In advanced disease, there is gross bowel wall thickening, proximal bowel dilatation, large regional nodes, mesenteric thickening and adherent bowel loops forming a soft-tissue mass in the right iliac fossa. Active inflammation is seen

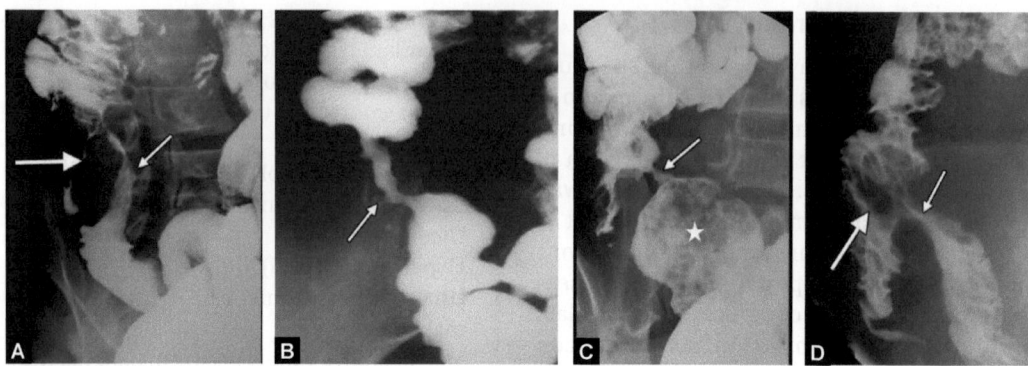

FIG. 2: Ileocecal tuberculosis on barium studies. **A,** Barium meal follow through (BMFT) image shows narrowing and mild mucosal irregularity (thin arrow) in the terminal ileum (string sign) with associated contracted cecum (thick arrow); **B,** BMFT image of another patient shows narrowing of terminal ileum which is emptying directly into ascending colon (thin arrow) with nonvisualization of cecum (Stierlin sign); **C,** BMFT image in a different patient shows fibrotic stricture in the terminal ileum (thin arrow) with proximal dilatation (star) and contracted cecum; and **D,** BMFT image of another patient shows mild gaping (thin arrow) and filling defect (thick arrow) in the region of ileocecal valve (Fleischner's sign) due to edema of the valve

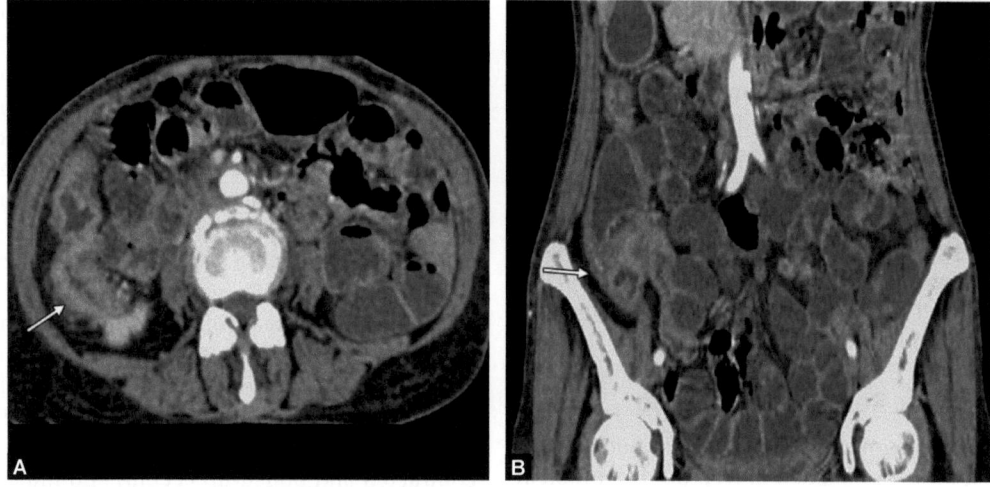

FIG. 3: Ileocecal tuberculosis. **A,** Axial; and **B,** coronal computed tomography enterography images showing wall thickening of terminal ileum, ileocecal junction, medial wall of cecum and ascending colon with surrounding fat stranding (arrow)

as abnormal mucosal enhancement with stratification of the bowel wall (Figs 4 and 5). Bowel obstruction is seen in 12–60% of patients with intestinal TB and occurs due to strictures or peritoneal adhesions.[28] Clumping of bowel loops may be seen with "cocoon" formation. Bowel perforation (in about 6% cases) occurs due to deep ulcers proximal to strictures and is seen as pneumoperitoneum, collections with air foci or with localized extraluminal air, in cases of sealed perforation.[29] Enteroenteric fistulae are uncommon in TB and may be seen as tethering of small bowel loops to a single point. Because of better contrast resolution, MRE can improve the detection of bowel abnormalities. Diffusion-weighted sequence can be used as an additional paradigm in which the involved areas of bowel and lymph nodes may show diffusion restriction (Fig. 6).

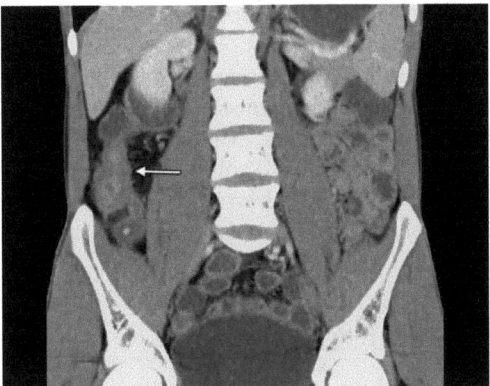

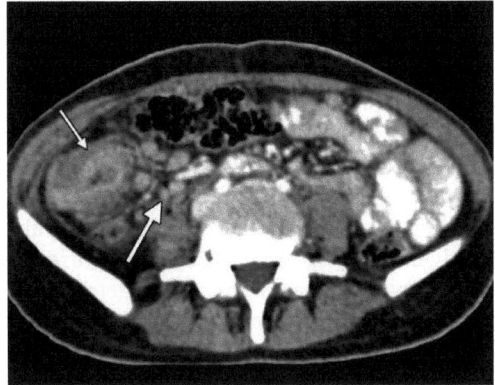

FIG. 4: Active inflammation in ileocecal tuberculosis: Coronal computed tomography enterography image shows abnormal mucosal enhancement with wall thickening involving terminal ileum, ileocecal junction, cecum and ascending colon with mural stratification (arrow)

FIG. 5: Ileocecal tuberculosis: Axial contrast-enhanced computed tomography image showing circumferential wall thickening involving the cecum (thin arrow) with surrounding fat stranding and enlarged lymph nodes (thick arrow). The earlier features are suggestive of tuberculosis

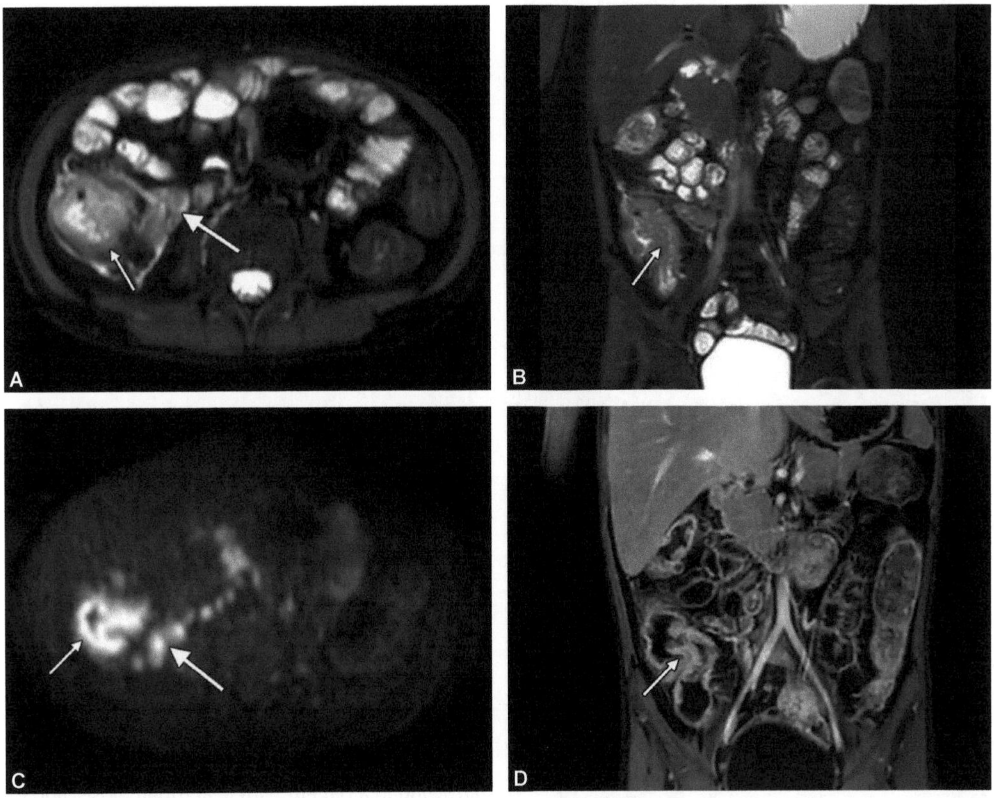

FIG. 6: Ileocecal tuberculosis. **A,** T2-weighted fat suppressed magnetic resonance enterography image in axial and **B,** coronal plane showing wall thickening involving the terminal ileum, ileocecal valve and cecum (thin arrow) with multiple enlarged lymph nodes in right iliac fossa mesentery (thick arrow); **C,** high B value image of diffusion-weighted sequence showing significant diffusion restriction in the involved bowel loops and the lymph nodes; and **D,** the postcontrast T1-weighted fat suppressed image in coronal plane showing thickening and diffuse enhancement of ileocecal junction

Multiple sites of involvement may also be seen in small bowel TB but this is more common in Crohn's disease. Focal, short segment (usually <3 cm) involvement is a much more common pattern of small bowel TB than diffuse, long segment abnormality (Figs 7 and 8). If single, the most common site of involvement is the terminal ileum with contiguous ileocecal valve involvement (Fig. 9). Fibrotic strictures of small bowel in TB are seen as symmetric bowel wall thickening (up to 1 cm) without mural stratification (Figs 10 and 11).

Associated mesenteric, periportal and retroperitoneal lymphadenopathy is seen in 90% cases.[4] Lower para-aortic lymph node involvement in TB is rare. Ascites is another common associated abnormality. Imaging plays an important role in response assessment after antituberculous therapy (ATT) (Fig. 12).

There is great degree of overlap between the clinical presentations, radiological features, operative findings, and even histology of TB and Crohn's disease. The Table 1 sums up some of the salient features which can categorize the abnormality into either of the category.

COLONIC AND ANORECTAL TUBERCULOSIS

The second most common site of involvement of GI-TB is colon, accounting for 9% of all cases of abdominal TB.[30] The right-sided colon is more commonly involved. Ascending colon is the next most commonly affected site. Involvement

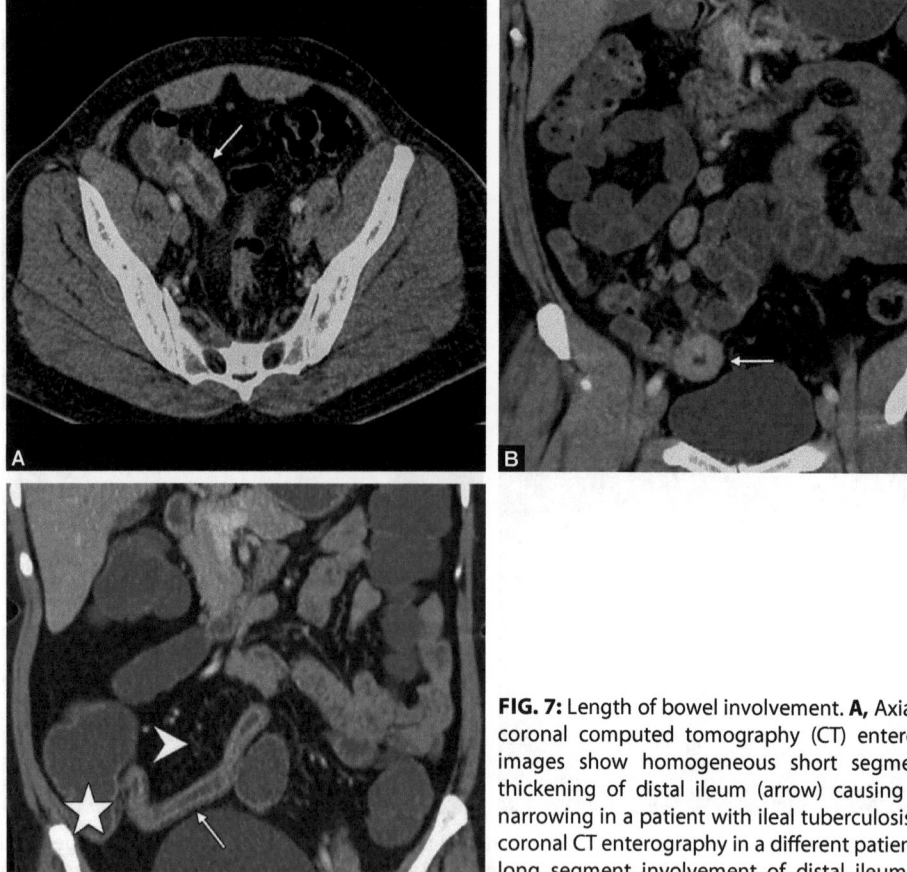

FIG. 7: Length of bowel involvement. **A,** Axial and **B,** coronal computed tomography (CT) enterography images show homogeneous short segment wall thickening of distal ileum (arrow) causing luminal narrowing in a patient with ileal tuberculosis; and **C,** coronal CT enterography in a different patient shows long segment involvement of distal ileum (arrow) with mural stratification and comb sign (arrow head) suggestive of Crohn's disease. The cecum (star) is normal

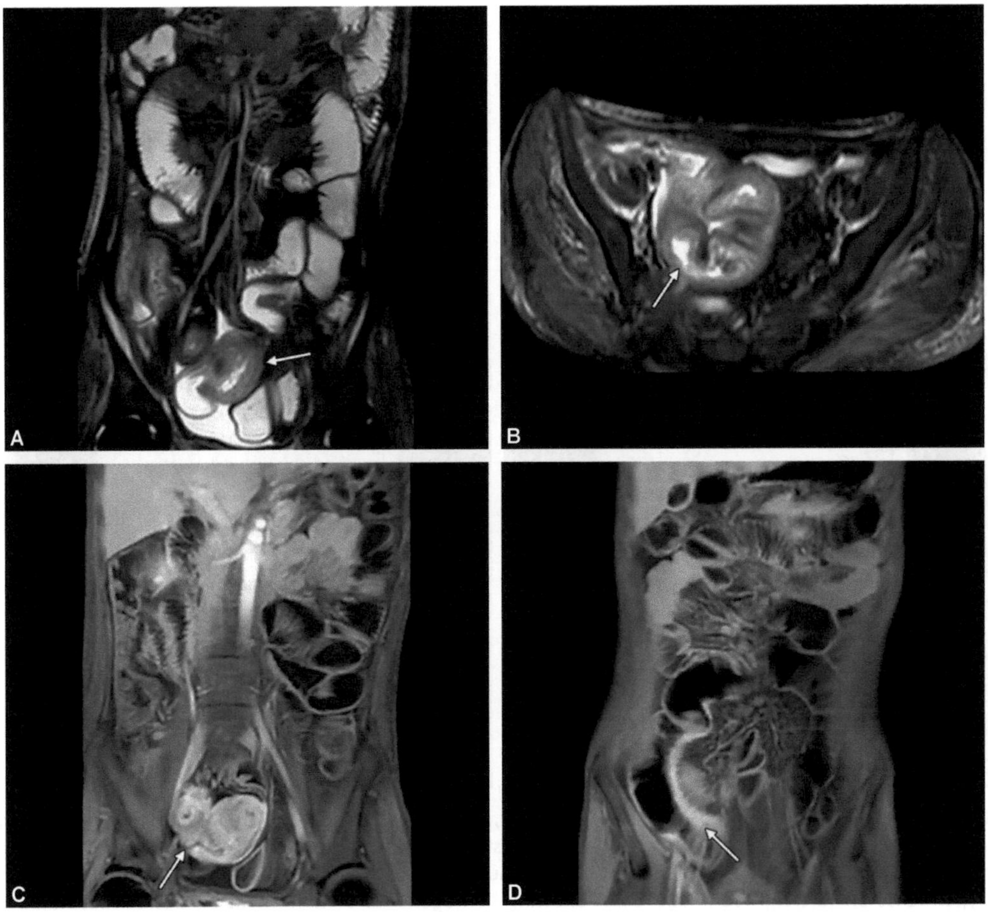

Imaging in Abdominal Tuberculosis

FIG. 8: Active Crohn's disease (CD). **A,** coronal magnetic resonance enterography and **B,** axial T2-weighted images showing segmental wall thickening of a pelvic ileal loop (arrow) which is showing T2 hyperintensity; and **C and D,** coronal postcontrast images show stratified mural enhancement, asymmetrical wall thickening involving the mesenteric border of terminal ileum with intense enhancement (arrow). These findings are typical for active inflammatory stage of CD

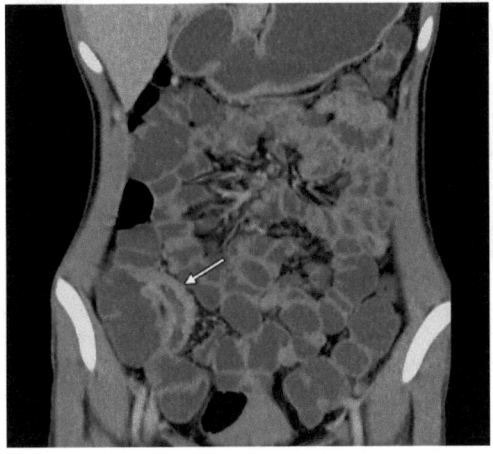

FIG. 9: Crohn's disease: Coronal computed tomography enterography image shows abnormal mucosal enhancement with wall thickening involving the terminal ileum (arrow) extending till the ileocecal junction. The cecum (C) is normal

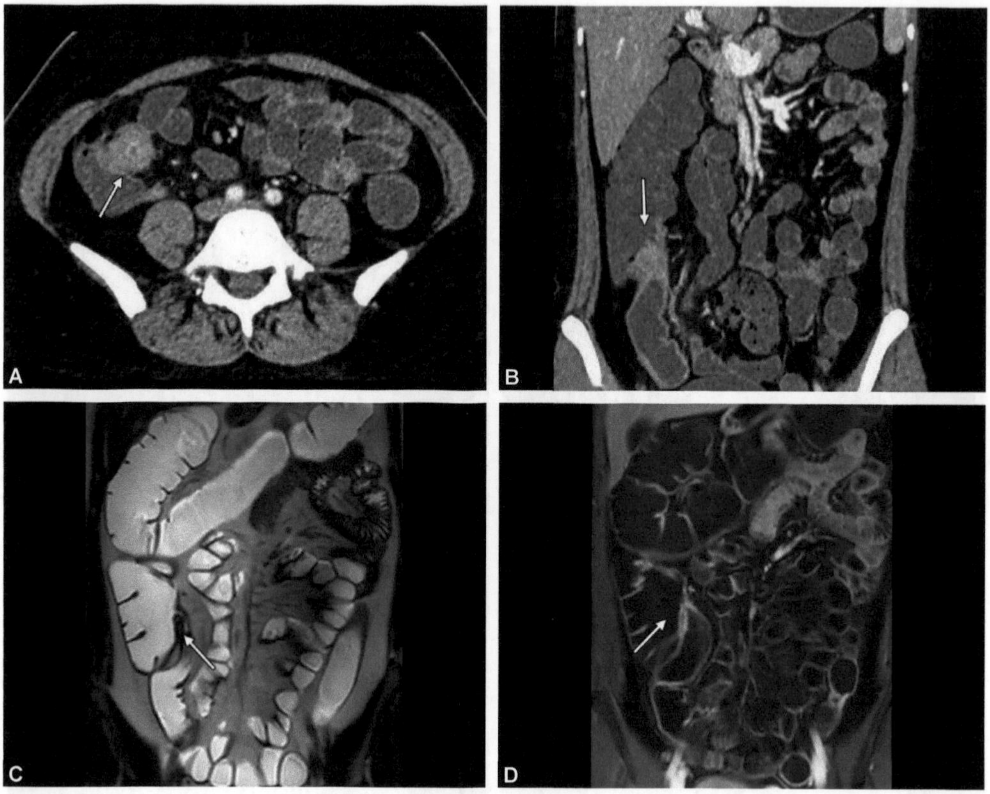

Imaging in Tuberculosis: Clinicopathological Correlation

FIG. 10: Fibrotic stricture in tuberculosis. **A and B,** Computed tomography enterography images; and **C and D,** magnetic resonance enterography images showing circumferential wall thickening involving the terminal ileum and ileocecal junction (thin arrow) causing mild proximal obstruction. The wall thickening is hypointense on T2-weighted image C and showing homogeneous enhancement on postcontrast image D suggestive of fibrosis

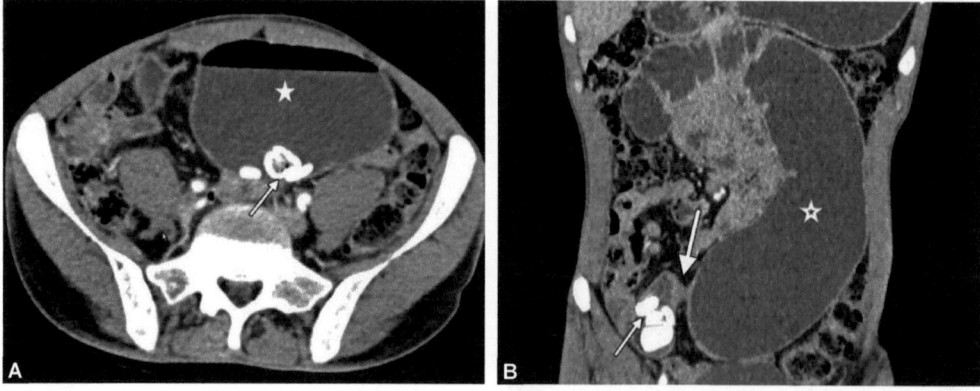

FIG. 11: Small bowel obstruction with enteroliths. **A,** Axial contrast-enhanced computed tomography image; and **B,** coronal multiplanar reconstruction show a short segment ileal stricture (tick arrow). There is marked proximal dilatation of small bowel with air-fluid level (star) suggestive of small bowel obstruction. Also noted is presence of multiple enteroliths (thin arrow)

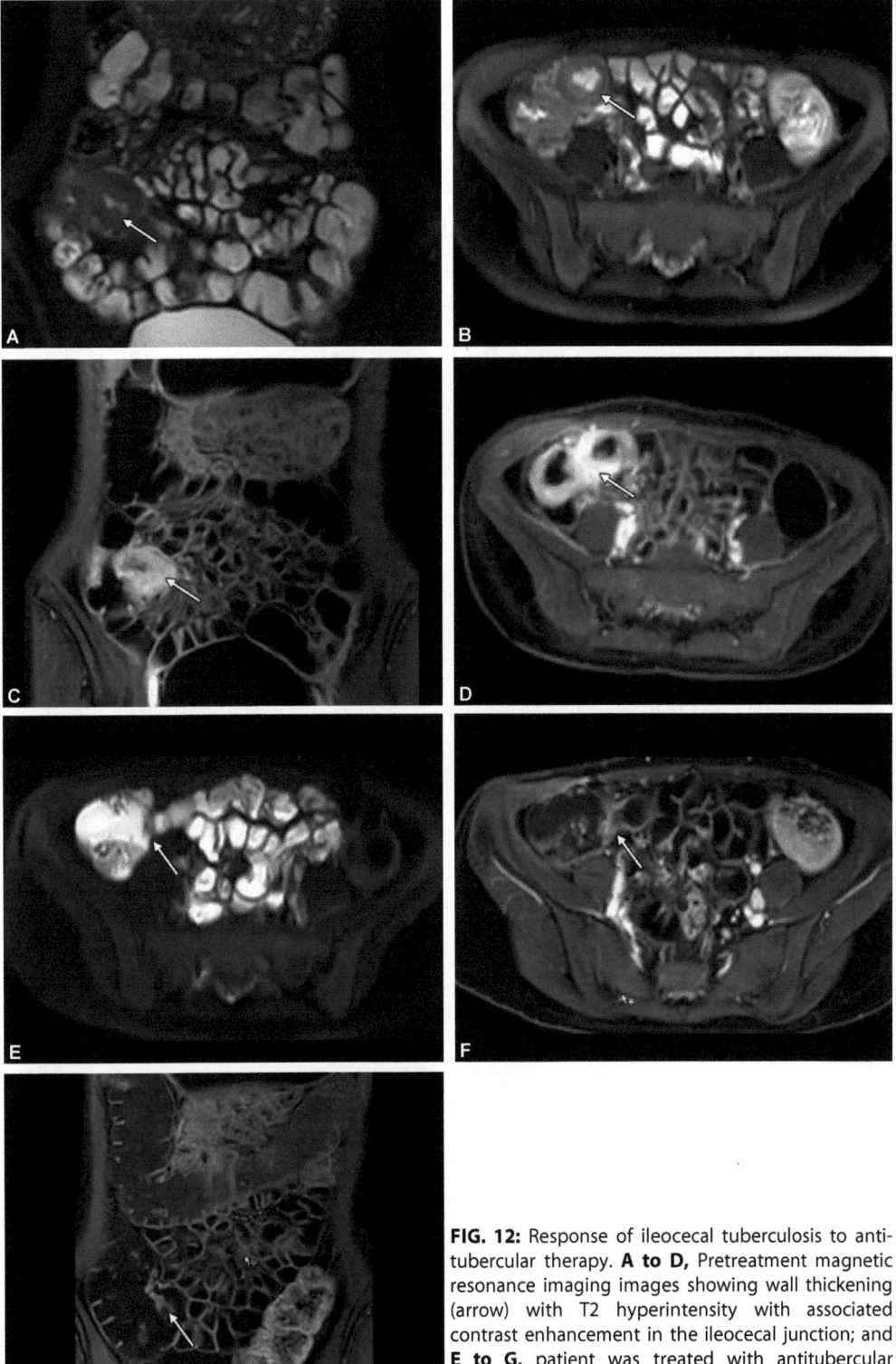

FIG. 12: Response of ileocecal tuberculosis to antitubercular therapy. **A to D,** Pretreatment magnetic resonance imaging images showing wall thickening (arrow) with T2 hyperintensity with associated contrast enhancement in the ileocecal junction; and **E to G,** patient was treated with antitubercular therapy and the follow-up images show complete resolution of the abnormality (arrow)

Table 1: Imaging features to differentiate tuberculosis from Crohn's disease		
Imaging features	Tuberculosis	Crohn's disease
Site of involvement	Ileocecal junction, cecum > ileum	Terminal ileum > cecum
Segments	One or two, short length	Multiple, with skip areas Long length
Strictures	Concentric and smooth	Eccentric, with sacculations
Mural thickening	Usually homogeneous	With stratification
Mesenteric changes	Uncommon	Common
Lymph nodes	Necrotic	Small, homogeneous, <1 cm
High-density ascites	Present	Absent
Fibrofatty proliferation	Uncommon	Common
Abscesses and fistulae	Rare	Common

of transverse, descending and sigmoid colon is much more common than stomach and duodenal TB.[31] Involvement of appendix is rare and may present with acute or recurrent appendicitis.

Involvement of colon is seen as short or long segment wall thickening, strictures, dilatation of colon, ulcerations, and polyps. Barium enema provides information on the luminal and wall abnormalities (Fig. 13).[31] Tubercular strictures usually show wall thickening of less than 1 cm and produce hourglass configuration unlike malignancy (apple core stricture). Computed tomography is superior in showing the extent and associated extraluminal findings (Figs 14 and 15).

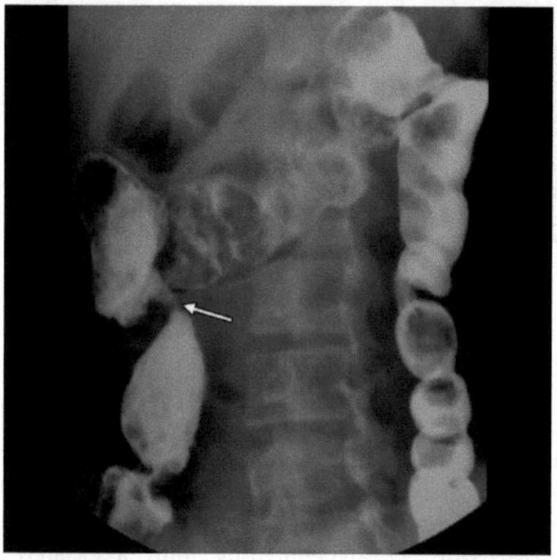

Anorectal involvement is rare and may present as anal fistulae, fissures, abscesses, proctitis and may result in rectal stricture formation. Rectal stricture is seen as symmetric circumferential wall thickening, which may be indistinguishable from malignancy (Fig. 16). In additional to fistula, anorectal TB may have atypical presentations in the form of pilonidal sinus, anal ulceration with inguinal adenopathy, recurrent perianal growth, anal strictures, and rectal submucosal tumor. Perianal TB is seen as complex perianal fistula formation, which is best demonstrated on MRI. Biopsy is needed for confirmation and differentiation from Crohn's disease.[4]

GASTRIC TUBERCULOSIS

Stomach is the least common part of GI tract to be affected by TB. Most common presenting complaints are dyspepsia, epigastric pain, weight loss and rarely upper GI bleed.[31] Antropyloric region is the most commonly affected, resulting in gastric outlet obstruction.[32] Barium studies may show dilated stomach with stricture in the antropyloric region, ulcers in mucosa and deformed pylorus.[33] Computed tomography shows thickening of antrum or pyloric region with distended stomach. Gastric outlet obstruction may be due to pyloric stricture or due to extrinsic compression by nodes.[33]

FIG. 13: Colonic tuberculosis: Barium enema showing short segment stricture in the ascending colon (arrow)

Imaging in Abdominal Tuberculosis

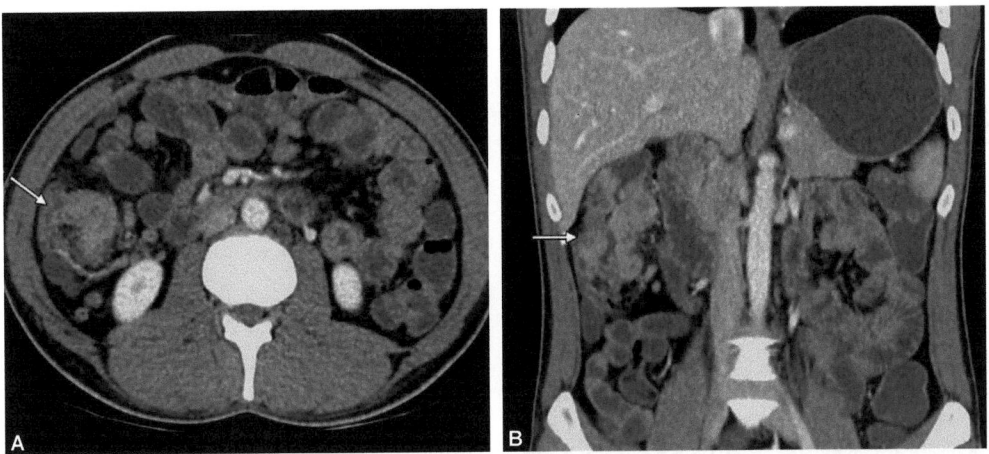

FIG. 14: Colonic tuberculosis. **A,** Axial; and **B,** Coronal computed tomography enterography images show abnormal mucosal enhancement with nodular wall thickening involving ascending colon (arrow) with adjacent necrotic mesenteric lymph nodes

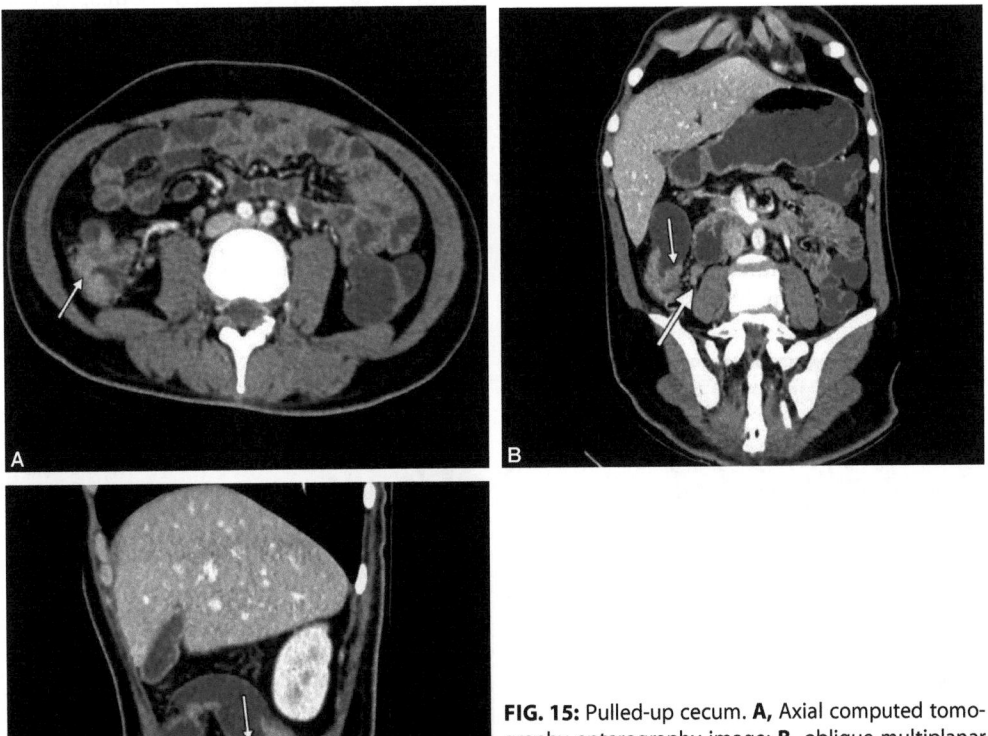

FIG. 15: Pulled-up cecum. **A,** Axial computed tomography enterography image; **B,** oblique multiplanar reconstruction (MPR); and **C,** sagittal MPR showing wall thickening and abnormal enhancement involving the cecum (thin arrow) with few enlarged regional lymph nodes (thick arrow). The cecum is contracted and has migrated cranially to the right lumbar region suggestive of pulled-up cecum in a patient with ileocecal tuberculosis

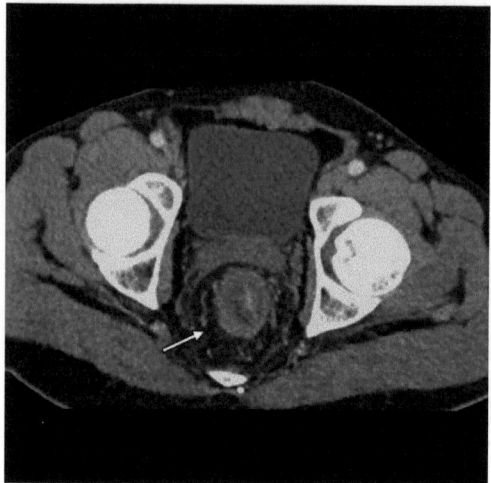

FIG. 16: Rectal tuberculosis: Axial contrast-enhanced computed tomography section shows circumferential wall thickening of rectum (arrow) with preserved mural stratification, fat stranding and prominent vascularity in the surrounding mesorectal fascia

Rarely, granulomatous gastritis can present with imaging appearance similar to linitis plastica.

DUODENAL TUBERCULOSIS

About 2% of cases of GI-TB involve duodenum.[31] Barium studies may show diffuse mucosal ulcerations, polyps, strictures, fistulization with biliary tree and widening of C-loop of duodenum due to associated lymphadenopathy.[34] Computed tomography may show circumferential wall thickening of the duodenum with luminal narrowing and proximal dilatation (Fig. 17). Second and third parts of the duodenum are most commonly involved, seen in 71% cases.[35]

ESOPHAGEAL TUBERCULOSIS

Tubercular involvement of the esophagus is very rare, forming less than 0.5% of cases of GI-TB. It most commonly occurs secondary to contiguous spread from mediastinal nodal disease.[31]

Middle third of esophagus is the most common site of involvement. Earliest findings seen on barium studies are mucosal nodularity and ulcerations.[36] Other findings are extrinsic compression by enlarged nodes, smooth strictures, ulcerations, traction diverticulum, and sinuses and fistulae. On CT scan, the involved segment shows symmetric wall thickening with luminal narrowing, which may be indistinguishable from malignancy.

PERITONEAL TUBERCULOSIS

Peritoneal TB which is constituted by involvement of peritoneum, mesentery, and

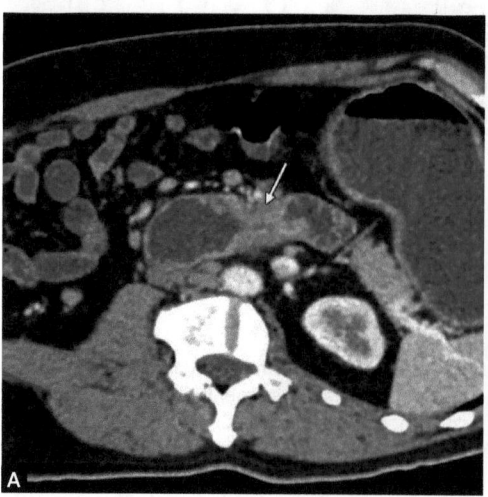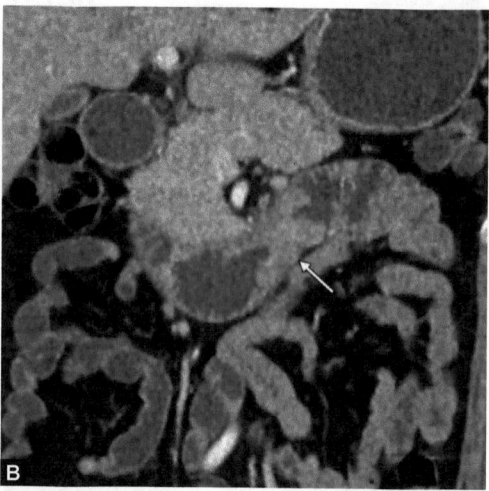

FIG. 17: Duodenal tuberculosis. **A,** Axial; and **B,** coronal computed tomography images showing short segment of wall thickening and luminal narrowing in the third part of duodenum (arrow) with mild proximal dilatation

omentum is the most common presentation of ATB.[37] Isolated involvement of peritoneum by TB is rare and it is usually associated with involvement of other abdominal structures such as nodes and GI tract.[35] The incidence of peritoneal disease is high in AIDS.[38] Peritoneal thickening and small nodules are the most common manifestation of peritoneal involvement. Thickening of peritoneum in the absence of nodules can be seen as smooth thickening ranging from 2 to 6 mm and when the thickening is superimposed with nodules, it gives an irregular appearance. Thickening and nodules are seen as hypoechoic structures on US, which are much better seen in the presence of ascites.[39,40] On CECT and contrast-enhanced MRI, peritoneal involvement is seen as smooth and diffusely enhancing peritoneal lining. Diffusion-weighted imaging can be used to detect tubercular peritoneal thickening and nodularity.

Ascites is a common association of peritoneal involvement and it can be seen in 30–100% of patients.[40,41] It may show multiple complete or incomplete fibrinous septae in the ascitic fluid sometimes giving a lattice appearance.[38] Computed tomography typically shows a high-density fluid [25–45 Hounsfield unit (HU)] because of high protein and cellular content.[41] Rarely, because of lymphatic obstruction patient can have chylous ascites which can be seen as fat-fluid level in the ascites.[42] The presence of chylous ascites and necrotic abdominal nodes have been considered to be diagnostic for ATB. In addition to imaging features, biochemical analysis of ascitic fluid is very helpful in characterizing the nature of fluid. Depending on the amount of ascites and the associated features tuberculous peritoneal involvement is usually classified into three types namely:

- Wet type
- Fibrotic-fixed type
- Dry-plastic type.[38,43]

Wet type is the most common variety (90% of cases) in which large amount of diffusely distributed or loculated ascites is seen (Fig. 18). Fibrotic-fixed type is a less common variety in which matted and tethered bowel loops, large omental, and mesenteric masses can be seen (Figs 19 and 20). Sometimes loculated ascites can also be present. Dry-plastic type is the rarest type, which is characterized by caseating nodules, dense fibrous peritoneal reaction, and adhesions. Another unusual type of peritoneal involvement of TB is cocoon formation or sclerosing encapsulating peritonitis (SEP)

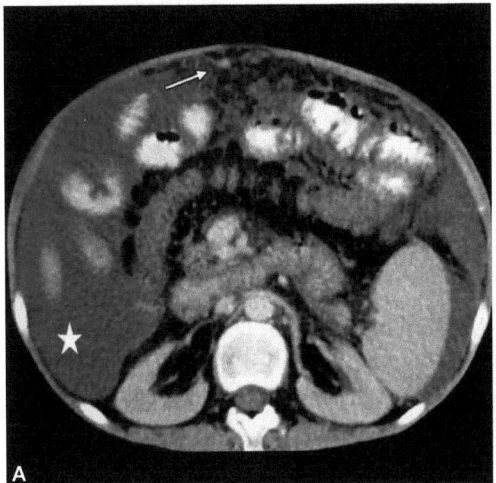 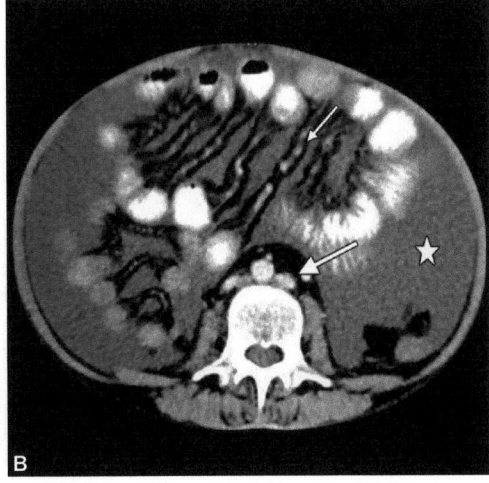

FIG. 18: Peritoneal tuberculosis (wet type): **A,** Contrast-enhanced computed tomography images of abdomen show gross ascites (star) and thickening of omentum (thin arrow) with fat stranding giving a smudged appearance; **B,** The ascitic fluid is seen to separate the leaves of the mesentery (thin arrow). These findings are suggestive of wet type of peritoneal tuberculosis. Incidental duplication of inferior vena cava (thick arrow) is seen

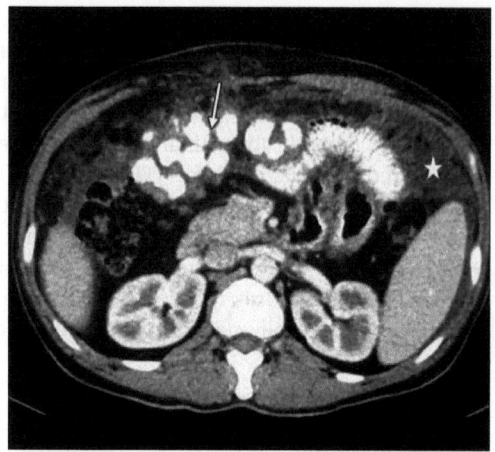

FIG. 19: Peritoneal tuberculosis (fibrotic-fixed type): Contrast-enhanced computed tomography image of abdomen in a patient who presented with a long standing abdominal pain and weight loss shows wall thickening, clumping of small bowel loops (arrow), omental thickening and loculated ascites (star). The earlier features are suggestive of fibrotic-fixed type of peritoneal tuberculosis

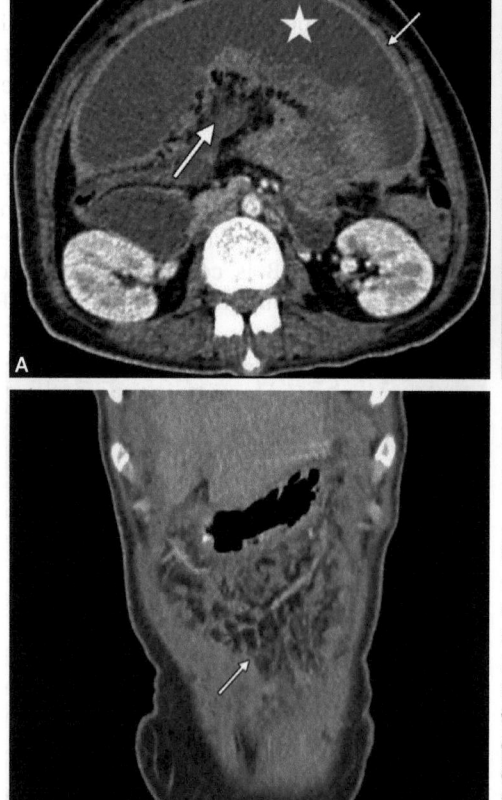

FIG. 20: Peritoneal tuberculosis. **A,** Axial contrast-enhanced computed tomography (CECT) image of abdomen showing loculated ascites (star) with smoothly thickened enhancing peritoneal lining (thin arrow) and associated omental thickening (thick arrow). The earlier features are suggestive of wet type of peritoneal TB; and **B and C,** CECT images of abdomen in a different patient showing minimal ascites (star) and omental thickening giving a smudged appearance (arrow) suggestive of fibrotic-fixed type of peritoneal tuberculosis

in which a part of bowel loop or abdominal viscera are encased within a fibrocollagenous membrane (Fig. 21).[44] Sclerosing encapsulating peritonitis usually involves a part of small bowel loop however, in rare occasions it can involve colon, stomach, liver, and spleen.[45] Ultrasound may show a clump of bowel loops surrounded by a thick wall, which may be associated with

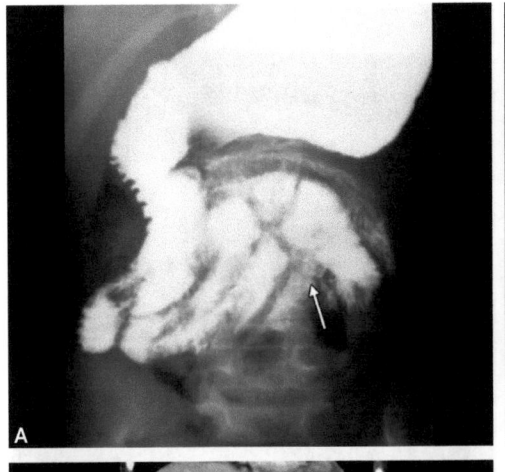
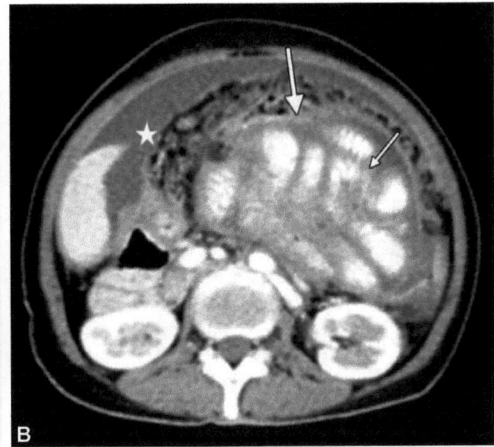
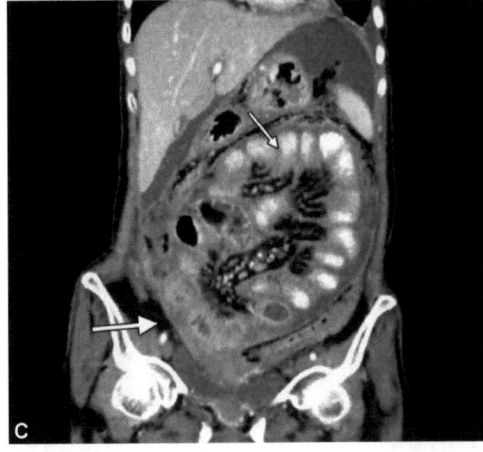

FIG. 21: Peritoneal cocoon formation. **A,** Barium meal follow through shows clumping and fixed position of the dilated small bowel loops (thin arrow) in the central abdomen; **B,** Contrast-enhanced computed tomography images in axial; and **C,** Coronal plane show clumping of dilated proximal small bowel loops which are encapsulated by a thick membrane (thick arrow) all around suggestive of sclerosing encapsulating peritonitis (cocoon formation). There is associated loculated ascites (star) seen

ascites. On BMFT study SEP is seen as clumping of bowel loops with no relative change in position of the involved loops. The loops may not separate even after external compression and move as a whole. On CT scan typical features such as a thick membrane, which can completely or partially encase the bowel loops, loculated ascites and bowel wall thickening may be seen.[45]

Involvement of mesentery is frequently seen on CT (up to 98%) and can manifest as mild fat stranding, thickening, diffuse infiltration, micronodules (<5 mm) or macronodules (>5 mm), abscess formation, or nodal enlargement.[37] Sometimes the deformed and thickened mesentery can cause tethering of bowel loops giving a stellate appearance.[38]

Omental involvement can be seen as simple diffuse thickening, thickening with fat stranding giving a smudged appearance, nodular lesion or sometimes omental caking. Smudged type is commonly seen with ATB, whereas omental caking can also be seen in peritoneal carcinomatosis (Fig. 22). Omental caking in TB is seen only in less than 20% of cases, whereas it is more common (up to 40%) in peritoneal carcinomatosis.[37]

The differential diagnosis of tuberculous involvement of peritoneum are peritoneal carcinomatosis secondary to ovarian (Fig. 23), gastric, colorectal, pancreatic, gallbladder cancers, mesothelioma, nontubercular infections, and lymphoma.

LYMPH NODAL TUBERCULOSIS

Lymph nodal involvement is one of the most common manifestations of ATB. The group of abdominal lymph nodes which are commonly involved in ATB are mesenteric, omental,

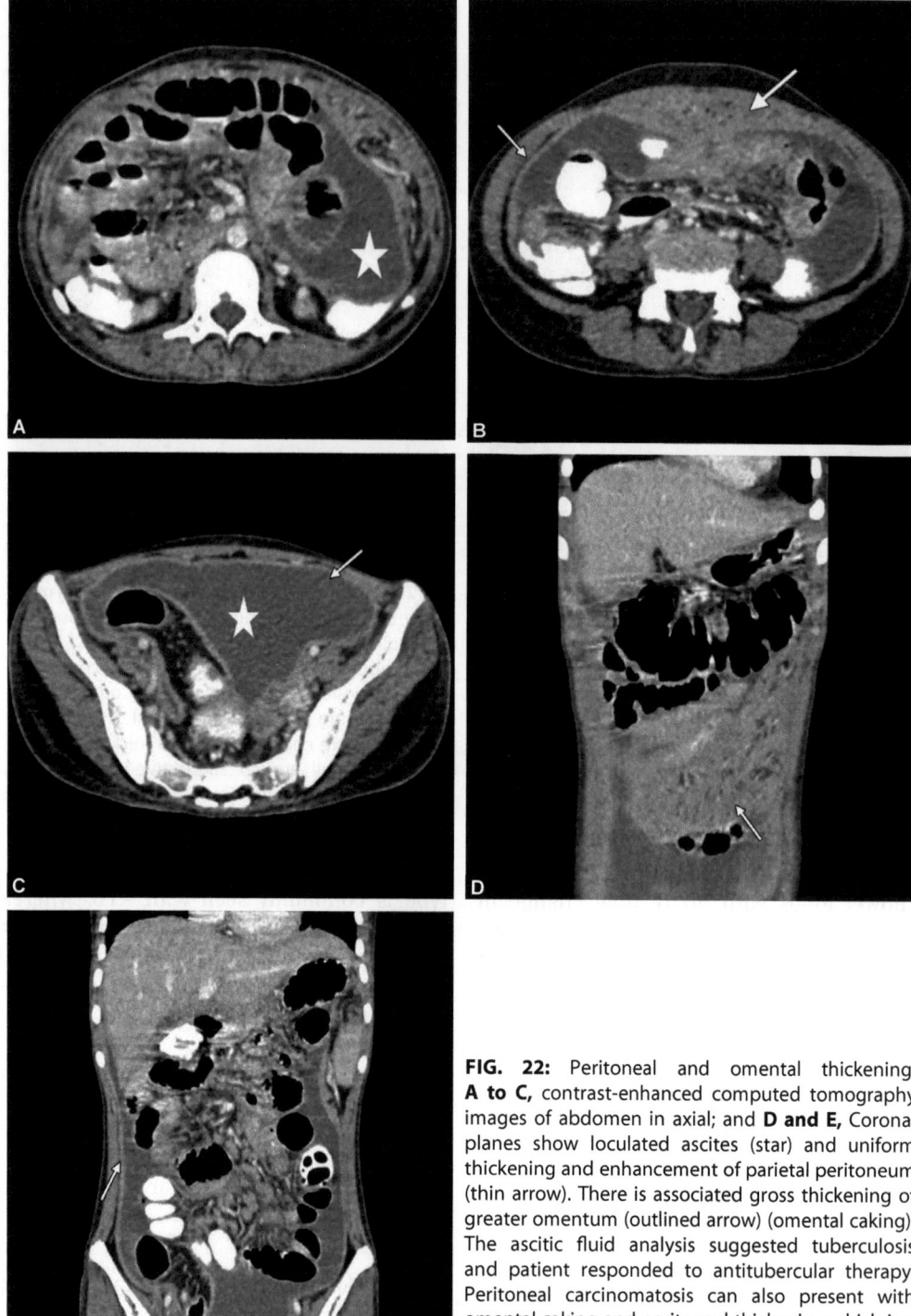

FIG. 22: Peritoneal and omental thickening. **A to C,** contrast-enhanced computed tomography images of abdomen in axial; and **D and E,** Coronal planes show loculated ascites (star) and uniform thickening and enhancement of parietal peritoneum (thin arrow). There is associated gross thickening of greater omentum (outlined arrow) (omental caking). The ascitic fluid analysis suggested tuberculosis and patient responded to antitubercular therapy. Peritoneal carcinomatosis can also present with omental caking and peritoneal thickening which is a close differential diagnosis

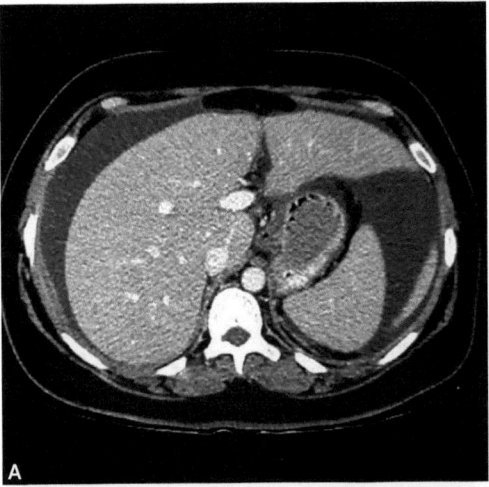
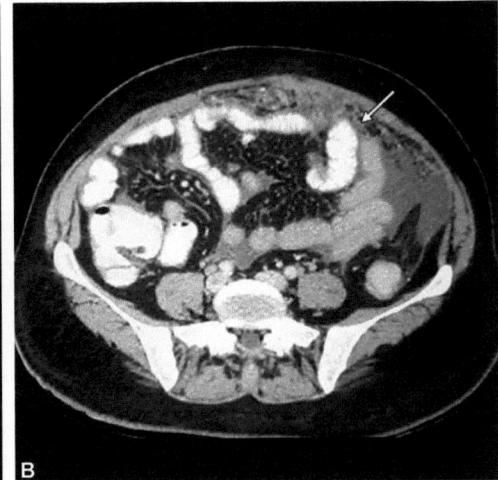
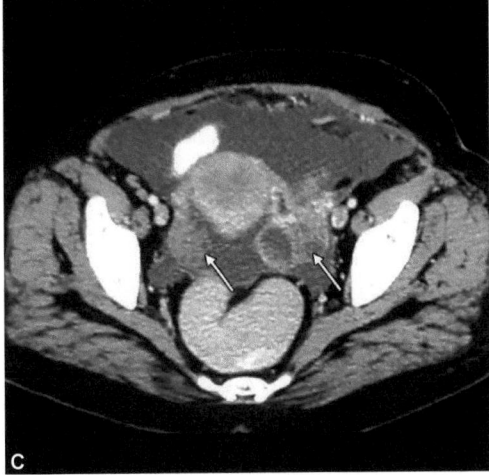

FIG. 23: Peritoneal carcinomatosis mimicking abdominal tuberculosis: contrast-enhanced computed tomography images of abdomen showing ascites and omental thickening (thin arrow) which can also be seen in abdominal tuberculosis (ATB). However, presence of heterogeneous masses in bilateral ovaries should favor the diagnosis of advanced ovarian malignancy. This case depicts the fact that ATB can very well mimic peritoneal carcinomatosis on imaging

peripancreatic, periportal, and upper para-aortic group.[46,47] These are the draining lymph node groups for the small bowel, right side colon, liver, and spleen which are the most common affected organs in ATB.

Depending on the stage of disease evolution the imaging appearance can vary. Nodal enlargement and peripheral enhancement with central necrosis is the most common appearance (Fig. 24). Homogeneous enhancement, heterogeneous enhancement, multiloculated appearance, and nonenhancement are the other types of manifestation on imaging. Nonenhancement is usually seen in immunocompromised individuals.[38,46]

Tuberculosis can present as multiple normal sized lymph nodes which is not typical for TB as it can occur in other infections also. On US, nodes are seen as hypoechoic lesion with or without central caseation which is seen as a relatively anechoic area. Calcification in lymph node which is a sign of healing can also be seen on US. Area of caseation is usually seen as T1 and T2 hypointensity on MRI which can help in better characterization.

Although, peripheral enhancement with central necrosis is a characteristic finding of tuberculous lymph node, it can also occur in pyogenic infections, malignancies, lymphoma, and Whipple's disease.[47,48]

Imaging in Tuberculosis: Clinicopathological Correlation

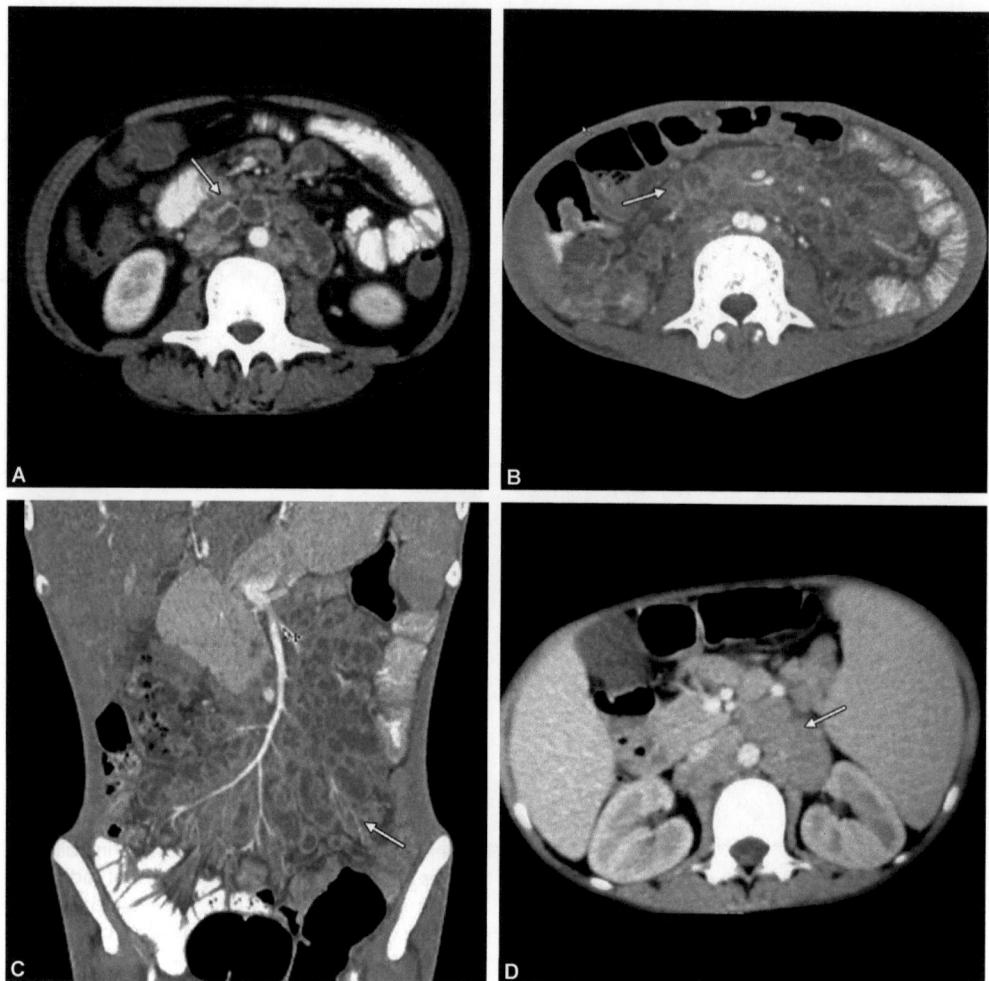

FIG. 24: Tuberculous adenitis. **A,** Abdominal contrast-enhanced computed tomography (CECT) image of a patient who presented with recurrent abdominal pain and fever shows multiple enlarged necrotic lymph nodes (arrow) in retroperitoneum and mesentery. Almost all nodes show central necrosis and a peripheral thin enhancing rim; **B,** CECT images of abdomen in axial and **C,** coronal plane in a different patient show extensive matted necrotic lymphadenopathy in mesentery. The small bowel loops with oral contrast are seen separately in the periphery; and **D,** CECT scan image of abdomen of another patient with lymphoma shows splenomegaly and multiple discrete enlarged lymph nodes in retroperitoneum without necrosis or calcification. The distribution and the morphology of nodes can be used to differentiate these two conditions

TUBERCULOSIS OF THE SOLID ORGANS

Tuberculosis can involve the solid organs of abdomen such as liver, spleen, and pancreas. Genitourinary TB will be covered in a separate chapter.

Hepatosplenic Tuberculosis

Hepatosplenic TB is an unusual antemortem diagnosis and it is usually seen in disseminated disease.[49,50] Hepatosplenic TB can manifest as two types: (i) micronodular and (ii) macronodular (Figs 25 to 27). Micronodular

Imaging in Abdominal Tuberculosis

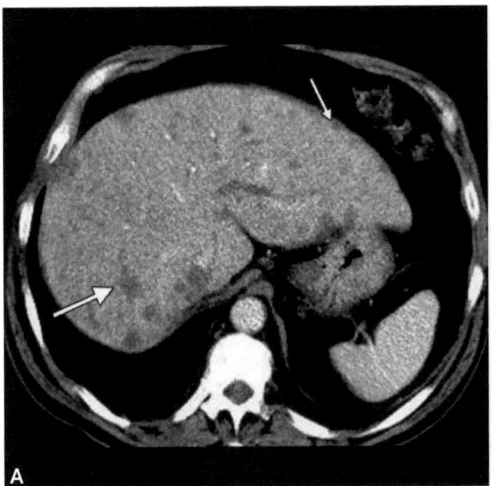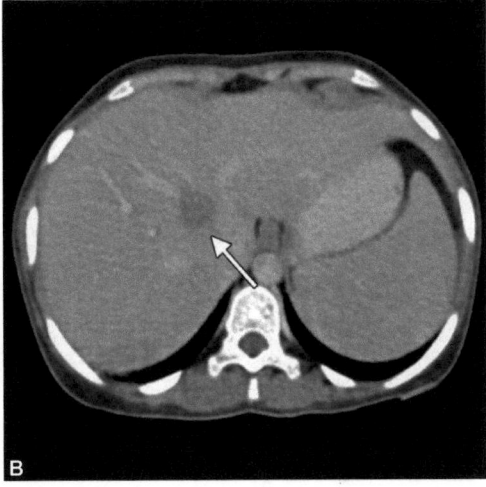

FIG. 25: Hepatic tuberculosis: Abdominal contrast-enhanced computed tomography (CECT) image shows multiple focal hypoenhancing lesions distributed in both the lobes of liver. Some of the lesions are tiny (<1 cm) (thin arrow) and others are more than a centimeter (thick arrow). Multiple enlarged necrotic lymph nodes and pulmonary infiltrates were also present (not shown). These liver lesions are suggestive of micronodular (thin arrow) and macronodular type (thick arrow) of tuberculous involvement of liver. The CECT of abdomen in a different patient who presented with disseminated tuberculosis shows a single focal lesion in left lobe (macronodular type) of liver with hepatosplenomegaly

type which is the most common, occurs as multiple miliary nodules and most of these nodules are tiny. Hence, they are not usually detected on imaging and manifest as nonspecific hepatosplenomegaly. Occasionally, it may appear as hypoechoic nodules on high-resolution US using linear probe, though they are not seen on other cross-sectional modalities highlighting the role of US in these patients (Fig. 28). In the macronodular type the lesions usually range from 1–3 cm and can be single or multiple. Solid lesions before liquefaction are seen as hypo to isoechoic lesions on USG and when there is caseation within the lesion it is manifested as anechoic area. It may also show multiple septations giving a honeycomb appearance.[51] On CECT, the solid lesions appear as hypodense focal nodules which can be difficult to differentiate from metastasis. Caseating lesions may show nonenhancing lesion with peripheral enhancement which can closely mimic pyogenic or amebic abscess. On MRI, these are seen as hypointense lesions on T1W and hyperintense on T2W images (Fig. 26). Diffusion-weighted imaging may show diffusion restriction in the areas of caseation necrosis which can be used to differentiate it from necrotic masses. In immunocompromised patients the lesions can be larger in size forming a tubercular abscess with no appreciable rim enhancement. Rarely, tubercular abscess can rupture into peritoneum leading to peritonitis.

Tuberculosis of Biliary Tract

Biliary tract involvement by TB is very rare and it can involve gall bladder and the ducts. The gall bladder involvement presents as cholecystitis showing wall thickening or mass lesion. There can be associated nodes in the vicinity. Mass lesion due to TB can closely mimic gall bladder carcinoma which necessitates sampling. Biliary TB can also present as obstructive jaundice which can be due to the stricture of the duct itself or extrinsic compression by enlarged lymph nodes. The noninvasive evaluation of

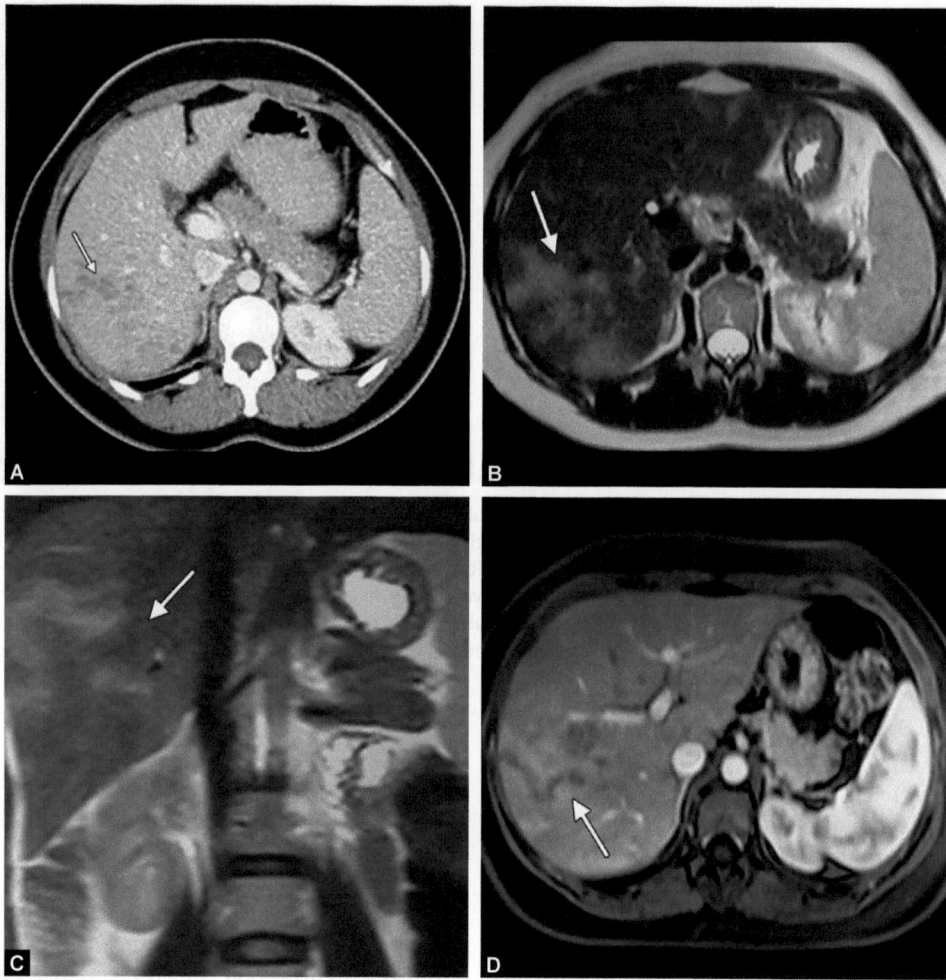

FIG. 26: Hepatic tuberculosis. **A,** Abdominal contrast-enhanced computed tomography (CECT) image of a young patient presented with abdominal pain and fever shows ill-defined hypoenhancing focal lesion (arrow) in the right lobe of liver; **B,** T2-weighted magnetic resonance imaging (MRI) images in axial and **C,** coronal plane show ill-defined hyperintense area in the same location. The morphology and extension is much better seen on MRI than CECT; and **D,** postcontrast T1-weighted fat suppressed image in axial plane shows an ill-defined serpiginous lesion with mild peripheral enhancement. Histopathology of the liver lesion showed tuberculosis and patient responded to antitubercular therapy

biliary involvement is best done using magnetic resonance cholangiopancreatography (MRCP) which can also depict the associated findings of liver parenchymal involvement. These findings are not characteristic of TB as these can also occur in sclerosing cholangitis. Presence of necrotic lymph nodes in the vicinity favors the diagnosis of TB in such situations.

Tuberculosis of Pancreas

Pancreatic TB is extremely rare and it is attributed to the protective effect of pancreatic juice from tuberculous bacilli.[52] Involvement is common in the head and body of pancreas and locoregional adenopathy is seen in up to 75% of patients.[53] The patterns of involvement

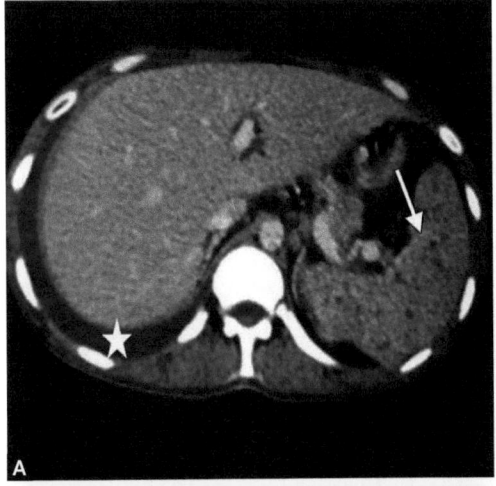
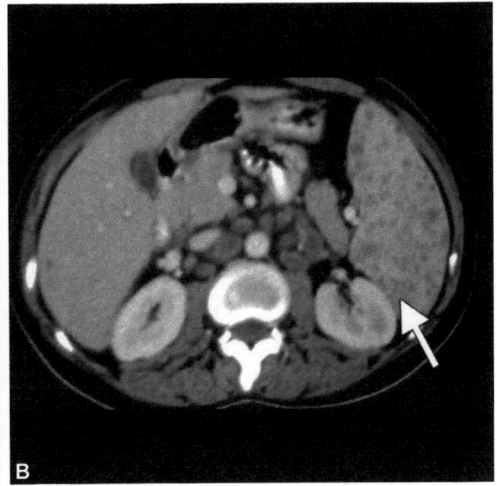
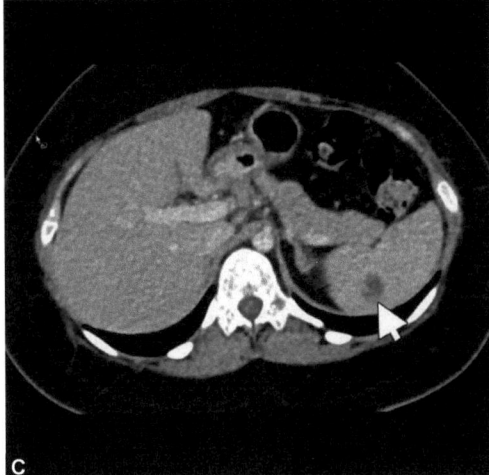

FIG. 27: Splenic tuberculosis. **A,** Contrast-enhanced computed tomography abdomen of three different patients with abdominal tuberculosis. Multiple tiny focal lesions in spleen (thin arrow in A) suggestive of micronodular type of tuberculous involvement. Right side pleural effusion (star) is seen in this patient; **B,** multiple focal lesions of varying sizes (thick arrow in B) seen in enlarged spleen with associated necrotic lymph nodes in retroperitoneum suggestive of micronodular and macronodular type of involvement of spleen; and **C,** A single focal lesion in spleen (>1 cm) (arrow head in C) suggestive of macronodular involvement

are diffuse involvement of entire pancreas and multiple or solitary focal lesions. Imaging features are nonspecific and on US the lesion can be seen as hypoechoic focal lesion. On CECT the lesion is usually seen as hypodense area with scattered cystic and necrotic areas (Fig. 29). Tiny calcifications and multiple necrotic lymph nodes can also be seen. It is challenging to differentiate pancreatic TB from pancreatic adenocarcinoma. There are reports highlighting the possible role of perfusion CT in the diagnosis of pancreatic TB.[52] Role of MRI is not very clear, however it can delineate the main pancreatic duct in relation to the mass.[54]

CONCLUSION

Tuberculosis is one of the most important health problems in developing countries like India. It is crucial to detect these patients early in the course of disease to treat them with effective multidrug regimen so as to reduce mortality and morbidity. Imaging plays a key role in diagnosis as the clinical picture is nonspecific. It is of paramount importance for the radiologists to be aware of the features of intestinal TB and differentiate it from Crohn's disease. The focus has shifted from barium studies to CT and MRI for this purpose.

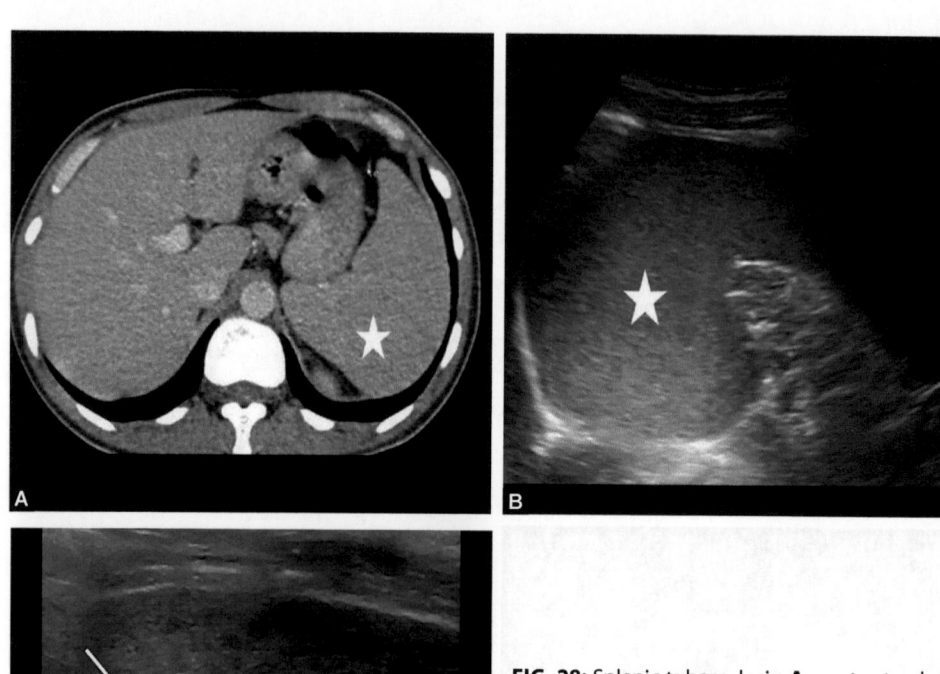

FIG. 28: Splenic tuberculosis. **A,** contrast-enhanced computed tomography image of a patient who presented with fever, weight loss and abdominal pain shows splenomegaly (star) without any appreciable focal lesion; **B,** ultrasound image using a convex probe shows enlarged spleen (star) with no focal lesion; and **C,** ultrasound image using high-resolution linear probe shows multiple tiny focal lesions (arrow) in spleen. These tiny splenic lesions represent the micronodular involvement by tuberculosis and they may be seen only on high-resolution ultrasound images as depicted in this patient

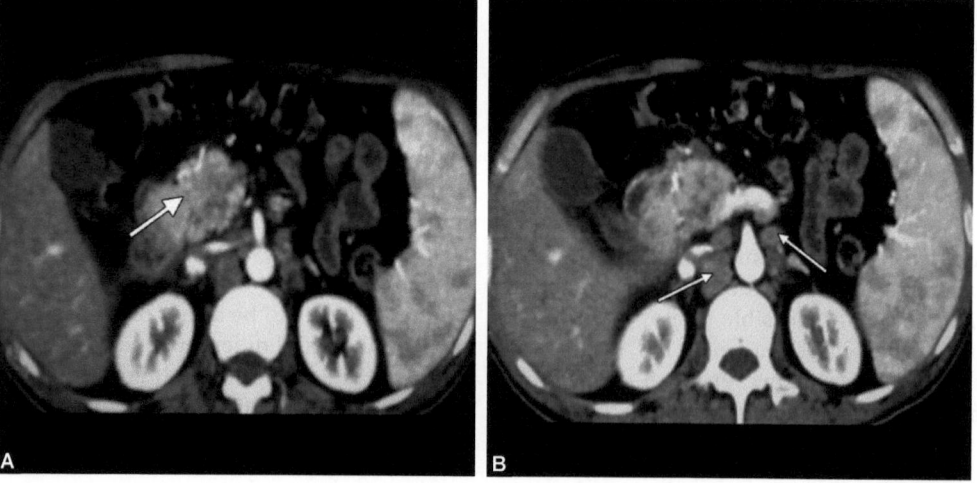

Continued

Continued

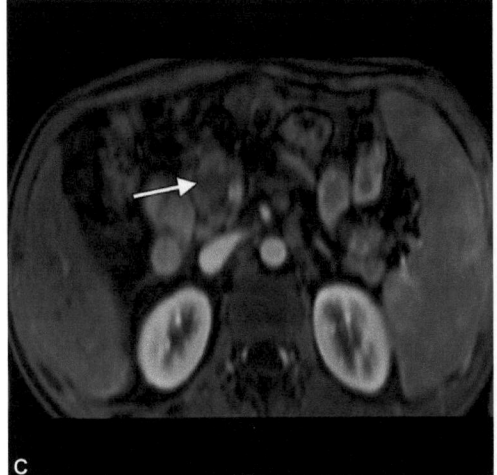
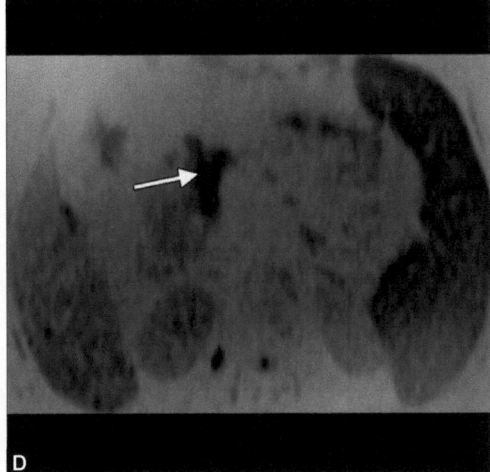
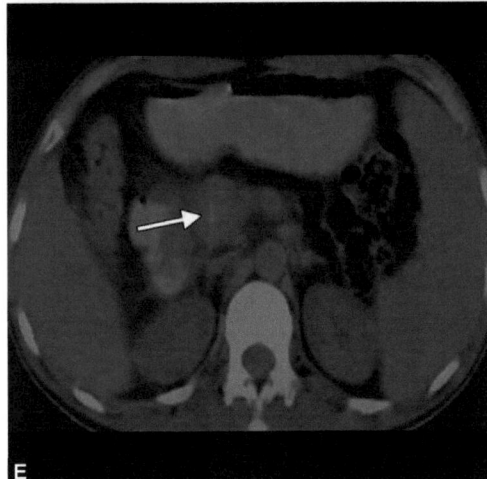

FIG. 29: Pancreatic tuberculosis. **A and B,** Abdominal contrast-enhanced computed tomography images show hypodense mass lesion (thick arrow) in the head of pancreas with multiple necrotic lymph nodes in retroperitoneum (thin arrow) and there is associated splenomegaly; **C and D,** post-contrast T1-weighted fat suppressed image also shows pancreatic focal lesion which is showing diffusion restriction on inverted grey scale image of diffusion-weighted sequence (B 1000); and **E,** tracer uptake on fluorodeoxyglucose positron emission tomography-CT scan. Based on the earlier imaging features this patient was diagnosed to have pancreatic carcinoma. However, endoscopic ultrasonography-guided fine-needle aspiration cytology revealed tuberculosis which is a rare entity and a close mimicker of pancreatic carcinoma *(For color version, see Plate 11)*

REFERENCES

1. Sircar S, Taneja VA, Kansra U. Epidemiology and clinical presentation of abdominal tuberculosis--a retrospective study. J Indian Med Assoc. 1996;94(9):342-4.
2. Lee WK, Van Tonder F, Tartaglia CJ, et al. CT appearances of abdominal tuberculosis. Clin Radiol. 2012;67(6):596-604.
3. Sood R. Diagnosis of abdominal tuberculosis: role of imaging. J Indian Acad Clin Med. 2001;2(3):169-77.
4. Sharma MP, Bhatia V. Abdominal tuberculosis. Indian J Med Res. 2004;120(4):305-15.
5. Balthazar EJ, Gordon R, Hulnick D. Ileocecal tuberculosis: CT and radiologic evaluation. AJR Am J Roentgenol. 1990;154(3):499-503.
6. Ramesh J, Banait GS, Ormerod LP. Abdominal tuberculosis in a district general hospital: a retrospective review of 86 cases. QJM. 2008;101(3):189-95.
7. Gulati MS, Sarma D, Paul SB. CT appearances in abdominal tuberculosis. A pictorial essay. Clin Imaging. 1999;23(1):51-9.
8. Balamurugan R, Venkataraman S, John KR, Ramakrishna BS. PCR amplification of the IS6110 insertion element of Mycobacterium tuberculosis in fecal samples from patients with intestinal tuberculosis. J Clin Microbiol. 2006;44(5):1884-6.
9. Amarapurkar DN, Patel ND, Rane PS. Diagnosis of Crohn's disease in India where tuberculosis is widely prevalent. World J Gastroenterol. 2008;14(5):741-6.
10. Horvath KD, Whelan RL. Intestinal tuberculosis: return of an old disease. Am J Gastroenterol. 1998;93(5):692-6.
11. Pereira JM, Madureira AJ, Vieira A, et al. Abdominal tuberculosis: imaging features. Eur J Radiol. 2005;55(2):173-80.
12. Vanhoenacker FM, De Backer AI, Op de BB, et al, Van Beckevoort D, et al. Imaging of gastrointestinal and

12. abdominal tuberculosis. Eur Radiol. 2004;14 Suppl 3: E103-15.
13. Kapoor VK. Abdominal tuberculosis. Postgrad Med J. 1998;74(874):459-67.
14. Minordi LM, Vecchioli A, Guidi L, et al. Multidetector CT enteroclysis versus barium enteroclysis with methylcellulose in patients with suspected small bowel disease. Eur Radiol. 2006;16(7):1527-36.
15. Rodgers PM, Verma R. Transabdominal ultrasound for bowel evaluation. Radiol Clin North Am. 2013;51(1):133-48.
16. Lee DH, Ko YT, Yoon Y, et al. Sonographic findings of intestinal tuberculosis. J Ultrasound Med. 1993;12(9):537-40.
17. Denton T, Hossain J. A radiological study of abdominal tuberculosis in a Saudi population, with special reference to ultrasound and computed tomography. Clin Radiol. 1993;47(6):409-14.
18. Gompels BM, Darlington LG. Ultrasonic diagnosis of tuberculous peritonitis. Br J Radiol. 1978;51(612):1018-9.
19. Pombo F, Rodriguez E, Mato J, et al. Patterns of contrast enhancement of tuberculous lymph nodes demonstrated by computed tomography. Clin Radiol. 1992;46(1):13-7.
20. Suri S, Gupta S, Suri R. Computed tomography in abdominal tuberculosis. Br J Radiol. 1999;72(853):92-8.
21. Ilangovan R, Burling D, George A, et al. CT enterography: review of technique and practical tips. Br J Radiol. 2012;85(1015):876-86.
22. Macari M, Megibow AJ, Balthazar EJ. A pattern approach to the abnormal small bowel: observations at MDCT and CT enterography. AJR Am J Roentgenol. 2007;188(5):1344-55.
23. Siddiqui MRS, Ashrafian H, Tozer P, et al. A diagnostic accuracy meta-analysis of endoanal ultrasound and MRI for perianal fistula assessment. Dis Colon Rectum. 2012;55(5):576-85.
24. Singhal A, Gulati A, Frizell R, Manning AP. Abdominal tuberculosis in Bradford, UK: 1992-2002. Eur J Gastroenterol Hepatol. 2005;17(9):967-71.
25. De Backer AI, Mortelé KJ, De Keulenaer BL, et al. CT and MR imaging of gastrointestinal tuberculosis. JBR-BTR. 2006;89(4):190-4.
26. Kapoor VK, Chattopadhyay TK, Sharma LK. Radiology of abdominal tuberculosis. Australas Radiol. 1988;32(3):365-7.
27. Nagi B, Sodhi KS, Kochhar R, Bhasin DK, Singh K. Small bowel tuberculosis: enteroclysis findings. Abdom Imaging. 2004;29(3):335-40.
28. Bhansali SK, Sethna JR. Intestinal obstruction: a clinical analysis of 348 cases. Indian J Surg. 1970;32:57-70.
29. Lee MJ, Cresswell FV, John L, et al. Diagnosis and treatment strategies of tuberculous intestinal perforations: a case series. Eur J Gastroenterol Hepatol. 2012;24(5):594-9.
30. Mukewar S, Mukewar S, Dua KS. Tuberculosis of the colon: endoscopic features with prospective follow-up after anti-tuberculosis treatment. Gastrointest Endosc. 2007;65(5):AB253.
31. Chong VH, Lim KS. Gastrointestinal tuberculosis. Singapore Med J. 2009;50(6):638-45.
32. Bandyopadhyay S, Bandyopadhyay R, Chatterjee U. Isolated gastric tuberculosis presenting as haematemesis. J Postgrad Med. 2002;48(1):72-3.
33. Amarapurkar DN, Patel ND, Amarapurkar AD. Primary gastric tuberculosis—report of 5 cases. BMC Gastroenterol. 2003;3:6.
34. Chavhan GE, Ramakantan R. Duodenal tuberculosis: radiological features on barium studies and their clinical correlation in 28 cases. J Postgrad Med. 2003;49(3):214-7.
35. Marshall JB. Tuberculosis of the gastrointestinal tract and peritoneum. Am J Gastroenterol. 1993;88(7):989-99.
36. Mokoena T, Shama DM, Ngakane H, et al. Oesophageal tuberculosis: a review of eleven cases. Postgrad Med J. 1992;68(796):110-5.
37. da Rocha EL, Pedrassa BC, Bormann RL, et al. Abdominal tuberculosis: a radiological review with emphasis on computed tomography and magnetic resonance imaging findings. Radiol Bras. 2015;48(3):181-91.
38. Akhan O, Pringot J. Imaging of abdominal tuberculosis. Eur Radiol. 2002;12(2):312-23.
39. Kedar RP, Shah PP, Shivde RS, et al. Sonographic findings in gastrointestinal and peritoneal tuberculosis. Clin Radiol. 1994;49(1):24-9.
40. Akhan O, Demirkazik FB, Demirkazik A, et al. Tuberculous peritonitis: ultrasonic diagnosis. J Clin Ultrasound. 1990;18(9):711-4.
41. Hulnick DH, Megibow AJ, Naidich DP, et al. Abdominal tuberculosis: CT evaluation. Radiology. 1985;157(1):199-204.
42. Prasad S, Patankar T. Computed tomography demonstration of a fat-fluid level in tuberculous chylous ascites. Australas Radiol. 1999;43(4):542-3.
43. Thoeni RF, Margulis AR. Gastrointestinal tuberculosis. Sem Roentgenol. 1979;14(4):283-94.
44. Puppala R, Sripathi S, Kadavigere R, et al. Abdominal cocoon secondary to disseminated tuberculosis. BMJ Case Rep. 2014;2014.
45. Jayant M, Kaushik R. Abdominal cocoon in a young man. World J Emerg Med. 2014;5(3):234-6.
46. Leder RA, Low VH. Tuberculosis of the abdomen. Radiol Clin North Am. 1995;33(4):691-705.
47. Yang ZG, Min PQ, Sone S, et al. Tuberculosis versus lymphomas in the abdominal lymph nodes: evaluation with contrast-enhanced CT. AJR Am J Roentgenol. 1999;172(3):619-23.
48. Li DK, Rennie CS. Abdominal computed tomography in Whipple's disease. J Comput Assist Tomogr. 1981;5(2):249-52.
49. Akgun Y. Intestinal and peritoneal tuberculosis: changing trends over 10 years and a review of 80 patients. Can J Surg. 2005;48(2):131-6.
50. Saluja SS, Ray S, Pal S, et al. Hepatobiliary and pancreatic tuberculosis: a two decade experience. BMC Surg. 2007;7:10.
51. Wilde CC, Kueh YK. Case report: Tuberculous hepatic and splenic abscess. Clin Radiol. 1991;43(3):215-6.
52. Yadav AK, Nadrajah J, Kandasamy D, et al. Volume perfusion computed tomography as an aid to diagnosis of pancreatic tuberculosis. Trop Gastroenterol. 2015;35(4):264-6.
53. Nagar AM, Raut AA, Morani AC, et al. Pancreatic tuberculosis: a clinical and imaging review of 32 cases. J Comput Assist Tomogr. 2009;33(1):136-41.
54. Kim SY, Kim MJ, Chung JJ, et al. Abdominal tuberculous lymphadenopathy: MR imaging findings. Abdom Imaging. 2000;25(6):627-32.

CHAPTER 13

Imaging in Urogenital Tuberculosis

Chandan J Das, Ankur Goyal

INTRODUCTION

Tuberculosis (TB) is one disease which can affect any organ system and can have variable imaging manifestations. Chest is the most frequent site of primary TB with entry of bacilli through the inhalation route. However, the bacteria have a propensity for dissemination by hematogenous route to almost any part of the body. Urogenital involvement is a common form of extrapulmonary TB (EPTB) and kidneys are the most frequently involved. The involvement of urinary system [including kidneys, ureter, and bladder (KUB)] and prostate usually occurs after hematogenous dissemination from the lungs to the kidneys followed by descending transmission of bacilli.[1] Involvement of the genital tract (urethra, epididymis, and testis) usually occurs via ascending route. Tuberculosis of these organs presents insidiously with nonspecific symptoms. Moreover, urogenital TB (UGTB) can mimic a variety of other diseases and thus it is important to be familiar with the imaging features to ensure prompt diagnosis.[2] Also, the choice of imaging modality should be judicious, keeping in view radiation exposure and cost issues. Imaging also plays an important role in the follow-up of these patients and detection of complications.

URINARY TRACT TUBERCULOSIS

Clinical Epidemiology

Urogenital TB commonly affects adults in the age group of 10–40 years. There is usually a long latent period (in years) between primary chest infection and secondary urogenital involvement.[3] Clinical manifestations are nonspecific and often constitutional features are also lacking. Increased urinary frequency, dysuria, flank pain or hematuria are the usual clinical features. Patients remain asymptomatic for a long time and sterile pyuria is commonly seen. The yield of 24-hour urine sediment for acid-fast bacilli (AFB) analysis as well as of culture studies is low; moreover, urinalysis does not give any information regarding the site or extent of disease.[3] Polymerase chain reaction-based assays are more accurate and provide a much faster way of diagnosis. Abnormal chest radiographs (CXRs) are seen in only one-third of the patients.

Pathogenesis (Fig. 1)

Tuberculosis infection of urinary tract results from hematogenous dissemination to the kidneys. The mycobacteria reach renal parenchyma via bloodstream and can then spread locally. Small renal cortical lesions develop, which can heal spontaneously. Tuberculosis bacilli can pass down the renal tubules, involving the calyces leading to papillary abscess formation and necrosis. These abscess cavities can enlarge, cavitate, and extend towards the capsule of the kidney (Fig. 1). Unlike bacterial urinary infections, TB of the urinary tract takes a descending route of infection. Infected material can enter the renal pelvis and then further descend to involve the epithelium of ureter. There is ureteritis which further leads to stricture formation. The stricture can result in upstream hydroureter and hydronephrosis. Finally, the

Imaging in Tuberculosis: Clinicopathological Correlation

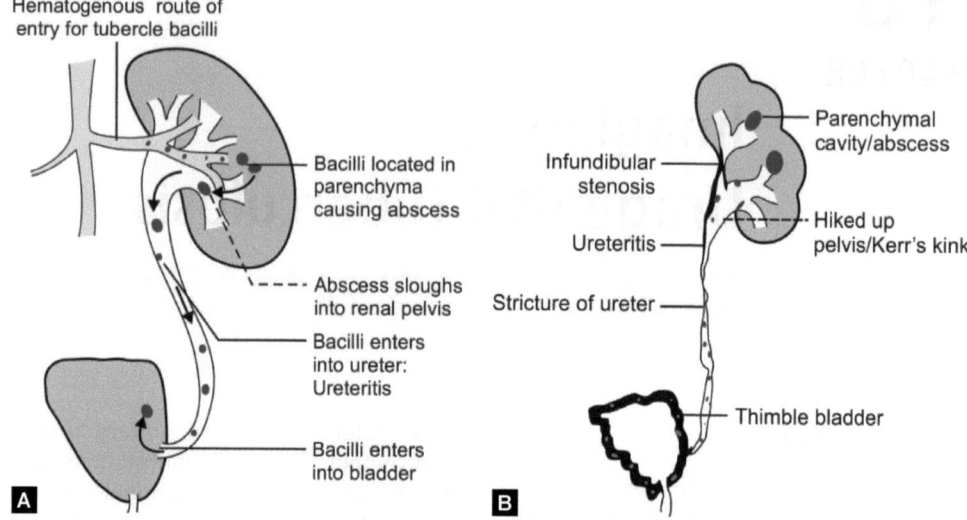

FIG. 1: A, Schematic diagram showing pathogenesis of tuberculosis of the urinary tract; **B,** Schematic diagram showing various morphological changes seen in urinary tract tuberculosis

infection can reach urinary bladder where initially there is mucosal edema (due to TB cystitis) and later on transmural involvement. Up to 10% of patients with renal TB have bladder contractures, commonly known as "thimble bladder".

Renal involvement is frequently unilateral (in 75%) and most common finding is presence of calcifications (seen in about 50%).[4] Complications of renal TB occur due to extension of infection/abscess to perinephric region and retroperitoneum, development of fistulae and formation of psoas abscess. End-stage renal failure, amyloidosis, and predisposition to squamous carcinoma due to chronic urothelial inflammation are other complications.

Imaging Diagnosis

- Radiographs (Fig. 2): Abdominal radiographs may point towards the presence of UGTB by incidental depiction of calcifications in the renal fossa, ureter, bladder or lymph nodes. Chest radiograph may show associated pulmonary TB and spine radiographs may show vertebral end plate destruction. Renal calcifications may be amorphous, granular, curvilinear and may be seen in lobar distribution. Ring-like calcifications occur as a result of papillary necrosis. Renal calculi are frequently seen and often have irregular shapes and orientation, conforming to the deformed renal pelvis. Lobar pattern of calcification is pathognomonic of end-stage renal TB. In the end stage, there is parenchymal scarring and calcification, so much so that it may give rise to putty kidney (homogenous dense calcification of caseous tissue greater than 1 cm in size). Involvement of the extraurinary sites may be evident in 20–50% cases on radiographs
- Sonography (Fig. 2): Being widely available, quick to perform and not involving ionizing radiation, sonography serves as a screening modality and also serves to guide percutaneous sampling and drainage procedures. Sonography is helpful in depicting the hydronephrosis, internal debris, urothelial thickening, hypoechoic parenchymal lesions, calcification, and perinephric abscesses.[5] The early calyceal changes however, may not be detected. The papillary lesions may be seen as ill-defined hypoechoic or echogenic lesions and may mimic masses. Calyceal dilatation is uneven and renal pelvis may appear contracted. Different patterns of involvement have been described on gray-scale sonography, based on the presence of dilatation of the

pelvicalyceal system (PCS), atrophy and calcification.[6] These include nephrectasia type, hydrops, empyema, atrophy, calcification, and mixed types
- Intravenous urography (IVU) (Fig. 3): Intravenous urography is the modality of choice for diagnosis of renal TB in early stages. This is one indication where a conventional imaging modality is the earliest to detect subtle changes in the papillary outlines. Sonography and computed tomography (CT) are useful for advanced disease, chronic

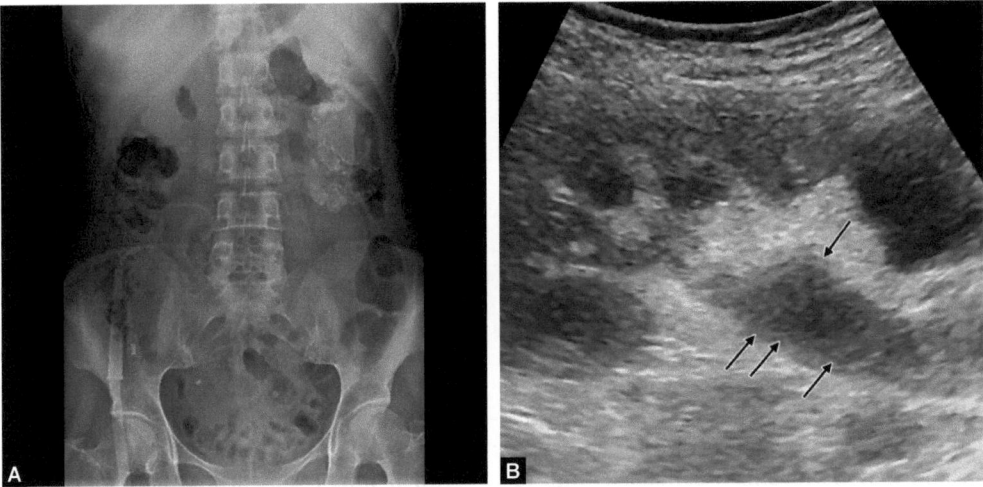

FIG. 2: Radiographs and sonography in urinary tract tuberculosis. **A,** Abdominal radiograph shows amorphous granular calcification in the left renal fossa, some of these calcifications are outlining the dilated calyces; and **B,** sagittal ultrasound section shows moderate hydronephrosis with dilated proximal ureter and presence of internal echogenic debris. Also there is urothelial thickening involving the pelvicalyceal system and ureter (arrows)

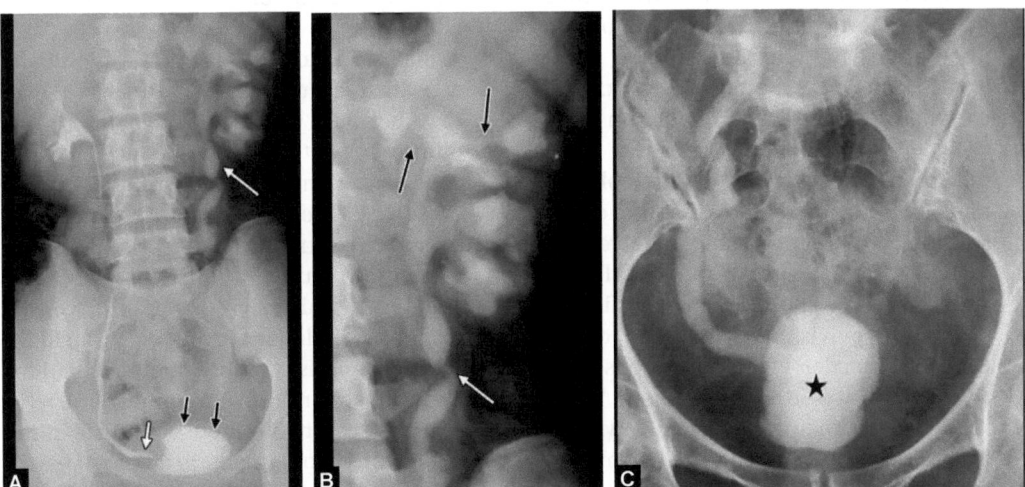

FIG. 3: Intravenous urography in urinary tuberculosis. **A,** 15-minute intravenous pyelography spot and **B,** zoomed image of left renal fossa in a patient with sterile pyuria. Left kidney is hydronephrotic, there is loss of papillary impressions with fuzzy outlines and infundibular stenosis in the upper polar region (long black arrows). Long white arrow demonstrates beaded appearance of the ureter with alternate areas of stricture and dilatation. Small black arrows in A depict bladder wall thickening and small capacity bladder. Short white arrow delineates the site of stricture at right vesicoureteric junction; and **C,** another patient, full bladder spot film demonstrates thimble bladder (star) with dilated right lower ureter

changes, and complications. Involvement of the urinary tract starts from hematogenous dissemination of the tubercular bacilli to the kidneys, where it results in formation of granulomas. The latter coalesce in the region of medullary pyramids with resultant distortion of the minor calyces. The erosion of the calyces gives rise to fuzzy irregular outline (feathery appearance) of the calyces on IVU, the earliest radiological sign of renal TB. Thus, IVU may be unremarkable in early stages when bacilli are lodged in the parenchyma. This loss of definition of minor calyx (*moth-eaten* appearance) may resemble papillary necrosis. Nontubercular causes of papillary necrosis usually cause ischemia; but in TB there is direct tissue destruction as well. The other imaging differentials for renal TB at this stage include transitional cell carcinoma, blood clots/pus in PCS and other infections (focal bacterial nephritis and xanthogranulomatous pyelonephritis). There may be localized caliectasis due to development of an infundibular stricture or the whole PCS may be dilated due to involvement of pelviureteric junction. When infundibulum is occluded, this results in complete cutoff of the calyx with failure of contrast excretion from it (known as phantom calyx).[7] The infundibular stump is seen, known as amputated calyx. Thus, various patterns of PCS dilatation (focal caliectasis, caliectasis without pelvic dilatation, or generalized hydronephrosis) may be seen depending on the site of stricture.[8] With increasing involvement, there is deformation of the entire collecting system due to wall thickening and fibrosis. "Hiked-up pelvis" may be seen due to cephalic retraction of the renal pelvis owing to involvement of its inferior margin. "Kerr's kink" denotes sharply angulated pelvic kink pointing in the direction of the involved calyx/infundibulum. The resultant stasis predisposes to calculi formation, which are the most common form of calcification encountered in renal TB. Due to deformity of the renal PCS, calculi also depict abnormal shapes, termed as "scarred calculi".[3] End-stage disease manifests either as (a) calcified fibrotic shrunken nonfunctioning kidney, or as (b) enlarged hydronephrotic sac with caseous material within due to obstructive uropathy (caseo-cavernous type). The latter may also develop lobar calcification along the rims, outlining the dilated calyces

Rest of the urinary system is involved as a result of passage of the tubercular bacilli form the renal PCS into the ureter. The initial response of ureters to bacilluria is atony which is seen as dilatation on the static IVU images. There may be irregularity of the ureteric wall due to mucosal erosions. Occasionally, filling defects may also be seen due to granulomas in the ureteric wall. Ureteric dilatation with wall irregularity, strictures and calcifications can be seen on urography.[8] Normal anatomical sites of narrowing show predilection for stricture formation. Nonuniform scarring results in beaded appearance due to interspersed areas of ureteric strictures. Severe wall thickening results in rigid shortened "pipe stem ureter" with narrow lumen. The renal changes secondary to obstructive uropathy may result in more severe damage than direct parenchymal involvement.[9] Ureteric stenting is commonly done to salvage the kidney.

Bladder involvement manifests initially as wall thickening and irregularity which may be focal (seen as filling defects) or diffuse. The latter results in reduced bladder capacity, the most common finding in TB cystitis.[10] Circumferential scarring and irregular contractures give rise to small capacity irregular "thimble bladder" and eventually wall calcification. Differential diagnosis of bladder involvement includes schistosomiasis, cystitis (due to radiation/cyclophosphamide) and malignancy (in case of focal involvement). Fibrosis in the region of trigone leads to gaping vesicoureteric junction with reflux.

- Multidetector computed tomography, and CT urography (Figs 4 to 7): Contrast-enhanced CT provides accurate depiction of abnormalities involving the renal parenchyma, perinephric-periureteric regions, and urothelial thickening. Computed tomo-

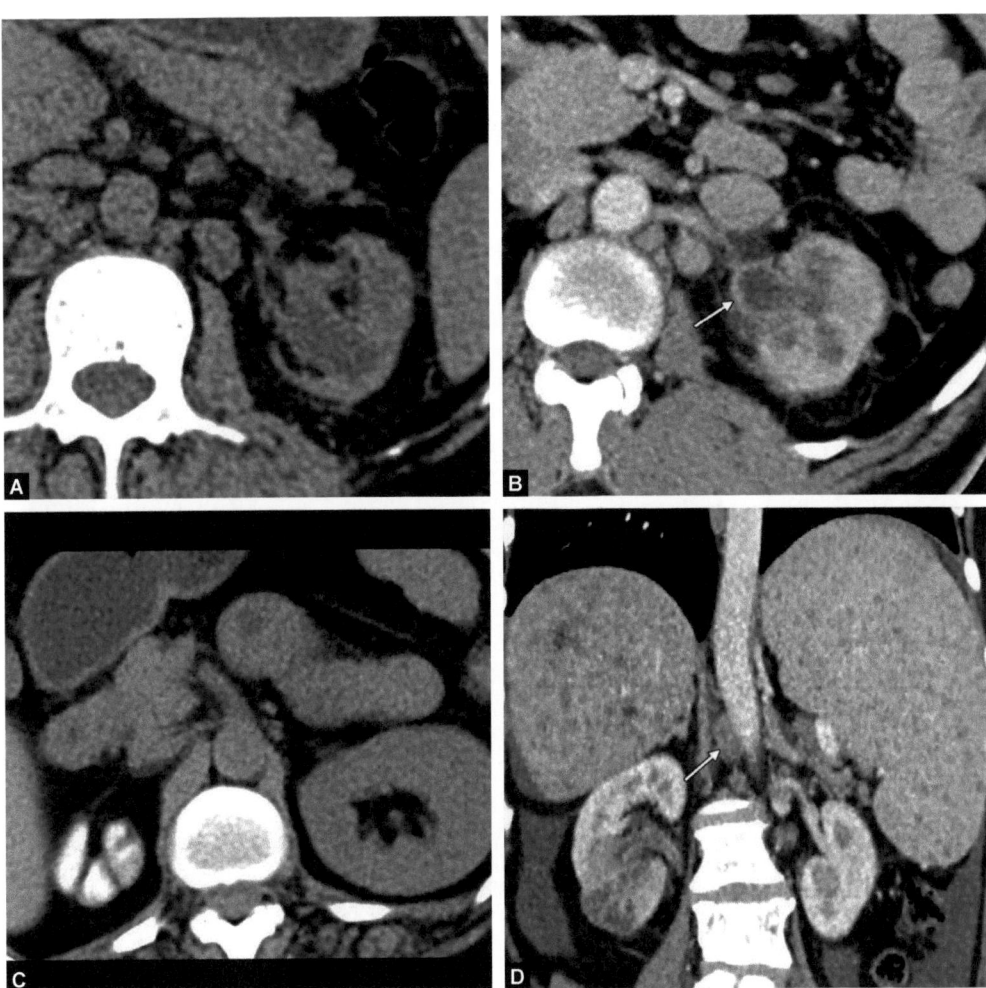

FIG. 4: Computed tomography (CT) in urinary tuberculosis (TB). **A,** Noncontrast and **B,** contrast-enhanced axial CT sections shows dilated left renal pelvis with wall thickening (arrow), mild irregularity and atrophy of renal parenchyma and perinephric fat stranding. There is caliectasis with irregular margins. Multiple enlarged retroperitoneal lymph nodes are seen; **C,** Another patient shows parenchymal calcification involving atrophic right kidney (sequelae of TB). Note made of compensatory enlargement of left kidney; and **D,** Different patient with disseminated TB. Right kidney shows ill-defined wedge-shaped hypodensity involving lower pole along with urothelial thickening. There is hepatosplenomegaly with multiple small ill-defined hypodense lesions, retroperitoneal lymphadenopathy (arrow) and ascites

graphy depicts the perirenal extension and other sites of tubercular involvement. The radiological changes described on IVU are usually also seen on CT urogram. With the advent of CT urography (delayed acquisition in excretory phase), CT is emerging as the investigation of choice for comprehensive evaluation of suspected EPTB. Coalescence of TB granulomas in the renal parenchyma may lead to formation of hypodense mass lesions. Cavitation within the renal parenchyma is seen as irregular hypodense lesions showing irregular pooling of contrast on delayed phase CT urogram images and may be seen to communicate with a deformed calyx. Papillary necrosis is also well seen on multidetector CT (MDCT) coronal projection images. Multidetector CT is a better modality to demonstrate ureteric involvement and may show periureteric

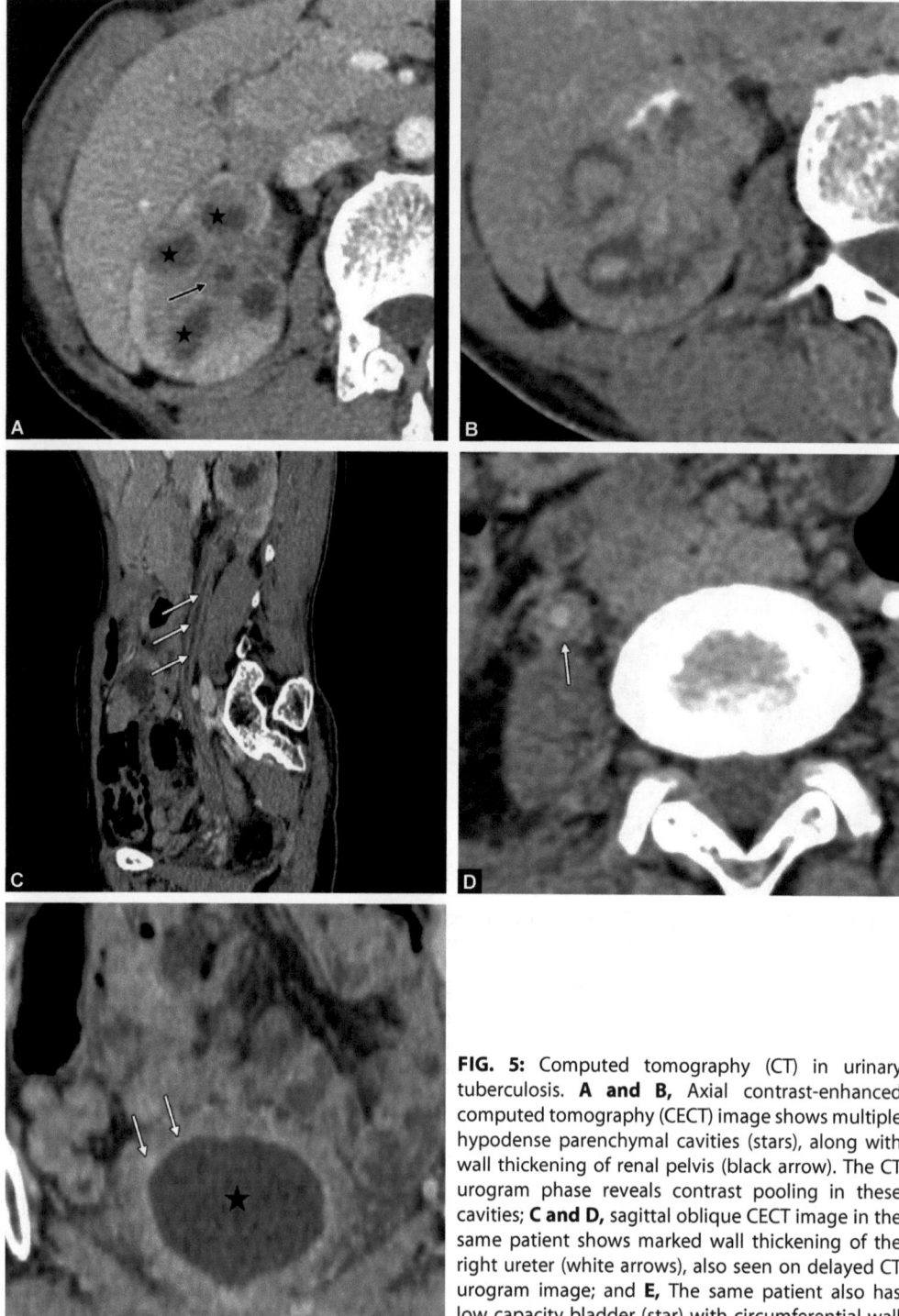

FIG. 5: Computed tomography (CT) in urinary tuberculosis. **A and B,** Axial contrast-enhanced computed tomography (CECT) image shows multiple hypodense parenchymal cavities (stars), along with wall thickening of renal pelvis (black arrow). The CT urogram phase reveals contrast pooling in these cavities; **C and D,** sagittal oblique CECT image in the same patient shows marked wall thickening of the right ureter (white arrows), also seen on delayed CT urogram image; and **E,** The same patient also has low capacity bladder (star) with circumferential wall thickening (white arrows)

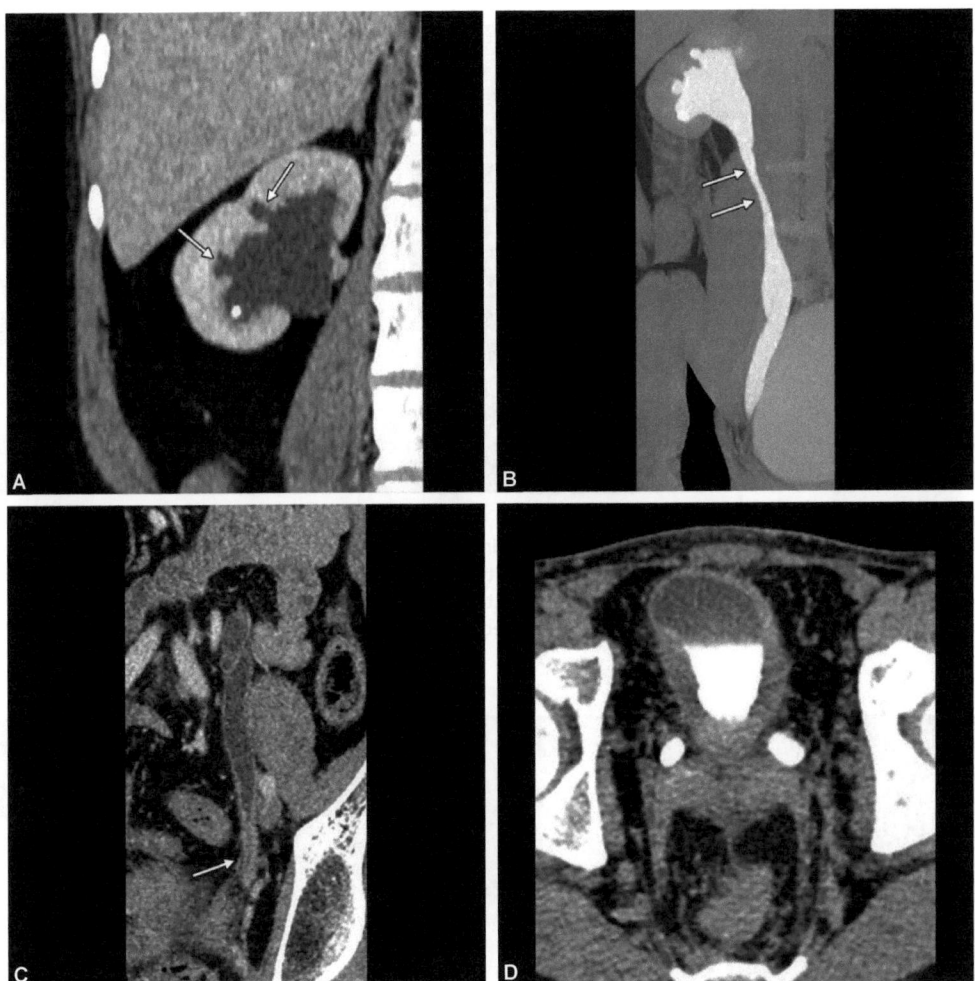

FIG. 6: Computed tomography in urinary tuberculosis (TB). **A,** Coronal contrast-enhanced computed tomography image in a patient with renal TB shows moderate hydronephrosis with irregular walls, tiny calculus and parenchymal cavities (arrows), communicating with pelvicalyceal system; **B,** maximum intensity projection image of delayed urogram phase also shows persistent mid-ureteric narrowing (arrows). Also there was narrowing at right vesicoureteric junction with dilatation of the intervening ureteric segment; **C,** another patient shows wall thickening of left lower ureter (arrow) with proximal dilatation; and **D,** different patient shows thimble bladder with dilated lower ureters

inflammatory changes and better depict wall thickening. Computed tomography is a highly sensitive imaging modality to detect urothelial thickening, an important characteristic of tubercular involvement. Calcification of the ureteric wall is also pathognomonic of tubercular involvement. The MDCT urography nicely delineates "thimble bladder" and early calcification. The MDCT is also an excellent modality to evaluate retroperitoneal lymph nodes in genitourinary TB (GUTB) and associated involvement of lung, vertebra, and other abdominal organs

- Magnetic resonance and magnetic resonance urography (Fig. 8): Though literature is sparse on the use of magnetic resonance imaging (MRI) in UGTB, it has potential to provide both structural and functional information without involving radiation.

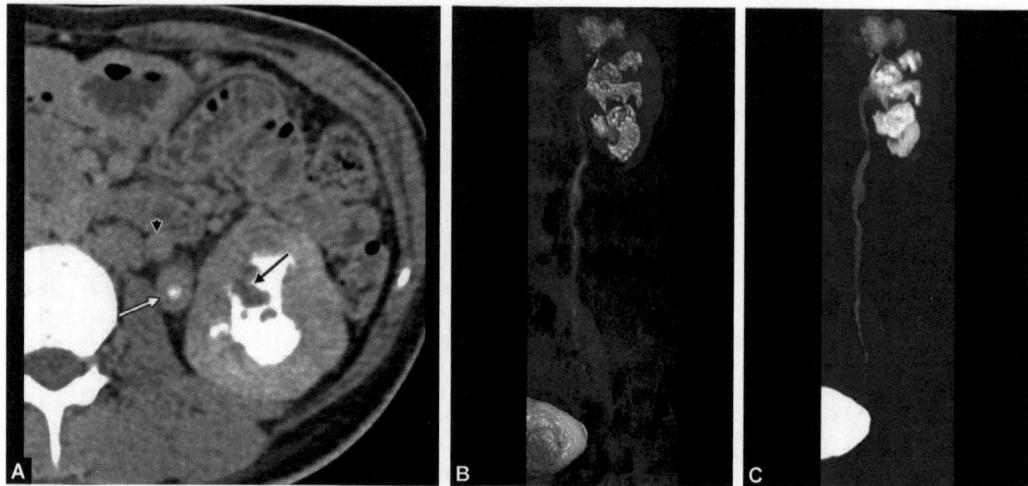

FIG. 7: Computed tomography (CT) urography. **A,** Axial urogram phase CT image demonstrates left hydronephrosis with irregular margins, hypodense filling defects (due to papillary sloughing) (black arrow), ureteric wall thickening (white arrow) and left paraaortic lymph node (black arrow head); **B,** coronal volume rendered image; and **C,** thick maximum intensity projection image better demonstrate irregular caliectasis with debris and multiple ureteric strictures resulting in beaded appearance *(For color version, see Plate 12)*

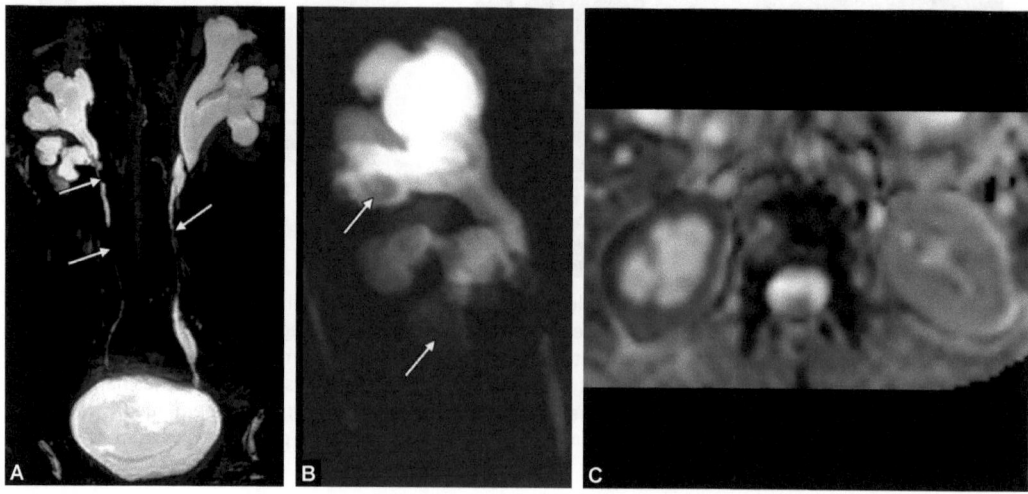

FIG. 8: Maximum intensity projection (MIP) in urinary tract tuberculosis (TB). **A,** Thick MIP generated from three dimensional restore sequence (magnetic resonance urogram) depicts bilateral hydronephrosis with multiple ureteric strictures (arrows); **B,** projectional magnetic resonance urogram image shows debris in the dilated calyces of right kidney (white arrows) as a result of papillary necrosis; and **C,** different patient with history of renal TB (right side), (post-treatment) axial apparent diffusion coefficient (ADC) map shows reduced ADC values of renal parenchyma of right kidney (suggested by dark signal) along with atrophy, suggesting renal parenchymal disease

The MR urography enables demonstration of PCS abnormalities without radiation and contrast. Heavily T2-weighted (T2W) images are the most commonly employed method of static urogram and are useful in demonstration of PCS, ureters and bladder lumen. Depending on the degree of caseation and calcification, the tuberculous parenchymal lesions can have variable signal intensity. Diffusion-weighted imaging (DWI) is a useful adjunct to conventional sequences and shows restricted diffusion in areas of abscess formation, pyonephrosis, and fibrosis. Contrast-enhanced MRI (CEMRI) along with delayed phase imaging provides functional information as well.

Box 1 summarizes the imaging features of urinary tract involvement by TB. Thus, TB should be considered in the setting of chronic renal inflammatory disease, especially when there is involvement of the urothelium, renal papillae, and periureteric/peripelvic inflammation.

> **Box 1: Imaging manifestations of TB involvement of KUB structures on various modalities**
>
> **Plain radiograph (X-ray KUB or abdomen)**
> - Renal calcifications in 24–44% of patients
> - Extensive parenchymal calcification (putty kidney)
> - Amorphous, granular, or curvilinear calcifications within the renal parenchyma
> - Focal globular/lobar calcification
> - Triangular ring-like calcifications due to papillary necrosis
> - Mesenteric lymph node and adrenal calcifications
> - Ureteric wall calcification
> - Presence of discrete calculi.
>
> **Intravenous urography**
> - Normal IVU in approximately 10–15% cases
> - Parenchymal scars in over 50% of patients
> - Fuzziness or feathery appearance of minor calyces (moth-eaten calices)—early finding
> - Irregularity of the papillary tips
> - Small cavities in the papillae or medulla
> - Infundibular stenosis and strictures
> - Localized caliectasis or incomplete opacification of the calix (phantom/amputated calyx)
> - Generalized hydronephrosis or caliectasis without pelvic dilatation
> - Sharp angulation of the renal pelvis (Kerr's kink and hike-up pelvis)
> - Dilatation and mucosal irregularity of ureter (sawtooth ureter)
> - Strictures and ureteral shortening (pipe-stem ureter)
> - "Beaded" or "corkscrew" ureter
> - Reduced bladder capacity (thimble bladder) with bilateral vesicoureteric reflux.
>
> *Continued*

> *Continued*
>
> **Sonography**
> - Hydronephrosis with echogenic debris
> - Uneven caliectasis
> - Intracalyceal filling defects
> - Wall thickening of pelvicalyceal system (PCS) (urothelial thickening)
> - Hypoechoic parenchymal lesions
> - Renal calcifications
> - Heteroechoic lesions with punctate calcifications and vascular cutoff
> - Septated ascites, omental thickening and evidence of TB in other abdominal organs
>
> **CECT + CT urography**
> - Renal, ureteric and nodal calcifications, in over 50% of cases
> - Hydronephrosis, uneven caliectasis, infundibular stricture, deformed renal pelvis
> - Parenchymal lesions containing either caseous or calcified material, usually adjacent to PCS
>   - These may have fluid attenuation (between 0 HU and 10 HU), along with septations
>   - Hypoenhancing (between 10 HU and 30 HU)—indicate debris and caseation
>   - Putty-like calcification, between 50 HU and 120 HU
>   - Calculi, greater than 120 HU.
> - Thickening of wall of PCS and/or ureter and/or bladder
> - Parenchymal cavities, communicating with PCS, showing contrast pooling on delayed phase
> - Wedge-shaped areas of hypoperfusion or focal ill-defined rounded lesions (findings resembling focal and diffuse forms of acute pyelonephritis)
> - Cortical thinning—focal or global and parenchymal scarring, perinephric inflammation
> - Fibrotic strictures of the infundibula, renal pelvis, and ureters
> - Dilated ureter with beaded/pipe-stem appearance, periureteric inflammation
> - Thimble bladder
> - Retroperitoneal necrotic lymph nodes, fibrosis and evidence of TB in other abdominal organs.
>
> **MRI + MR urography**
> - Similar to CT, except for calcifications
> - DWI can demonstrate evolving abscesses
> - DWI may evaluate residual parenchyma and serve as a surrogate marker to detect CKD.
>
> CECT, contrast-enhanced computed tomography; DWI, diffusion-weighted imaging; HU, Hounsfield unit; IVU, intravenous urography; KUB, kidneys, ureter, and bladder; MRI, magnetic resonance imaging; TB, tuberculosis

ADRENAL TUBERCULOSIS (FIG. 9)

Granulomatous involvement of the adrenals is frequently bilateral (90%), resulting in asymmetric enlargement of the glands or mass lesions.[1] Tuberculosis and histoplasmosis are the most common causes of granulomatous involvement. Although the contour of the gland may be preserved initially, later on it may be lost. There may be areas of calcification and larger masses may have necrotic centers. Other differential diagnoses of bilateral adrenal masses include metastases and hemorrhage. Tubercular involvement usually results in chronic adrenal insufficiency and in the end stage there may be atrophy and dense calcification.

MALE GENITAL TUBERCULOSIS (FIG. 10)

Clinical Epidemiology and Pathogenesis

The incidence of male genital TB (MGTB) is relatively low and there are difficulties in establishing the true diagnosis. The MGTB is important to detect because it leads to infertility, if left untreated. Besides, isolated TB epididymo-orchitis may mimic testicular cancer. The MGTB is associated with renal TB in two-third cases or with pulmonary TB in one-third cases, so plain chest radiography, IVU, and ultrasonography (USG) of the urinary tract should be performed on every patient.[11] The most common

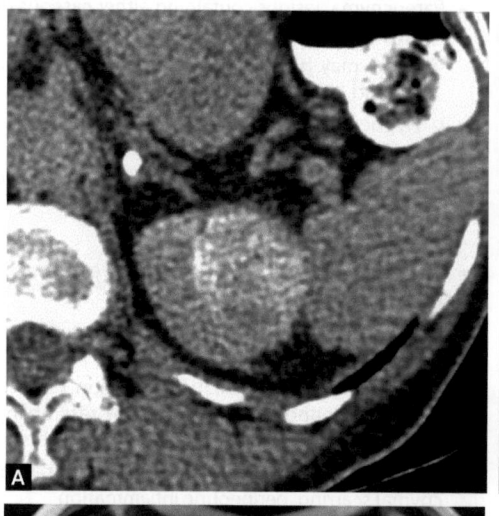
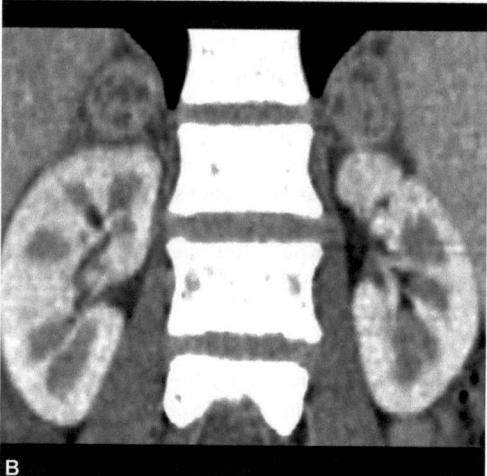
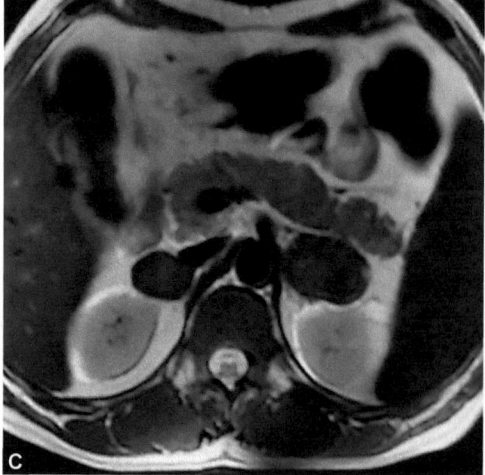

FIG. 9: Imaging in adrenal tuberculosis (TB). **A,** A 30-year-old female patient with history of taking antituberculosis therapy for disseminated Koch's shows punctate calcification in left adrenal, suggesting sequelae of TB; **B,** Another patient shows heterogeneously enhancing bilateral adrenal masses. Biopsy revealed TB; and **C,** A 29-year-old male patient with chronic adrenal insufficiency was found to have well-defined masses in both adrenals, hypointense on T2W sequence, indicating granulomatous involvement

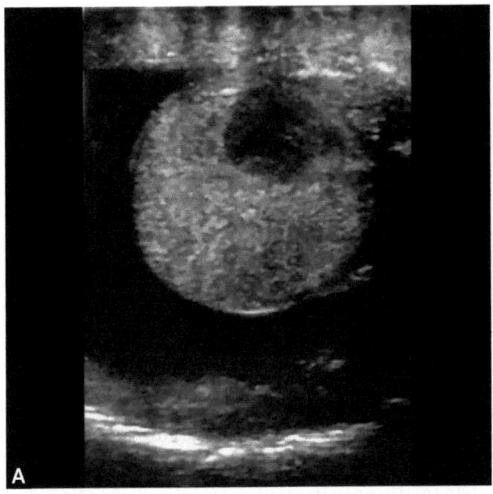 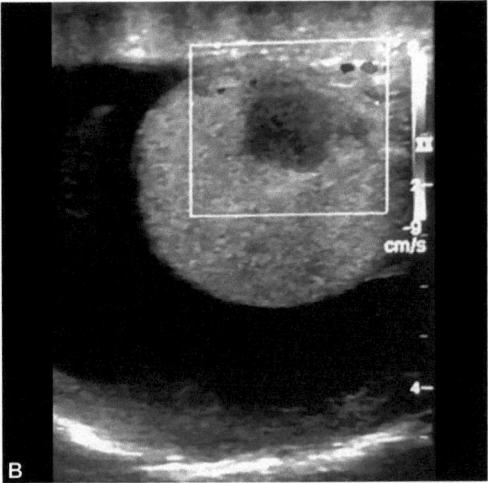

FIG. 10: Imaging in male genital tract tuberculosis. **A,** Gray-scale sonography image shows hypoechoic lesion in the right testis with hydrocele; and **B,** no significant vascularity is seen within. Ultrasonography-guided fine-needle aspiration cytology revealed necrosis with epithelioid cell granulomas, suggestive of tuberculous orchitis

sites for MGTB are the epididymis and the prostate, followed by the seminal vesicles and testicles.[12] Epididymis is usually involved via hematogenous spread of infection. Infection of the male genitalia is also believed to originate from renal foci. Hematogenous spread to these sites is also possible in cases of miliary infection. Tuberculosis epididymo-orchitis may occur following intravesical bacillus Calmette-Guérin (BCG) therapy for urothelial cancer of the bladder. Testicular involvement is usually the result of direct extension from the epididymis and scrotal involvement suggests extratesticular extension of the disease process.[13] In prostate TB, hematogenous spread is more frequent than through the urinary/genital system.[14] If the epididymal infection is extensive and abscess formation occurs, it can rupture through the scrotal skin, giving rise to a permanent sinus.

Acute infection of epididymis and testicles presents as a painful scrotal mass, which initially cannot be distinguished clinically from pyogenic epididymo-orchitis. Recurrent hematospermia though rare, should raise suspicion of TB epididymo-orchitis.[15] Also infertility may occur due to obstruction of the epididymis or vas deferens. Prostate TB is usually asymptomatic and sometimes, the diagnosis is made after histopathological examination (HPE) of transurethral resection of the prostate chips.[16] It may present with symptoms such as, dysuria, frequency, hematuria, and hematospermia. Penile TB is rare and presents as ulcer on the glans or skin.

Imaging Diagnosis

Confirmation of the MGTB diagnosis may be made by detection of AFB or positive cultures from pus or biopsy specimens or by demonstration of caseating granulomas on histology. Ultrasonography has traditionally been the diagnostic method of choice for investigation of TB epididymo-orchitis. However, the appearance mimics bacterial epididymo-orchitis. It may appear as homogeneous or heterogeneously hypoechoic lesions (Fig. 10).[17] Tuberculosis leads to chronic epididymo-orchitis which is seen as enlargement and heterogeneity of epididymis and testis. On transrectal USG, prostatic disease may appear as irregular hypoechoic lesions in the peripheral zone.[1]

On contrast-enhanced CT scan, TB of the prostate or seminal vesicles can be seen as low attenuating peripheral enhancing lesions due to necrosis and caseation, with or without calcification.[8] Tuberculosis may involve the prostate gland in men where it can cause chronic prostatitis and abscesses. The former manifests as nonspecific enlargement and heterogeneity of the gland, while latter is seen as rim-enhancing fluid collection which can extend into periurethral and periprostatic regions. Areas of abscess formation appear hypoechoic on transrectal sonography.

Magnetic resonance imaging of the prostate shows diffuse radiating streaky low signal intensity lesion (watermelon skin sign) on T2W images and may be specific for TB of the prostate.[18] Tuberculosis epididymo-orchitis presents as low signal intensity on T2WI sequence (due to chronic inflammation or fibrosis), and high signal intensity on T1WI sequence in most cases.[19,20] However, this appearance is nonspecific. Similarly, seminal vesicles may also be involved, and there may be enlargement with loss of normal fluid signal intensity. Later on, there may be dystrophic calcification in the involved structures.

Urethral involvement is uncommon, manifests as strictures commonly involving the bulbomembranous junction. Periurethral abscess and fistulas may also be seen.

FEMALE GENITAL TUBERCULOSIS (FIG. 11)

Clinical Epidemiology and Pathogenesis

The history of female genital TB (FGTB) dates back to 1943 with the accidental finding of tuberculous lesions by Sutherland in specimens of endometrium, obtained during routine investigations for sterility and menstrual disorders. Female genital TB is a common type of EPTB in India and constitutes 9–19% cases.[21] The exact incidence of FGTB is not known due to underreporting as it frequently presents without symptoms, requiring high index of suspicion for diagnosis. Involvement of the female genital tract can occur via dissemination from the fallopian tubes or via ascending infection. The most common site of involvement is the fallopian tube, followed by uterus.[22] The FGTB produces devastating effects by causing irreversible damage to fallopian tubes which is difficult to cure both by medical and surgical methods.[23] The FGTB poses a diagnostic dilemma because of its varied clinical presentations and lack of sensitive and specific diagnostic methods. The fallopian tubes and endometrium are the prime sites of involvement.[24] Menstrual symptoms are the most common presentation of genital TB followed by infertility.

Imaging Diagnosis

One-third to half of the patients of genital TB have positive findings on CXR. These findings may suggest active disease but more frequently represent sequelae of old infection. Hysterosalpingography (HSG) is the investigation of choice for evaluation of tubal patency in patients presenting with infertility. Bilateral salpingitis usually presents with infertility and is commonly due to hematogenous dissemination of infection.[1,9] Findings in TB salpingitis include tubal block, strictures, hydrosalpinx, rigid pipe-stem tube and loculated spill of contrast (due to peritubal adhesions). Involvement of the fallopian tube and adnexa commonly gives rise to complex tubo-ovarian (TO) mass lesions and dilated tubes (filled with pus—pyosalpinx or secretions—hydrosalpinx). The latter is seen as a tubular anechoic or hypoechoic aperistaltic channel with incomplete septations on sonography. The TO masses are seen as unilocular/multilocular cystic lesions with peripheral contrast enhancement on enhanced CT or MRI. The MRI better demonstrates involvement of the tubes and fluid component of TO abscesses shows restricted diffusion on DWI. Fluorodeoxyglucose-positron emission tomography (FDG-PET)/CT may be a useful investigation in detecting the presence, laterality and activity of tubercular TO masses.

Tuberculosis endometritis manifests as mucosal irregularity and narrowing of the endometrium which in the later stages may give rise adhesions (Asherman syndrome) and T-shaped narrowed and distorted endometrial cavity on HSG.[25]

UROGENITAL TUBERCULOSIS IN IMMUNOCOMPROMISED HOST

Immunocompromised patients usually present with predominance of systemic features.

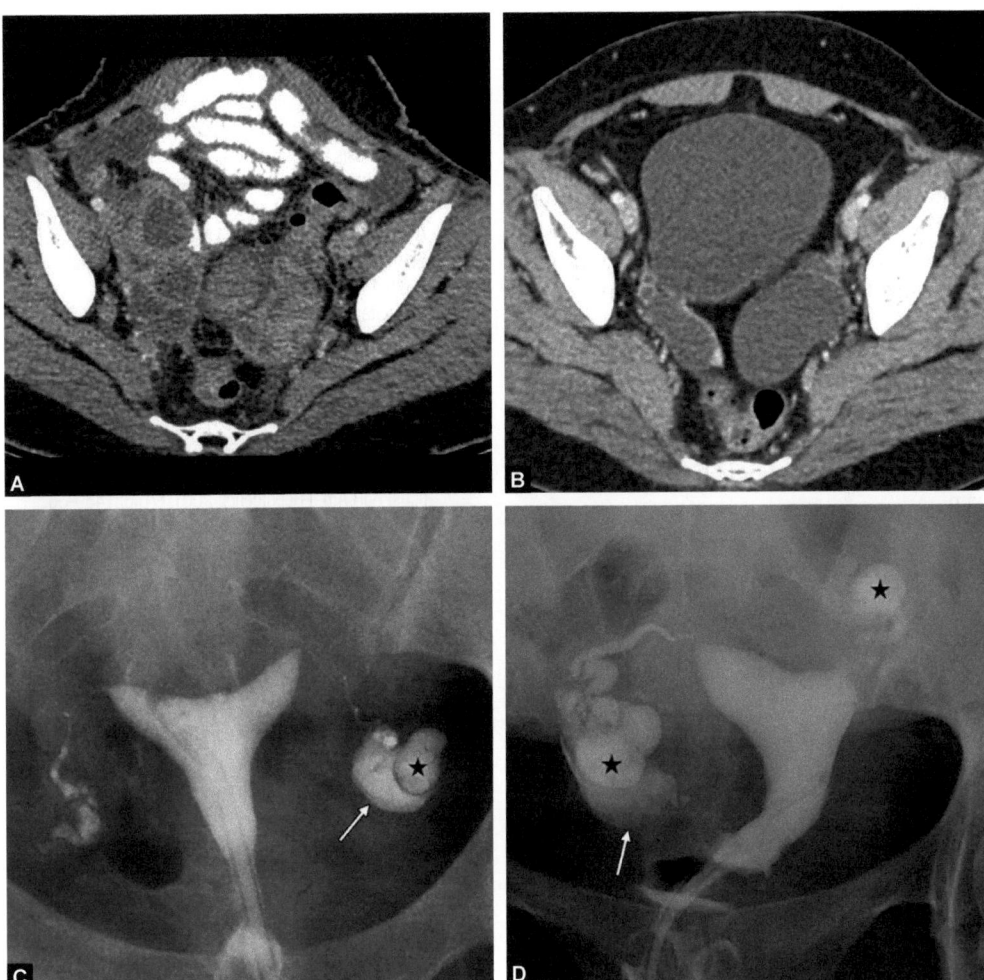

FIG. 11: Imaging in female genital tract tuberculosis. **A,** Axial contrast-enhanced computed tomography (CECT) image depicts bilateral multilocular cystic mass lesions in a young female presenting with infertility, along with ascites. Aspiration revealed necrosis with acid-fast bacilli; **B,** axial CECT image in a different patient shows fluid attenuation tubular structures in pelvis, corresponding to bilateral hydrosalpinx; **C,** another patient who underwent hysterosalpingography (HSG) for secondary infertility, shows right-sided tubal block, loculated spill (arrow) on left side (suggesting peritubal adhesions) and left hydrosalpinx (star); and **D,** a different patient on HSG demonstrates bilateral hydrosalpinx (star), right-sided loculated spill and no contrast spill on left side

Caseous changes and collecting system involvement is less frequent.[26] Hematogenous dissemination is more severe, leading to multiple foci of parenchymal involvement and miliary dissemination. The most common causative organism of kidney and urinary tract TB is the *Mycobacterium tuberculosis*, and occasionally *Mycobacterium bovis* can also be responsible. The MTB has an important impact on kidney transplant recipients, particularly during the 1st year after surgery. Tuberculosis of the urinary tract is easily overlooked and thus late diagnosis results in greater morbidity. Thus TB in immunocompromised host behaves as severe bacterial infection with hematogenous dissemination and multisystem involvement. Few studies[27] have however found no significant difference in the clinical presentation or mortality of GUTB in those affected with human immunodeficiency virus (HIV) and the rest.

CONCLUSION

Genitourinary TB is often difficult to diagnose and the only positive finding on laboratory evaluation may be sterile pyuria. The wide variety of imaging modalities provides a viable option to detect the disease early and to differentiate from other differential diagnoses. The increasing incidence of this disease across all age groups and irrespective of immune status makes TB a universal concern. The clinical profile of recurrent or persistent urinary tract infections that do not respond to conventional antibiotic therapy, accompanied with imaging evidence of urothelial/renal calcification and deformity of the collecting system, should lead one to suspect UGTB.

REFERENCES

1. Engin G, Acunaş B, Acunaş G, et al. Imaging of extrapulmonary tuberculosis. Radiographics. 2000;20(2):471-88.
2. Harisinghani MG, McLoud TC, Shepard JA, et al. Tuberculosis from head to toe. Radiographics. 2000;20(2):449-70.
3. Merchant S, Bharati A, Merchant N. Tuberculosis of the genitourinary system-Urinary tract tuberculosis: Renal tuberculosis-Part I. Indian J Radiol Imaging. 2013;23(1):46-63.
4. Burrill J, Williams CJ, Bain G, et al. Tuberculosis: a radiologic review. Radiographics. 2007;27(5):1255-73.
5. Matos MJ, Bacelar MT, Pinto P, et al. Genitourinary tuberculosis. Eur J Radiol. 2005;55(2):181-7.
6. Rui X, Li XD, Cai S, et al. Ultrasonographic diagnosis and typing of renal tuberculosis. Int J Urol. 2008;15(2):135-9.
7. Brennan RE, Pollack HM. Nonvisualized ("phantom") renal calyx: causes and radiological approach to diagnosis. Urol Radiol. 1979;1(1):17-23.
8. Wang LJ, Wong YC, Chen CJ, et al. CT features of genitourinary tuberculosis. J Comput Assist Tomogr. 1997;21(2):254-8.
9. Bhalla AS, Gupta AK, Sharma R. Tubercular infection of the urinary tract. In: Khandelwal N, Chowdhury V, Gupta AK (Eds). Diagnostic Radiology: Genitourinary Imaging, 3rd edition. New Delhi: Jaypee Brothers Medical Publishers (P) Ltd; 2009. pp. 120-37.
10. Leder RA, Low VH. Tuberculosis of the abdomen. Radiol Clin North Am. 1995;33(4):691-705.
11. Rajpal S, Dhingra VK, Malik M, et al. Tuberculous epididymo-orchitis treated with intermittent therapy: A case report. Indian J Allergy Asthma Immunol. 2002;16(1):51-4.
12. Medlar EM, Spain DM, Holliday RW. Post-mortem compared with clinical diagnosis of genito-urinary tuberculosis in adult males. J Urol. 1949;61(6):1078-88.
13. Das P, Ahuja A, Gupta SD. Incidence, etiopathogenesis and pathological aspects of genitourinary tuberculosis in India: A journey revisited. Indian J Urol. 2008;24(3):356-61.
14. Sporer A, Auerbach O. Tuberculosis of prostate. Urology. 1978;11(4):362-5.
15. Türkvatan A, Kelahmet E, Yazgan C, et al. Sonographic findings in tuberculous epididymo-orchitis. J Clin Ultrasound. 2004;32(6):302-5.
16. Richens J. Genital manifestations of tropical diseases. Sex Transm Infect. 2004;80(1):12-7.
17. Muttarak M, Peh WC, Lojanapiwat B, et al. Tuberculous epididymitis and epididymo-orchitis: sonographic appearances. AJR Am J Roentgenol. 2001;176(6):1459-66.
18. Wang JH, Sheu MH, Lee RC. Tuberculosis of the prostate: MR appearance. J Comput Assist Tomogr. 1997;21(4):639-40.
19. Michaelides M, Sotiriadis C, Konstantinou D, Pervana S, Tsitouridis I. Tuberculous orchitis US and MRI findings. Correlation with histopathological findings. Hippokratia. 2010;14(4):297-9.
20. Jung YY, Kim JK, Cho KS. Genitourinary tuberculosis: comprehensive cross-sectional imaging. AJR Am J Roentgenol. 2005;184(1):143-50.
21. Goel G, Khatuja R, Radhakrishnan G, et al. Role of newer methods of diagnosing genital tuberculosis in infertile women. Indian J Pathol Microbiol. 2013;56(2):155-7.
22. Wong A, Dhingra S, Surabhi VR. AIRP best cases in radiologic-pathologic correlation: Genitourinary tuberculosis. Radiographics. 2012;32(3):839-44.
23. Varma TR. Genital tuberculosis and subsequent fertility. Int J Gynaecol Obstet. 1991;35(1):1-11.
24. Singh N, Sumana G, Mittal S. Genital tuberculosis: a leading cause for infertility in women seeking assisted conception in North India. Arch Gynecol Obstet. 2008;278(4):325-7.
25. Chavhan GB, Hira P, Rathod K, et al. Female genital tuberculosis: hysterosalpingographic appearances. Br J Radiol. 2004;77(914):164-9.
26. Figueiredo AA, Lucon AM, Júnior RF, et al. Urogenital tuberculosis in immunocompromised patients. Int Urol Nephrol. 2009;41(2):327-33.
27. Nzerue C, Drayton J, Oster R, et al. Genitourinary tuberculosis in patients with HIV infection: clinical features in an inner-city hospital population. Am J Med Sci. 2000;320(5):299-303.

CHAPTER 14

Tuberculosis of Bones and Joints

Mahesh Prakash, Karthik Rayasam

INTRODUCTION

Tuberculosis (TB) continues to be a major health concern in developing nations like India. Global incidence rate of TB has increased because of expanding human immunodeficiency virus pandemic.[1] Musculoskeletal involvement is seen in 1-3% patients infected with TB.[2] Spondylitis is the most common form of musculoskeletal TB and accounts for approximately 50% cases. Tubercular arthritis which involves both bones and synovial joints is the second most common site of infection followed by osteomyelitis.[3] Early diagnosis and timely treatment are essential to avert deleterious joint and bony deformities.

CLASSIFICATION OF EXTRASPINAL MUSCULOSKELETAL TUBERCULOSIS

Extraspinal TB can be broadly classified into four categories as depicted in flowchart 1.

ETIOLOGY

Mycobacterium tuberculosis is the main causative organism. Atypical mycobacteria like *M. kansasii* and *M. avium* complex accounts for approximately 1-4% cases. They produce low virulence indolent infection resistant to standard antibiotics.[4]

PATHOGENESIS

Mode of Spread

Musculoskeletal TB mostly results from hematogenous spread of mycobacterial from primary focus of infection or by reactivation.[2] Direct inoculation of organism into the wound site also results in infection in rare instances.[5-7] Dormant infection can also be reactivated by injuries.[8]

Tubercular Osteomyelitis

Isolated bone involvement is seen in approximately 15% cases, concomitant osseous and articular involvement is seen in 85% cases. Marked inflammation and exudative reaction is seen. Enlargement of the infected focus results in caseation and liquefactive necrosis. Sequestrum and periosteal reaction are not so common as compared to pyogenic infections. Diaphyseal involvement occurs in few cases with associated cortical destruction and formation of abscesses

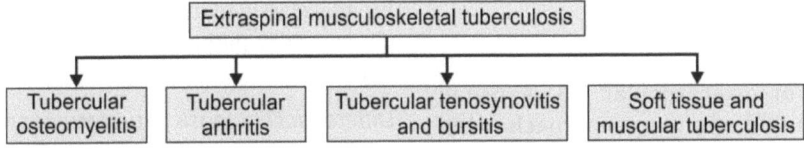

FLOWCHART 1: Classification of extraspinal musculoskeletal tuberculosis

that track along the fascial planes. Plaques of bone and calcification present in the wall of the abscesses/sinus suggest chronic tubercular osteomyelitis.

Tubercular Arthritis

Tubercular joint infection may occur through subsynovial vessels from hematogenous dissemination or from epiphyseal (adult) or metaphyseal (children) lesions that erode into the joint. Pyogenic arthritis rarely spreads through transphyseal route which is typical of TB.[9] Spread of granulation tissue erodes the free margin of cartilage, damaging it, causing its separation from subchondral bone thereby causing erosion of exposed bone and cartilage. These changes appear radiologically as marginal erosions in weight bearing joints, that are characteristic of TB. "Kissing sequestra" is a term described for wedge-shaped necrotic foci on either sides of joint. "Rice bodies" is a colloquial term for foci of necrosed cartilage and fibrin accumulation in the synovial cavity and bursae.

Tubercular Tenosynovitis

Formation of tubercles, caseative necrosis, tendon sheath effusion, and, tendon thickening and rupture are the pathological changes of tubercular tenosynovitis. Synovial sheath infection usually occurs with nontubercular mycobacteria, following surgery and wounds.

CLINICAL FEATURES

Apart from systemic symptoms like fever, weight loss, nocturnal sweating, regional symptoms depends on the anatomical site involved. Tubercular arthritis can lead to pain, swelling, weakness, muscle wasting, and deformities. Tubercular dactylitis produces swelling of the hands and feet. Tubercular tenosynovitis is associated with soft tissue swelling.

DIAGNOSIS

Diagnosis of osteoarticular TB is usually through multidisciplinary approach which includes clinical, radiological, and histological examinations and culture which facilitate accurate diagnosis.

Radiography

Based on the evolution of primary TB, it takes up to 3 years after the primary infection for the development of joint and bone TB.[10] There is a latent period of 3–14 months for the disease to manifest on plain radiographs.

Tubercular Osteomyelitis

Plain film findings include metaphyseal lesions, swelling of soft tissue, limited periosteal reaction, osteolysis/erosions, osteoporosis with minimal or no reactive changes.[11] Sclerosis is less frequently seen. Tubercular sequestra are relatively uncommon.

Multifocal tubercular osteomyelitis

Also known as osteitis tuberculosa multiplex cystica. Multiple skeletal sites are involved in children, whereas single site is involved in adults. On plain radiographs, the lesions are usually lytic, well-defined without sclerosis in children whereas lesions are smaller and may show reactive sclerotic margins in adults.

Differential diagnosis of extraspinal tubercular osteomyelitis

Tuberculosis is often called as "great mimicker" as it mimics wide range of pathologies. The differential diagnosis includes pyogenic osteomyelitis, fungal osteomyelitis, Brodie's abscess and rarely neoplasms like nonossifying fibroma, enchondroma, and bone cysts. Brown tumors, eosinophilic granulomas, disseminated sarcoidosis, cystic angiomatosis, lymphoma, and metastases are the differential diagnosis of multifocal TB.

Plain radiographic views should include routine anteroposterior and lateral projections of the involved region along with additional views depending on the site involved.

Tubercular Arthritis

The tubercular involvement of joints can be broadly classified into following stages based on clinico-radio-pathological features as depicted in table 1.

Differential diagnosis of tubercular arthritis

Pyogenic arthritis, fungal arthritis, rheumatoid arthritis (pauciarticular type), and juvenile idiopathic arthritis.

Table 1: Stages of articular tuberculosis		
Stage	Pathology	Radiological findings on plain film
Synovitis	• Joint effusion • Synovial hypertrophy • Trabecular/bony destruction	• Soft tissue swelling, juxta-articular osteopenia, osteolytic lesions, and feathery sequestrum
Arthritis	• Granulomatous inflammation of articular margins • Cartilage involvement	• Hazy articular margins with washed out appearance • Phemister triad • Juxtra-articular osteopenia • Marginal erosions • Gradual joint space narrowing
Advanced arthritis	• Collapse of bones	• Subluxation, dislocation of joints along with deformities
Fibrosis and healing	• Remineralization occurs	• Appearance of distinct articular margins • Fibrous ankylosis (bony ankylosis is uncommon in tubercular arthritis)

Ultrasonography

Ultrasound can be the first line modality in investigating tenosynovial infections. Ultrasound-guided aspiration/percutaneous biopsy is helpful in differentiating infectious and non-infectious forms of tenosynovitis. Ultrasound is good to demonstrate joint effusions, synovial thickening, cortical bone irregularity, and associated soft tissue changes. It is very useful in regions complicated by orthopedic instrumentation which therefore may not be well seen with computed tomography (CT) or magnetic resonance imaging (MRI).

Computed Tomography

It is of value in demonstrating bony lesions before they are evident on plain films. Computed tomography is more appropriate than MRI in detecting cortical bone destruction and calcification in abscesses.[12]

Nuclear Medicine

Technetium (Tc)-99m-methylene diphosphonate scan may be useful in differentiating osteomyelitis from cellulitis. In patients with osteomyelitis, there is increase in accumulation of radionuclide evident on all three phases of scan. 111-Indium labeled white blood cell scan is also helpful in differentiating cellulitis from osteomyelitis.[13]

Positron Emission Tomography/Computed Tomography

The value of fluorodeoxyglucose-positron emission tomography (FDG-PET)/CT in evaluation of skeletal TB is promising.[14] It is useful in detecting multifocal infection and sites of active inflammation. But it lacks specificity to be used as routine diagnostic tool. It has a potential role in monitoring treatment response, following appropriate period of anti-TB medication, follow-up 18F-FDG-PET/CT can show complete normalization of FDG uptake in the skeletal lesions.[15]

Magnetic Resonance Imaging

Coils and Imaging Planes

Body coil or large field of view phased array coils are used for pelvis and femora and smaller surface coils are used for joints and extremities. Axial and coronal images are used for lesions near hip, foot, shoulder, and wrist. Lesions near knee, ankle, and elbow are evaluated best with axial and sagittal imaging.[16]

Pulse Sequences

In pelvis and extremities, the protocols include T1, short T1 inversion recovery and postcontrast T1-weighted images. Short T1 inversion recovery and T2 fat-suppressed sequences are usually helpful for better delineation of bone marrow edema and fluid collections.

Role of Gadolinium

It allows differentiation of cellulitis from abscess or an abscess from bone marrow edema. Gadolinium enhanced sequences may alone sometimes depict epiphyseal growth plate involvement.[17]

Role of Diffusion-weighted Imaging

Diffusion-weighted imaging (DWI) when used in conjunction with routine MRI sequences can improve the diagnostic confidence levels and aid in further characterization, provide additional information as well as define the extent of the disease. In tubercular osteomyelitis, due to increased inflammatory cells in the marrow, there is bright signal in diffusion-weighted images with a resultant decrease in apparent diffusion coefficient values. On DWI, intraosseous abscess is bright whereas sequestrum, devitalized tissue and air appear dark. Infectious tenosynovitis exhibit diffusion restriction as compared to mechanical tenosynovitis.[18]

Whole Body Magnetic Resonance Imaging

It can be used in suspected cases of multifocal infection.[19]

Synovial Imaging

Synovial hypertrophy is most commonly seen in tubercular arthritis. Synovial thickening is typically iso to hypointense on T2-weighted images but may not be seen in all cases. Enhancement of synovial rim and erosions is seen on postcontrast images. Caseating granulomas give a hypointense signal to synovium on T2-weighted images.

Magnetic resonance imaging can detect bone marrow inflammation, intraosseous abscesses, sequestrum, cortical destruction, cloaca and sinus tract formation.

Differentiation of Subacute or Chronic Abscess from Tumor by Penumbra Sign

It consists of thin intermediate signal intensity rim along the periphery of bone or soft tissue abscess on T1-weighted images. It is highly suggestive of abscess and this finding is related to granulation tissue layer along its wall.

Magnetic resonance imaging is helpful to identify associated joint or osseous involvement in tubercular tenosynovitis and precise extent of soft tissue involvement.

TUBERCULAR OSTEOMYELITIS

Any bone can be affected, usually bones of extremities are involved. Active pulmonary TB is seen only in few patients although a pulmonary focus is very often presumed.

Plain radiographs show swelling of soft tissues, very little periosteal reaction (layered and extensive periosteal reaction may occur in young children with multiple bone lesions or dactylitis), osteolysis with very less reactive changes, periarticular osteopenia, and erosions. Sclerosis is predominantly seen in adults.

The spectrum of radiographic appearances is wide ranging from localized well circumscribed expansile lesion to diffuse uniform honeycomb-like areas of destruction that are usually associated with pathological fractures. Intraosseous thrombosis leads to large sequestra. Tibia is commonly involved (Fig. 1).

Multifocal skeletal TB is defined as osteoarticular lesions that occur simultaneously at two or more locations (Fig. 2).[20] Multiple diaphyseal cystic lesions are seen in osteitis tuberculosa multiplex cystica.

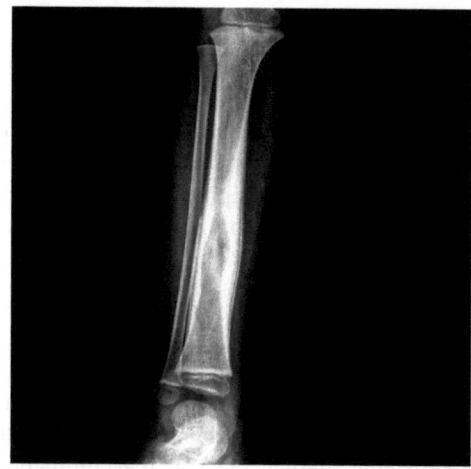

FIG. 1: Tubercular osteomyelitis of tibia. Plain radiograph reveals an ill-defined lytic lesion in the medullary cavity associated with sclerosis and periosteal reaction

Computed tomography and MRI reveal bone destruction along with adjacent soft tissue changes. Presence of eccentric lesion with associated focal breach in cortex with juxtacortical enhancing soft tissue abscesses are strong predictors of tuberculous involvement (Fig. 3).

Multiple fractures, myeloma, eosinophilic granuloma, fibrous dysplasia, chronic recurrent multifocal osteomyelitis are the list of differential diagnoses.

TUBERCULOSIS OF LONG BONES

Long bone involvement may occur in two forms: (i) diaphyseal (cystic type) and (ii) metaphyseal type. Radiologically there is well-defined lesion in metaphysis of long bones and can involve epiphysis and joints. Cystic variety commonly involves children with lesion involving diaphysis with or without its expansion. Sequestrum may be seen in the lesion. Magnetic resonance imaging shows altered signal in marrow with irregular marginated lesion. The lesion may breach the cortex and communicate with soft tissue abscess adjacent to it. Contrast-enhanced images depict the intraosseous and soft tissue abscesses better.

TUBERCULOSIS OF FLAT BONES

Ribs

Ribs are involved in less than 2% cases. Mechanism of rib TB include either hematogenous spread or direct extension from adjacent lymphadenitis or parenchymal lung disease. The

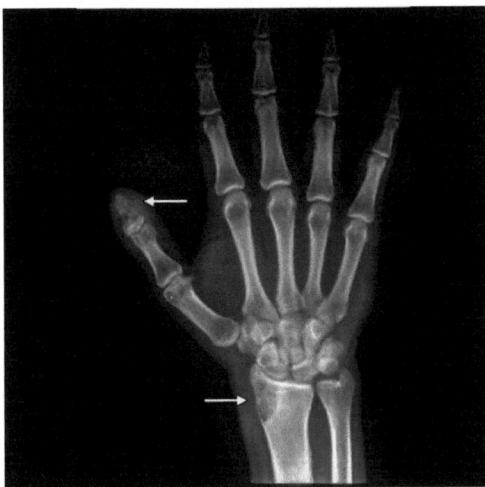

FIG. 2: Multifocal tuberculosis: Plain radiograph shows lytic lesion in the distal phalanx of the thumb with associated soft tissue as well as a well-defined lytic lesion in the distal radius (arrow)

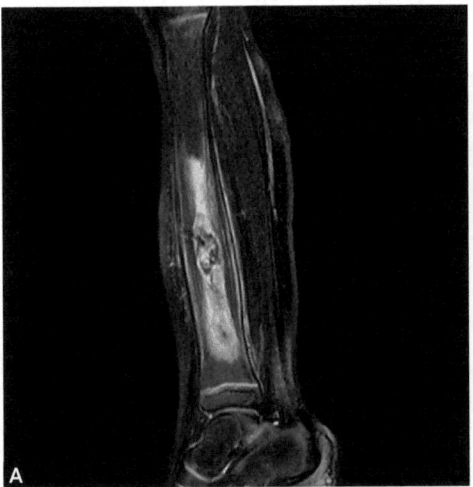 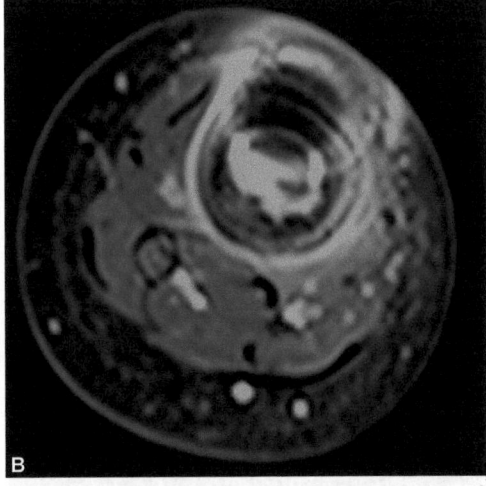

FIG. 3: Tubercular osteomyelitis (magnetic resonance imaging of Fig. 1). **A,** T2-weighted fat-suppressed (FS) sagittal; and **B,** postcontrast axial T1W FS image shows large intramedullary abscess in the tibia with associated periosteal reaction and focal cortical breach in the anterior cortex with juxtacortical enhancing soft tissue collection

location of rib is not classical as any part of the rib may be involved.[21] Bony expansion with ill-defined lytic lesions are seen with associated soft tissue abscesses (Fig. 4).

Scapula

Tubercular involvement of scapula is rare. Any part of scapula is involved by the infection. Plain X-ray may miss the lesion. MRI is useful to detect and characterize the lesion better (Fig. 5).

Pelvic Bones

Involvement of iliac bone, ischial tuberosity, and ischiopubic rami is rare. Radiographs reveal irregular cavitatory areas of bony destruction with little sclerosis or periosteal reaction. Involvement of pubic symphysis or sacroiliac joint can occur. Computed tomography/MRI provide anatomical details about soft tissue lesion/abscesses/fistulous tracts and osseous defects (Fig. 6).

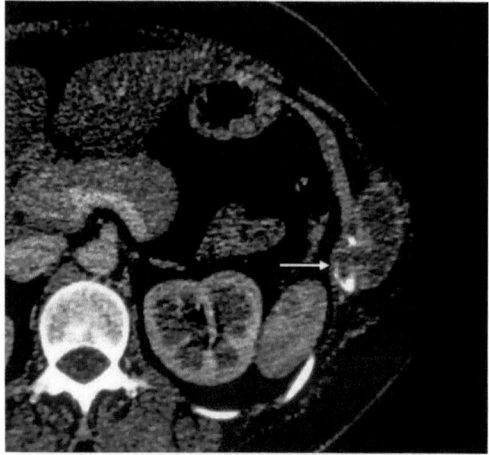

FIG. 4: Rib tuberculosis: Axial contrast-enhanced computed tomography image shows lytic destruction (arrow) in the posterior aspect of left tenth rib with associated peripherally enhancing collection adjacent to it

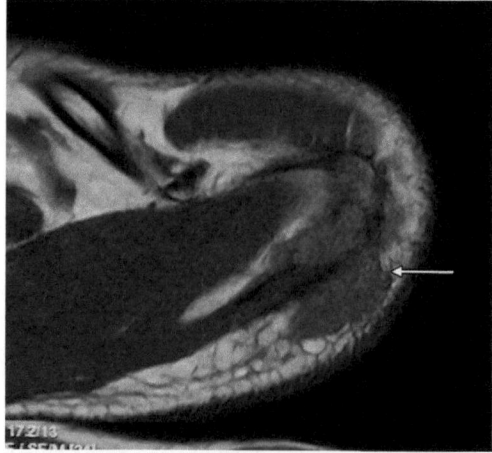

FIG. 5: Scapular tuberculosis: Axial T1-weighted non-fat-suppressed magnetic resonance imaging image shows ill-defined lesion in the superior aspect of the scapula with adjacent soft tissue (arrow)

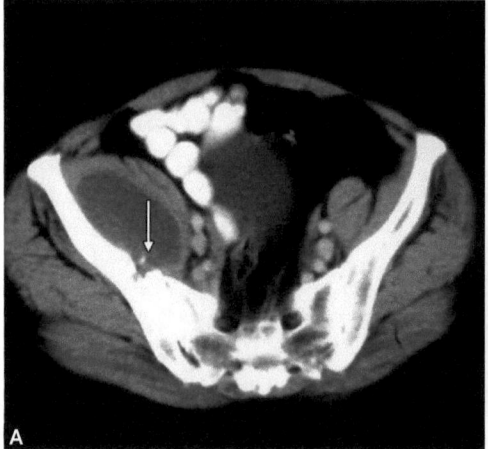
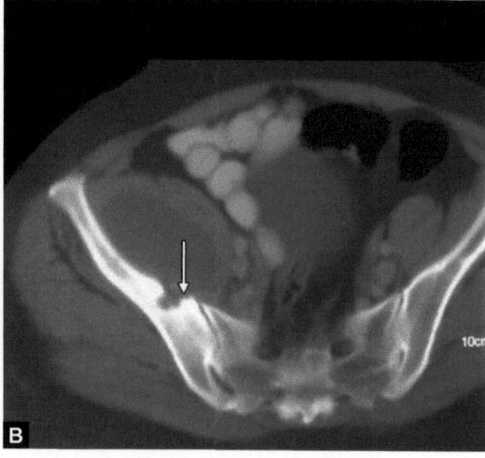

FIG. 6: Iliac bone tuberculosis with abscess. **A,** Axial contrast-enhanced computed tomography images of pelvis soft tissue window; and **B,** Bone window shows well-defined large abscess in the right iliacus muscle with associated small lytic lesion in the ilium (arrow)

Sternum

Isolated sternal TB constitutes less than 1% cases of TB osteomyelitis.[22] Sternal involvement may be secondary to direct extension from lymph nodal disease or as a part of hemato-lymphatic dissemination. Ultrasonography can depict the superficial soft tissue abscess (Fig. 7) and can guide drainage or tissue sampling. Computed tomography scan is used to determine anatomical localization, osseous destruction, and soft tissue abnormalities (Fig. 8). Magnetic resonance imaging can detect osseous and soft tissue involvement more precisely. Complications include fistula formation, spontaneous fracture of sternum, extension of abscess into the mediastinum, pleural cavity, and subcutaneous tissues.

Calvarium

Only 0.2–1.3% of tuberculous osteomyelitis involves the cranial bones.[23] Most cases are reported in children and young adults with male preponderance. Calvarial TB presents as painless scalp swelling, subgaleal collection, discharging sinuses, and osteolytic lesions involving frontal and parietal bones sometimes associated with overlying cold abscess (Pott's puffy tumor). Brain parenchymal involvement as confirmed by CT scan.

TUBERCULOSIS OF SHORT BONES

Tubercular Dactylitis

It is a rare condition that is most commonly seen in children less than 5 years of age.[24] Tuberculosis dactylitis represents 2–4% cases

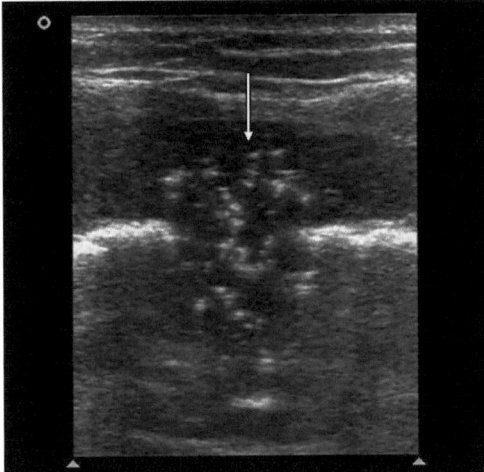

FIG. 7: Sternal tuberculosis: Ultrasound image shows destruction of mid part (arrow) of sternum with associated presternal and mediastinal collection with multiple echogenic foci

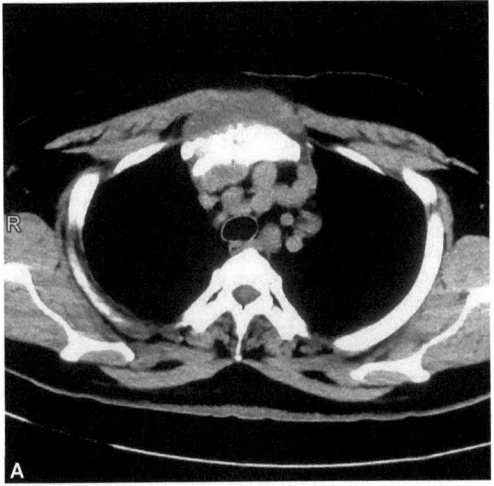
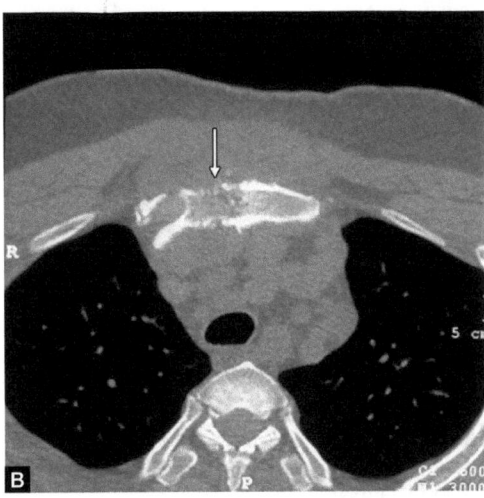

FIG. 8: Sternal tuberculosis. **A,** noncontrast computed tomography (CT) soft tissue window; and **B,** bone window shows lytic destruction involving the right side of sternum (arrow) with associated soft tissue extending into presternal and prevascular spaces. Note made of mediastinal lymphadenopathy

of osteoarticular TB. Bones of hands are more commonly involved than the feet. Proximal phalanges of second and third fingers of hand are most frequently reported locations. There is radiological clinical discordance due to indolent course of the disease. Mono-ostotic involvement is common, but multiple peripheral lesions may occur in 25% cases.

On plain radiography, the typical lesion causes diffuse soft tissue swelling, cystic bone expansion and thinning of cortex leading to classical radiological description of "spina ventosa" (spine—thorn like, ventosa—inflated with air). Associated joint disease is rare.[25]

At an early stage, simple cortical osteopenia is seen. A geode or articular pinching is more suggestive. Geodes are associated with bone destruction, fusiform bony expansion, most marked in the diaphysis. Periosteal reaction and sequestra are uncommon. Enchondroma, osteoid osteoma, syphilitic dactylitis, sarcoidosis, and pyogenic osteomyelitis are differential diagnosis for tubercular dactylitis. Uncommonly the lesions can be eccentric with periosteal reaction mimicking pyogenic osteomyelitis (Fig. 9).

Tubercular Arthritis

Hip Joint

Tuberculosis of hip constitutes 15–20% of osteoarticular TB.[26] The focus of infection may start as extra-articular or intra-articular. Lesions can arise in acetabulum, synovium, femoral epiphysis or metaphysis or spread to hip from lesions in the ischium or greater trochanter. Disease usually presents in the first 3 decades but no age is immune. Pain in the hip region, limp, restriction of movements is present in almost all the cases.

Clinicoradiological classification as proposed by Tuli is as follows:[27] Stage 1 disease is synovitis with joint effusion manifesting as haziness of articular margins and osteoporosis. Stage II disease is early arthritis, there is cartilaginous destruction leading to bony erosions in femoral head, acetabulum or both. Stage III disease is advanced arthritis, there is destruction of articular cartilage, ligaments, bones, and capsule leading to reduction in joint space (Fig. 10). Stage IV disease is associated with subluxation/dislocations (Fig. 11).

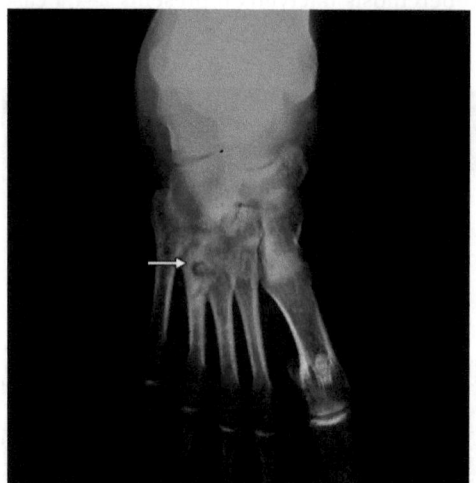

FIG. 9: Metatarsal tuberculosis: Plain radiograph of foot shows lytic lesion in the base of the fourth metatarsal (arrow)

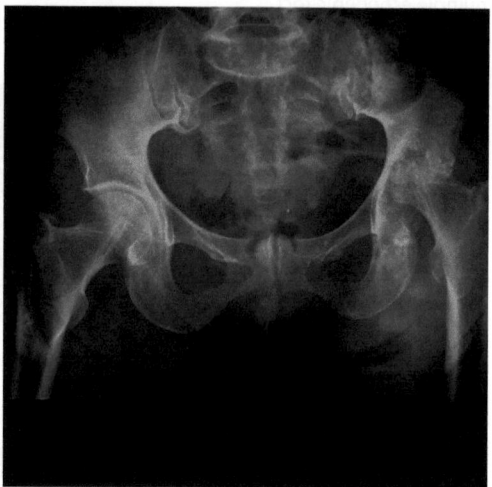

FIG. 10: Hip tuberculosis: Radiograph of pelvis shows destruction of left femoral head, joint space reduction, and superior migration of femoral head and associated partial joint ankylosis

Radiological classification for hip TB on plain radiographs as laid down by Shanmugasundaram is of seven types:[28]
1. Normal (joint space is normal, cysts or cavities in articular bones)
2. Wandering acetabulum (acetabulum roof is affected and proximal migration of femoral head)
3. Dislocating type (hip gets dislocated/subluxated)
4. Perthe's type (sclerotic hip) (Fig. 12)
5. Protrusio acetabuli (medial acetabular erosion)
6. Atrophic type (decreased joint space)
7. Mortar and pestle type (there is destruction of either femoral head/acetabulum leading to marked mismatch of the articular surfaces).

Ultrasonography can detect joint effusion and synovitis. Computed tomography can delineate cortical erosions and lytic lesions before they appear on plain X-ray. Magnetic resonance imaging is sensitive in detecting marrow edema, effusion, synovial thickening, cartilage destruction and soft tissue changes in and around the joint (Fig. 13).

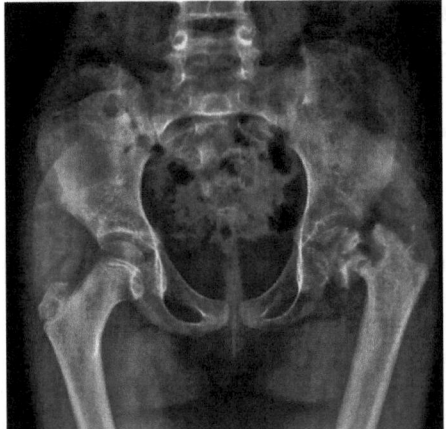

FIG. 11: Hip tuberculosis: Radiograph of pelvis shows fragmentation of femoral head with associated subluxation of upper end of femur

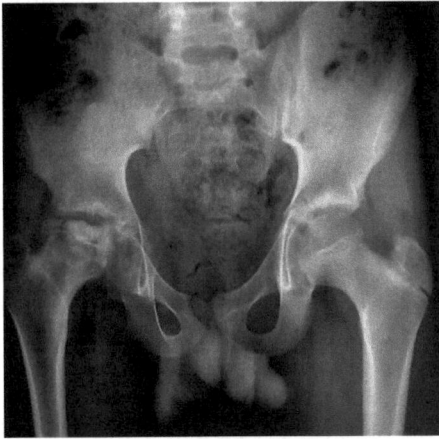

FIG. 12: Hip tuberculosis (Perthe's type appearance): Radiograph of pelvis shows partial collapse, sclerosis, and irregularity of right femoral epiphysis with associated acetabular margin irregularity

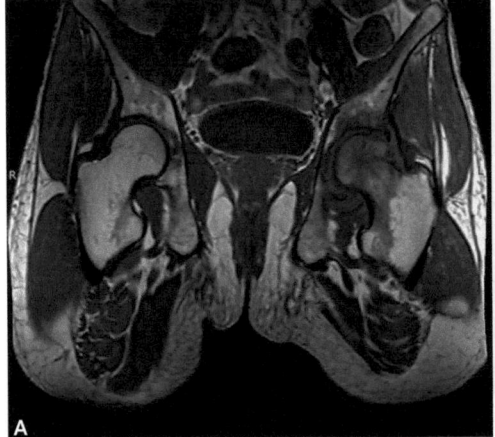
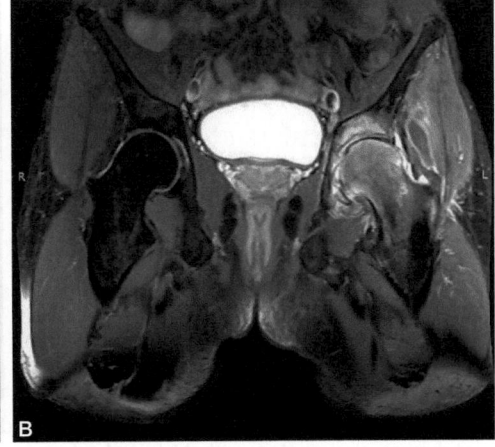

FIG. 13: Hip tuberculosis. **A,** Coronal non-fat-suppressed (FS) T1-weighted (T1W); and **B,** FS postcontrast T1W shows diffuse synovial thickening in the left hip joint with mild joint effusion and altered signal intensity and erosions seen in the left femoral head and acetabulum

Differential diagnosis of tubercular arthritis includes transient synovitis, Legg-Calve-Perthes disease, osteoid osteoma of neck of femur, avascular necrosis, rheumatoid arthritis, and infective arthritis.

Knee Joint

Knee joint is involved in approximately 10% of osteoarticular TB. The focus of infection is mainly synovial with local extension eroding the bone or subchondral bone of distal femur and tibia. Patellar TB is rare and accounts of less than 0.1% of osteoarticular TB.

In synovitis stage, there is joint effusion (Fig. 14), osteoporosis, epiphyseal enlargement (in children leading to growth and maturation) with associated widening of intercondylar notch. Joint effusion can become purulent with destruction of articular surfaces leading to bone erosions and classical Phemister triad. In the next stage, there are caseating cavities with destruction and deformity of joint. Magnetic resonance imaging depicts the articular as well as extra-articular changes very well. Knee is the most common joint where MRI depicts iso- to hypointense synovium on T2W images and provides clues to the diagnosis of TB (Fig. 15).

The differential diagnosis include juvenile idiopathic arthritis, pigmented villonodular synovitis (PVNS), and hemophilia.

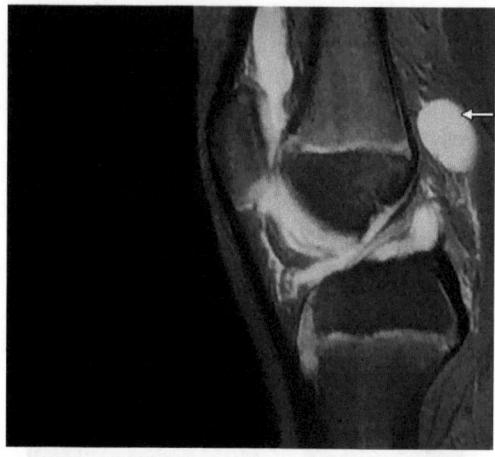

FIG. 14: Knee tuberculosis: Sagittal fat-suppressed T2-weighted images show joint effusion with synovial thickening in the left knee. An enlarged popliteal lymph node is also seen posteriorly (arrow)

Ankle and Foot Joints

Ankle joint is involved in 1–6% cases of osteoarticular TB.[29] Chronic septic arthritis is the usual presentation. Radiographic features appear only about 2–5 months after the onset of the disease.

In the synovitis stage, there is swelling around the malleoli and tendoachilles insertion. Areas of lytic destruction of lower end of tibia and fibula (Fig. 16) are seen. In advanced stage,

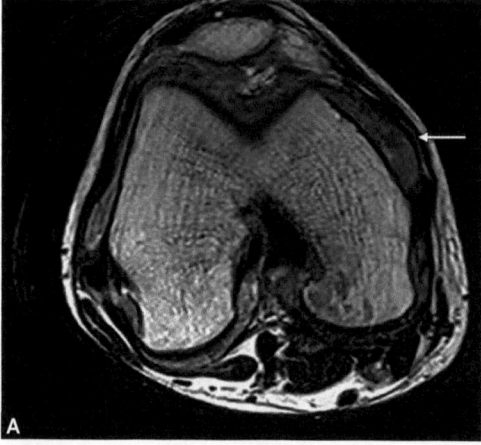
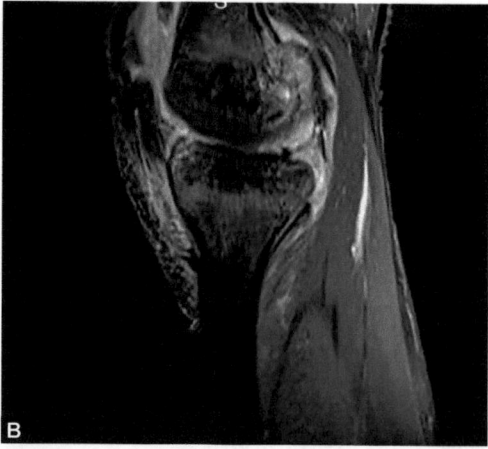

FIG. 15: Knee tuberculosis. **A,** Axial T2-weighted; and **B,** sagittal fat-suppressed postcontrast T1-weighted images show cortical erosions with thickened enhancing hypointense synovium (arrow) and soft tissue changes around the right knee

gross destruction and pathological anterior dislocation is seen.

In the foot region, calcaneum, subtalar and midtarsal joints (Fig. 17) can be affected. Radiographs reveal osteolytic lesion with or without coke-like sequestrum. MRI depicts associated soft tissue changes and abscesses (Fig. 18). Involvement of Os calcis leads to surrounding arthritis of talonavicular and naviculocuneiform joints. Metatarsal bones can be involved leading to tubercular dactylitis.

In a recent study, authors evaluated MRI features in 17 patients with ankle and foot TB.[30] The most common abnormality found was synovial thickening. Signal abnormality was frequently noted in talus bone. Presence of erosions, intraosseous abscesses, and tenosynovitis together on MRI favored a diagnosis of TB (Fig. 19).

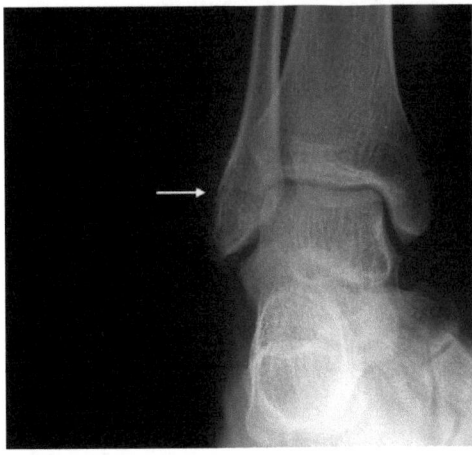

FIG. 16: Ankle tuberculosis: Plain radiograph of ankle joint shows cortical lytic lesion (arrow) with associated periosteal reaction and soft tissue involving the lateral malleolus

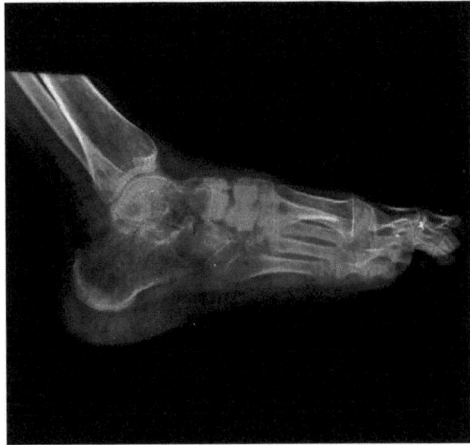

FIG. 17: Midtarsal tuberculosis: Radiograph of foot shows diffuse osteopenia with lytic sclerotic lesions involving the midtarsal bones

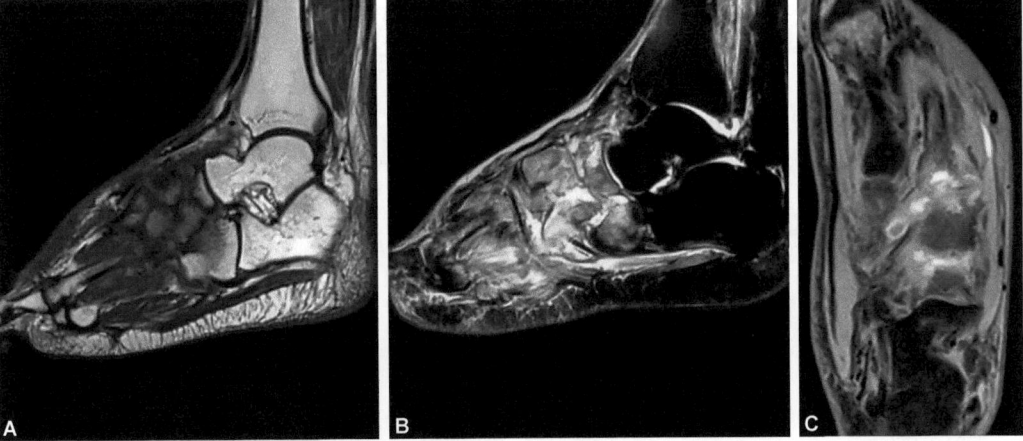

FIG. 18: Foot tuberculosis (magnetic resonance imaging of Fig. 17). **A,** T1-weighted (T1W); **B,** T2W fat-suppressed; and **C,** postcontrast images shows diffuse altered signal intensity involving the midtarsal bones and proximal metatarsals with synovitis and ill-defined enhancing soft tissue extending into interosseous and intermuscular planes

Shoulder

Shoulder is a relatively uncommon site for tubercular infection. In adults, the dry variant (caries sicca) which is associated with numerous pitted erosions in humerus without any collections or abscesses has been described, whereas in children, fulminant variety with cold abscesses and sinuses formation is more common.

The radiological manifestations depends on the stage of disease. In the initial stage, there are articular margin erosions with osteolytic lesions involving the humerus or glenoid or both (Fig. 20). In advanced cases, fibrous ankylosis and inferior subluxation of head occurs.

The differential diagnosis include rheumatoid arthritis, posttraumatic shoulder arthropathy, infective arthritis, etc.

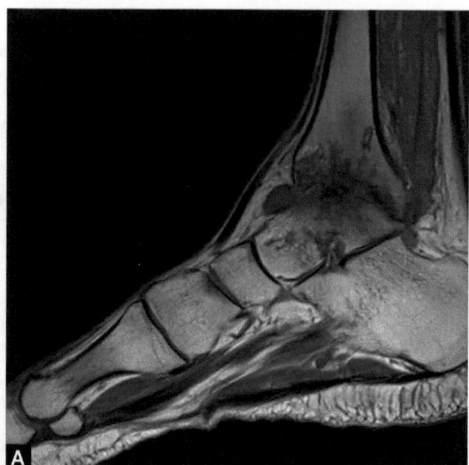
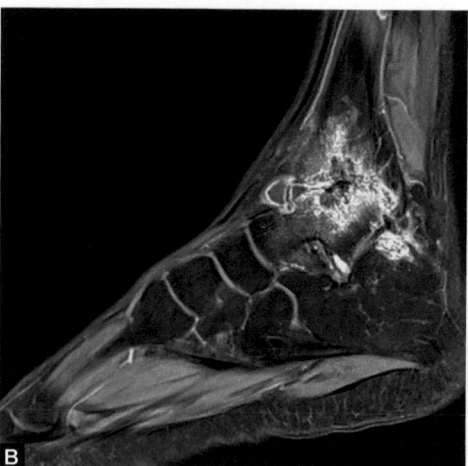

FIG. 19: Ankle tuberculosis. **A,** Sagittal non-fat-suppressed (FS) T1W; and **B,** Sagittal FS postcontrast T1-weighted show advanced arthritic changes in the tibiotalar joint with cartilage destruction, erosions, and synovial thickening with enhancement. Peripherally enhancing collection seen in the anterior recess of joint. Similar changes are seen involving the posterior subtalar joint

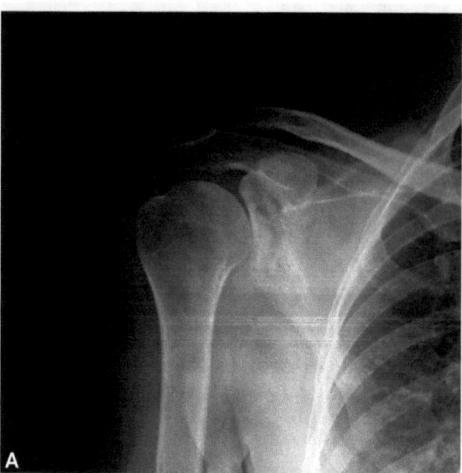
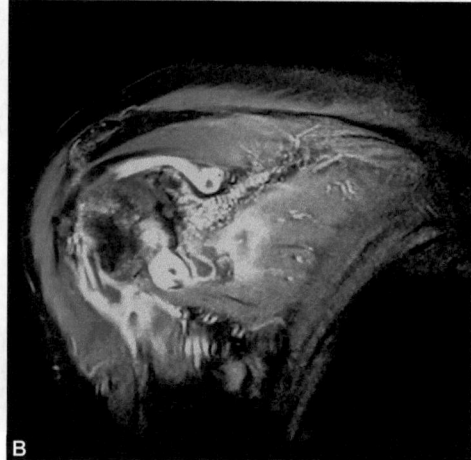

FIG. 20: Shoulder tuberculosis. **A,** Plain radiograph shows ill-defined lytic sclerotic areas predominantly involving the right glenoid fossa; and **B,** contrast-enhanced magnetic resonance imaging shows ill-defined lytic areas in the humeral head and glenoid with marked synovial thickening and enhancing intra-articular collections

Elbow

Elbow joint involvement is relatively rare and accounts for nearly 8% of tubercular arthritis. Clinical differentiation from other causes of monoarticular arthritis particularly inflammatory arthritis is challenging. A female preponderance has been reported in large series. The disease originates in the olecranon or lower end of humerus. Pure synovial involvement is uncommon.

Plain radiographs reveal rarefaction, haziness of articular margins involving humerus, and ulna in articular type while lytic lesions are seen in olecranon process or coronoid process in extra-articular type.

Magnetic resonance imaging reveals flexor and extensor tendon sheath synovial thickening. T2 hypointense synovium is characteristic of tubercular arthritis. Rice bodies are seen as T2 hypointense foci in the joint effusion. Periostitis is a common feature in children and most commonly affects the ulna. Other MRI findings include intraosseous abscesses, effusion (Fig. 21) and soft tissue abscesses. In a recent study, the authors described the MRI features in TB of elbow joint in 14 patients. The combination of bone erosion/synovial thickening, soft tissue/osseous abscess, and T2W hypointense synovium are more suggestive of TB.[31]

Wrist and Carpus

Tubercular involvement of carpus is rare, and the proximal row of carpal bones are involved along with concomitant involvement of tendon sheaths. The metacarpals are usually spared which may be used as differentiating feature from rheumatoid arthritis.

Radiographic features include osteopenia, bone erosions (Fig. 22) or cavitation, gross destruction, and eventual joint ankylosis.[32] Magnetic resonance imaging findings include thickened synovium and tenosynovitis. Enhancement of synovium is seen on postgadolinium images (Fig. 23). Carpal tunnel syndrome occurs as a result of tubercular tenosynovitis. Flexor tendon sheaths and radioulnar bursae have been reported as common sites of tenosynovitis.

Differential diagnosis include rheumatoid arthritis, juvenile idiopathic arthritis, PVNS and nontubercular mycobacterial infections, etc. Hypointense synovium on T2-weighted images along with central erosions, bone chips, and rim enhancing abscesses may differentiate tuberculous arthritis from other types of monoarticular inflammatory arthritis (including rheumatoid arthritis).[33]

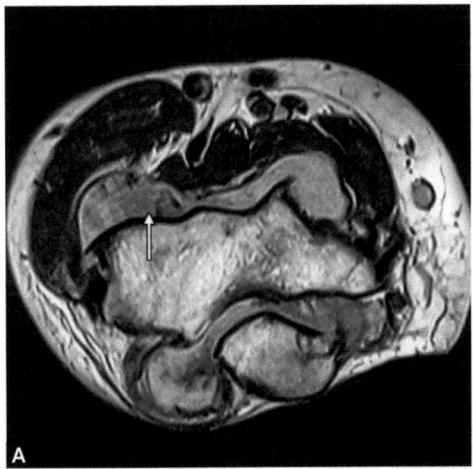 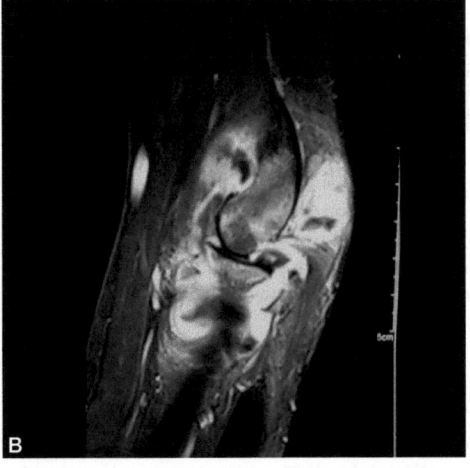

FIG. 21: Elbow tuberculosis. **A,** Axial proton density-weighted non-fat-suppressed (FS); and **B,** sagittal FS T1-weighted postcontrast images show diffuse iso to hypointense synovial thickening (arrow) along with effusion involving the elbow joint. Multiple erosions are seen in humerus and radial head

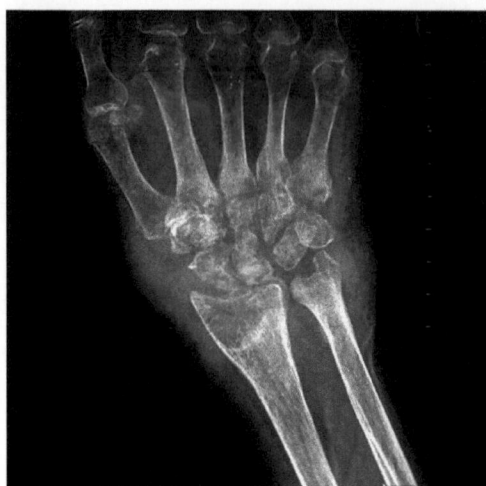

FIG. 22: Wrist tuberculosis: Plain radiograph shows diffuse osteopenia, bone erosion involving multiple carpal bones, and large lytic lesion in the distal end of radius

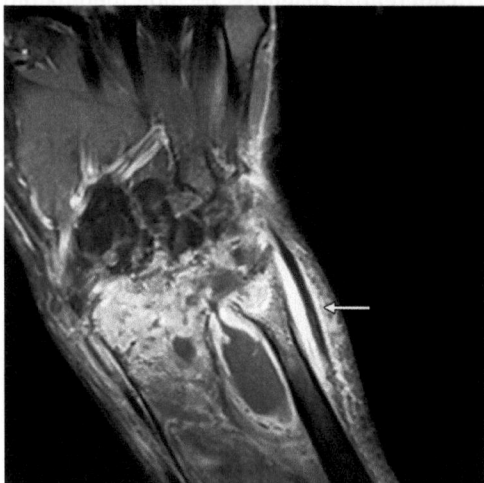

FIG. 23: Wrist tuberculosis (magnetic resonance imaging (MRI) of Fig. 22): MRI coronal T1-weighted postcontrast image shows extensive erosions involving multiple proximal row of carpal bones, distal radius, and ulna with synovial thickening and intra-articular enhancing collection with adjacent tenosynovitis (arrow)

Sacroiliac Joint

Approximately 10% cases of skeletal TB occurs in sacroiliac joint.[34] The joint is a synchondrosis and the hyaline cartilage is thinner on iliac surface which explains the predominance of sclerosis and erosions on iliac side. The disease is unilateral and occurs in young adults, children are less commonly affected.

Magnetic resonance imaging can demonstrate early bone marrow changes, joint effusion, cartilage destruction, deep soft tissue fistulae, sinus tracts, and abscesses. In early stages of disease, capsular distension is evident along with bone edema and lytic lesions. Widening of joint space (Fig. 24) and marginal erosions are seen. Associated periarticular tuberculous abscess can be seen, showing a smooth, thin enhancing rim (in contrast pyogenic abscess possesses a thick and irregular enhancing rim). In more advanced stages, there is joint destruction, sclerosis of margins, and feathery sequestra formation.

Tubercular sacroiliitis should be differentiated from a number of rheumatic and non-rheumatic conditions. Rheumatic conditions most commonly include ankylosing spondylitis followed by other seronegative spondyloarthropathies. Nonrheumatic conditions usually involves osteomalacia, neoplasms, and osteitis condensans ilii. Clinical history and human leukocyte antigen B27 positivity are of value in differentiating TB and ankylosing spondylitis. On MRI, in tubercular sacroiliitis, unilateral joint involvement, presence of blood degradation products, inflammation, necrosis, and fibrosis can be seen which are seldom seen in other proliferative arthropathies. Para-articular abscesses have thin, smooth, and enhancing walls on MRI. In contrast, ankylosing spondylitis shows bilateral symmetrical joint involvement, synovial enhancement correlating with disease

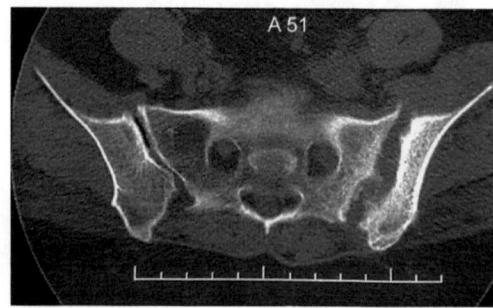

FIG. 24: Sacroiliac joint tuberculosis: Axial no-contrast computed tomography bone window shows widening of the left sacroiliac joint, with articular surface irregularity and erosion

activity, interspinous ligament enhancement, enthesopathic changes along with edema.[35] Definitive diagnosis is however obtained by fine-needle aspiration cytology/biopsy.

Tubercular Bursitis and Tenosynovitis

Primary tubercular tenosynovitis is very uncommon usually involving the flexor sheaths of the hand. It may occur due to hematogenous spread or periarticular extension of the disease.

Synovial effusion is predominant feature of acute suppurative tenosynovitis whereas tendon and synovial thickening are seen in chronic tenosynovitis.

Ultrasound is the first-line modality, MRI better delineates soft tissue, osseous, and joint involvement.

Three forms of TB tenosynovitis have been described:
1. Hygromatous: Presence of tendon sheath fluid without sheath thickening
2. Serofibrinous: Thickening of tendon and synovial sheath with rice bodies
3. Fungoid: Heterogeneous mass of soft tissues involving tendon and tendon sheaths.

Though primary bursitis is rare, secondary bursal involvement is a well documented condition. The bursa of greater trochanter, subgluteal, subacromial, and radioulnar bursae are most commonly affected.

Plain radiography may reveal soft tissue swelling, calcification, osteopenia, (due to hyperemia) and focal lytic bone lesions. On MRI, two patterns have been described—uniform bursal distension (Fig. 25) or multiple small abscesses. The bursal contents may contain T2 hypointense caseous necrotic material and fibrous tissue.

TUBERCULOSIS OF MUSCLES

Musculofascial involvement is usually seen in immunocompromised patients.[3] Muscular involvement usually occurs from local lymph nodal spread or extension of osteoarticular infection.[36] Isolated muscular TB is very rare. Granulomatous inflammation and abscesses

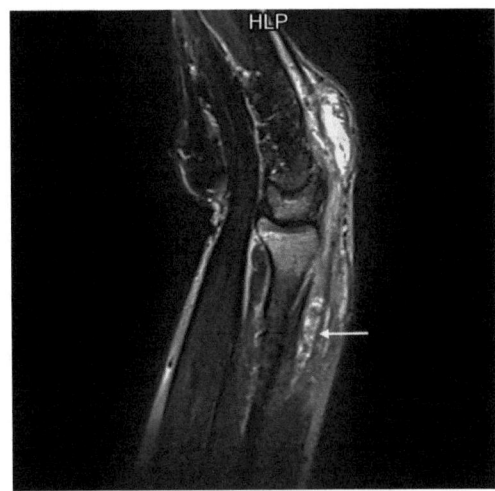

FIG. 25: Tubercular tenosynovitis- Sagittal T2-weighted (T2W) image shows tenosynovitis of the extensor tendon sheath with associated hypointense septae and rice bodies (arrow)

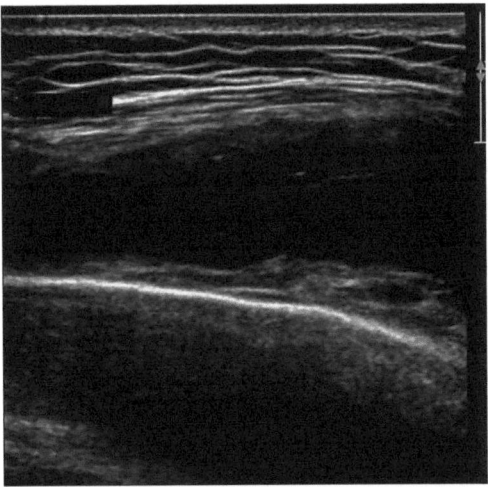

FIG 26: Tuberculosis of muscles—ultrasound image of right chest wall shows collection with septae in the anterior chest wall muscles. Fine-needle aspiration cytology confirmed the diagnosis

are usually seen in the chest wall region (Fig. 26) adjacent to sternum and costovertebral joints. On MRI, muscular involvement is visible as soft tissue mass lesion which is hyperintense on T2-weighted images and shows peripheral enhancement on postcontrast images.

NONTUBERCULAR MYCOBACTERIAL INFECTION

Atypical mycobacterial infections are usually seen in elderly and immunocompromised patients. Involvement of musculoskeletal system occurs in 5–10% patients with atypical mycobacterial infection.[37] Most osseous infections are caused by *M. kansasii* and *M. scrofulaceum* followed by *M. avium* intracellular and *M. fortuitum*.

Preferential involvement of metaphysis and diaphysis, multiple sites of involvement, discrete lytic areas with marginal sclerosis, and less marked osteopenia are the radiological findings.

CONCLUSION

Extraspinal osteoarticular TB involves various anatomical sites. Unfortunately the findings on imaging are not specific in many cases, as TB mimics a wide range of pathologies. Typical radiographic and MRI features in different joints may provide clues in the appropriate clinical setup. High degree of clinical suspicion and appropriate radiological methods are often the first step in diagnostic workup of bone and joint TB.

REFERENCES

1. World Health Organization (WHO). (2009). WHO Report on Global Tuberculosis Control: Epidemiology, Strategy, Financing. [online] Available from www.reliefweb.int/sites/reliefweb.int/files/resources/878BDA5E2504C9F4492575 84001B5E60-who_mar2009.pdf. [Accessed May, 2017].
2. Tuli SM. General principles of osteoarticular tuberculosis. Clin Orthop Relat Res. 2002;(398):11-9.
3. Vanhoenacker FM, Sanghvi DA, De Backer AI. Imaging features of extraaxial musculoskeletal tuberculosis. Indian J Radiol Imaging. 2009;19(3):176-86.
4. Wolinsky E. Nontuberculous mycobacteria and associated diseases. Am Rev Respir Dis. 1979;119(1):107-59.
5. Abdelwahab IF, Kenan S, Hermann G, et al. Tuberculous gluteal abscess without bone involvement. Skeletal Radiol. 1998;27(1):36-9.
6. Dhillon MS, Tuli SM. Osteoarticular tuberculosis of the foot and ankle. Foot Ankle Int. 2001;22(8):679-86.
7. Heycock JB, Noble TC. Four cases of syringe-transmitted tuberculosis. Tubercle. 1961;42(1):25-7.
8. Peh WC, Cheung KM. Progressive shoulder arthropathy. Ann Rheum Dis. 1995;54(3):168-73.
9. Teo HE, Peh WC. Skeletal tuberculosis in children. Pediatr Radiol. 2004;34(11):853-60.
10. Wallgren A. The time-table of tuberculosis. Tubercle. 1948;29(11):245-51.
11. De Vuyst D, Vanhoenacker F, Gielen J, et al. Imaging features of musculoskeletal tuberculosis. Eur Radiol. 2003;13(8):1809-19.
12. Gupta P, Prakash M, Sharma N, et al. Computed tomography detection of clinically unsuspected skeletal tuberculosis. Clin Imaging. 2015;39(6):1056-60.
13. Schauwecker DS. Osteomyelitis: diagnosis with In-111-labeled leukocytes. Radiology. 1989;171(1):141-6.
14. Yago Y, Yukihiro M, Kuroki H, et al. Cold tuberculous abscess identified by FDG PET. Ann Nucl Med. 2005;19(6):515-8.
15. Cho YS, Chung DR, Lee EJ, et al. 18F-FDG PET/CT in a case of multifocal skeletal tuberculosis without pulmonary disease and potential role for monitoring treatment response. Clin Nucl Med. 2014;39(11):980-3.
16. Helms CA, Major NM, Anderson MW, et al. Musculoskeletal MRI, 2nd edition. Philadelphia: Saunders; 2008.
17. Guillerman RP. Osteomyelitis and beyond. Pediatr Radiol. 2013;43 Suppl 1:S193-203.
18. Kumar Y, Khaleel M, Boothe E, et al. Role of Diffusion Weighed Imaging in Musculoskeletal Infections: Current Perspectives. Eur Radiol. 2017;27(1):414-23.
19. Pugmire BS, Shailam R, Gee MS. Role of MRI in the diagnosis and treatment of osteomyelitis in pediatric patients. World J Radiol. 2014;6(8):530-7.
20. Dlimi F, Abouzahir M, Mahfoud M, et al. Multifocal bone tuberculosis: A case report. Foot Ankle Surg. 2011;17(4):e47-50.
21. Asnis DS, Niegowska A. Tuberculosis of the rib. Clin Infect Dis. 1997;24(5):1018-9.
22. Saifudheen K, Anoop TM, Mini PN, et al. Primary tubercular osteomyelitis of the sternum. Int J Infect Dis. 2010;14(2):e164-6.
23. García-García C, Ibarra V, Azcona-Gutiérrez JM, et al. Calvarial tuberculosis with parenchymal involvement. Travel Med Infect Dis. 2013;11(5):329-31.
24. Yochum TR, Row LJ. Infection: Non suppurative osteomyelitis (tuberculosis). In: Yochum TR, Row LJ (Eds). Yochum and Rowe's Essentials of Skeletal Radiology, 2nd edition. Lippincott: Williams and Wilkins; 1986.
25. Sbai MA, Benzarti S, Sahli H, et al. Osteoarticular tuberculosis dactylitis: Four cases. Int J Mycobacteriol. 2015;4(3):250-4.
26. Saraf SK, Tuli SM. Tuberculosis of hip: A current concept review. Indian J Orthop. 2015;49(1):1-9.
27. Tuli SM. Tuberculosis of the Skeletal System (Bones, Joints, Spine and Bursal Sheaths), 4th edition. New Delhi: Jaypee Brothers Medical Publishers (P) Ltd; 2010. pp. 69-110.
28. Shanmugasundaram TK. A clinicoradiological classification of tuberculosis of the hip. In: Shanmugasundaram TK (Ed). Current Concepts in Bone and Joint Tuberculosis. India: Proceedings of Combined Congress of International Bone and Joint Tuberculosis Club and the Indian Orthopedic Association; 1983. p. 60.

29. Samuel S, Boopalan PR, Alexander M, et al. Tuberculosis of and around the ankle. J Foot Ankle Surg. 2011;50(4):466-72.
30. Prakash M, Gupta P, Sen RK, et al. Magnetic resonance imaging evaluation of tubercular arthritis of the ankle and foot. Acta Radiol. 2015;56(10):1236-41.
31. Prakash M, Gupta P, Dhillon MS, et al. Magnetic resonance imaging findings in tubercular arthritis of elbow. Clin Imaging. 2016;40(1):114-8.
32. Hsu CY, Lu HC, Shih TT. Tuberculous infection of the wrist: MRI features. AJR Am J Roentgenol. 2004;183(3):623-8.
33. Sawlani V, Chandra T, Mishra RN, et al. MRI features of tuberculosis of peripheral joints. Clin Radiol. 2003;58(10):755-62.
34. Ramlakan RJ, Govender S. Sacroiliac joint tuberculosis. Int Orthop. 2007;31(1):121-4.
35. Prakash J. Sacroiliac tuberculosis – A neglected differential in refractory low back pain – Our series of 35 patients. J Clin Orthop Trauma. 2014;5(3):146-53.
36. De Backer AI, Mortelé KJ, Vanhoenacker FM, et al. Imaging of extraspinal musculoskeletal tuberculosis. Eur J Radiol. 2006;57(1):119-30.
37. Theodorou DJ, Theodorou SJ, Kakitsubata Y, et al. Imaging characteristics and epidemiologic features of atypical mycobacterial infections involving the musculoskeletal system. AJR Am J Roentgenol. 2001;176(2):341-9.

CHAPTER 15

Cardiovascular Tuberculosis

Munish Guleria, Sanjeev Kumar, Gurpreet S Gulati

INTRODUCTION

Cardiovascular involvement occurs in 1–2% of the patients with tuberculosis (TB).[1] The present discussion is subdivided into cardiac and vascular TB as distinct entities.

CARDIAC TUBERCULOSIS

Tuberculosis can affect all three layers of the heart. Pericardial involvement is the most common, with the long-term sequelae of constrictive pericarditis (CP), usually associated with pericardial calcification. Almost two-third of the cases of CP in India are tubercular.[2] Tubercular myocardial involvement is rare, mostly seen in association with pericardial disease. Isolated myocardial TB happens in 0.14–0.3% of patients.[3,4] Endocardial involvement is extremely rare,[5] as is coronary vessel involvement.[6]

Pathogenesis

Tubercular bacilli spreads to the heart and pericardium by direct extension from the tracheobronchial tree, the mediastinal or hilar lymph nodes, the sternum or the spine. Peribronchial or lymphatic spread can also occur. The spread may also take place by a hematogenous route from a focus in the lung during the primary tuberculous infection.[7]

TUBERCULOUS PERICARDITIS

Tuberculous pericardial involvement can manifest as acute pericarditis, pericardial effusion, cardiac tamponade, and CP.

Classification of tuberculous pericardial involvement:
- Acute pericarditis
- Pericardial effusion:
  - With or without tamponade
- Constrictive pericarditis:
  - Acute, subacute, chronic
  - Effusive-constrictive, pericardial abscess
  - Pericardial calcification:
    - With/without hemodynamic effects.

Tuberculous pericarditis rarely presents as acute condition, mostly in immunocompromised patients and in TB endemic areas. Tuberculosis remains an uncommon cause of large pericardial effusion and cardiac tamponade is distinctly rare.

Constrictive pericarditis is caused by pericardial fibrosis and calcification. Pericardial calcification occurs in about 50% of the patients. This leads to stiff pericardium, restricting the diastolic heart filling and producing right-sided heart failure.

The clinical picture of CP is often nonspecific and can be difficult to differentiate from restrictive cardiomyopathy (RCM), heart failure and hepatic disease. Imaging plays a vital diagnostic and prognostic role in tubercular pericardial disease.

Imaging

Acute Pericarditis

Chest radiograph: Chest radiograph is mostly normal in acute pericarditis. Rarely, cardiomegaly can be present if there is associated pericardial effusion. Pericardial calcification appears late in the course of the disease process.

A left pleural effusion is usually associated with pericarditis, but is a nonspecific finding.[8]

Echocardiography

The echocardiogram may be normal when there is no or little pericardial effusion. Pericardial fluid exceeding 50 mL is considered abnormal and it generally corresponds to a pericardial width of more than 4 mm.[9] Small fibrinous pericardial effusion may be seen as a partially echo-free space surrounding the heart during the acute phase.

Pericardial Effusion and Cardiac Tamponade

Chest radiograph: It is frequently characterized by cardiomegaly, particularly in the presence of a pericardial effusion. A "water bottle" configuration of the cardiac silhouette may be seen (Fig. 1).[10] At least 200–250 mL of fluid must be present for the radiologic appearance of enlarged cardiac silhouette; therefore, the absence of an enlarged cardiac silhouette does not exclude a small pericardial effusion.[8]

Echocardiography

Normally there is absence of the echolucent space surrounding the heart on echocardiogram. With a small pericardial effusion (<100 cc) there is about 1 cm of echolucent space around the heart. With a large effusion (>500 cc), the echolucent space increases to over 2 cm and may consequently be associated with features of tamponade.[11]

The most useful echocardiographic signs of cardiac tamponade are inspiratory shift of the ventricular septum toward the left ventricle, right ventricular diastolic collapse and right atrial compression. Echocardiogram can be used to guide a pericardiocentesis needle for diagnostic or therapeutic purposes.[12]

Constrictive Pericarditis

Chest radiograph: Radiograph is mostly abnormal in hemodynamically significant CP. Cardiac size is usually normal or only mildly enlarged. Characteristic flattening of the right cardiac contour is seldom present. Bilateral pleural effusions are usual. Dilatation of the superior vena cava and azygos vein may be seen.

In cases with left-sided constriction, left atrial enlargement and pulmonary venous hypertension are seen. Frequently, there is upper pulmonary flow redistribution and Kerley B lines may be evident.

Shaggy and thick calcification of the pericardium is usually specific for tubercular CP. Pericardial calcification is much easier to visualize on the lateral projection than in the posteroanterior view and is very evident on fluoroscopy. A rim of calcium appears surrounding the heart, with preference over the right atrium and right ventricle especially right atrioventricular (AV) groove region and the diaphragmatic wall (Fig. 2).[13]

Other probable causes of cardiac calcification to be considered in the differential diagnosis include calcified left ventricular aneurysm, calcified intracardiac thrombus, coronary calcifications and valvular calcifications.[14]

Echocardiography and Doppler Study

The thickened pericardium can be appreciated by echocardiography. Two-dimensional (2D)-echo demonstrates small ventricular cavities, normal systolic function, biatrial enlargement and increased vena cava and hepatic veins diameter. The variation in intracardiac flow velocities yields an expiratory septal bulge toward the left ventricle, fairly characteristic of constrictive physiology.[9]

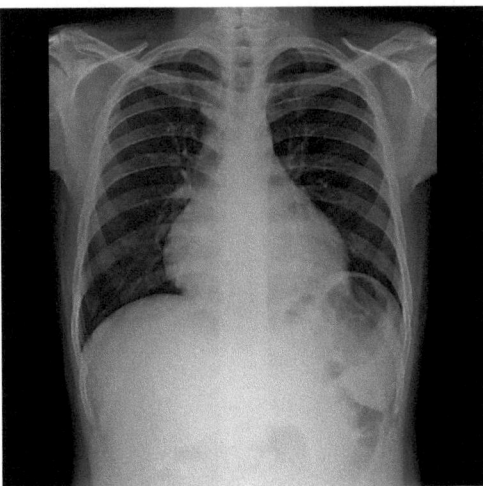

FIG. 1: Chest radiograph posteroanterior (PA) view showing globular enlargement of heart producing typical "water bottle" appearance

Imaging in Tuberculosis: Clinicopathological Correlation

On Doppler study, there are restrictive mitral and tricuspid inflow velocities with respiration. Constrictive physiology is differentiated from the RCM by demonstrating reciprocal respiratory changes between transmitral and transtricuspid flow (or between pulmonary vein and hepatic vein flow) using simultaneous respirometry in constriction. Hepatic veins show decreased diastolic forward flow with expiration and increase in diastolic flow reversal.[15-17] Tissue Doppler may also aid in differentiating CP from RCM, since tissue velocities are usually preserved in the former and impaired in the latter.[18]

Transesophageal echocardiography (TEE) provides an adequate means of detecting pericardial thickening, visualizing right atrial tethering and evaluating the hemodynamics of constrictive physiology.[15]

It is important to distinguish between CP and RCM since the former is treated surgically, while the latter is treated medically. Pericardial thickening can be difficult to detect with echocardiography, and therefore computed tomography (CT) and magnetic resonance (MR) imaging are frequently done to confirm the diagnosis. CT is much more sensitive for the detection of calcium; MR imaging is better at distinguishing between small pericardial effusions and pericardial thickening as well as for evaluation of functional abnormalities.[16,17]

Cardiac and Chest Computed Tomography

Modern advances in CT technology have helped yield images of the heart with high spatial resolution and reduced motion artifacts. Prospectively electrocardiogram (ECG)-triggered or retrospectively ECG-gated multidetector CT (MDCT) is equivalent to cardiac MR (CMR) for demonstrating pericardial thickening and effusion, and is superior for identifying calcification. Nongated delayed contrast-enhanced (CE) CT thorax identifies the associated lung lesions.[15]

FIG. 2: Chest radiograph posteroanterior view showing mild cardiomegaly with curvilinear calcification along the left diaphragmatic surface of heart

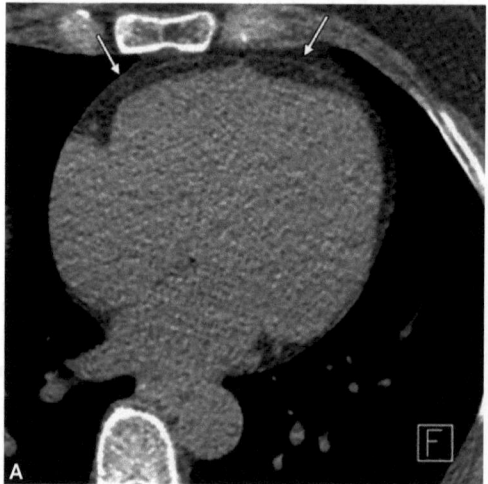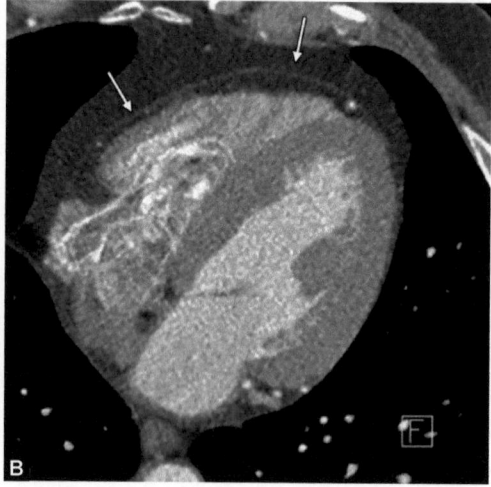

FIG. 3: Axial computed tomography images. **A,** Noncontrast; **B,** contrast-enhanced showing the pericardium as a thin white line between black epicardiac and pericardiac fat (arrows)

The pericardium is typically seen as a 1–2 mm thick layer with a small amount of interposed fluid (Fig. 3). A thickness more than 3 mm is considered abnormal, best appreciated anterior to the right ventricle. Computed tomography can identify areas of the pericardium that are more or less thickened, and as such serve as a tool for surgical planning by helping the surgeon in choosing the optimal surgical approach (Figs 4 and 5).[19]

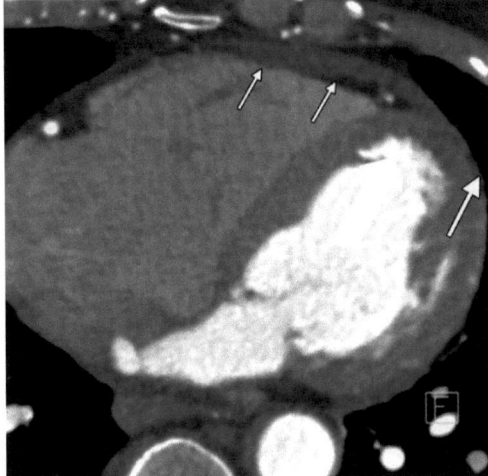

FIG. 4: Contrast-enhanced axial computed tomography image showing some pericardial fluid anterior to right ventricle (arrows) mimicking as thickened pericardium

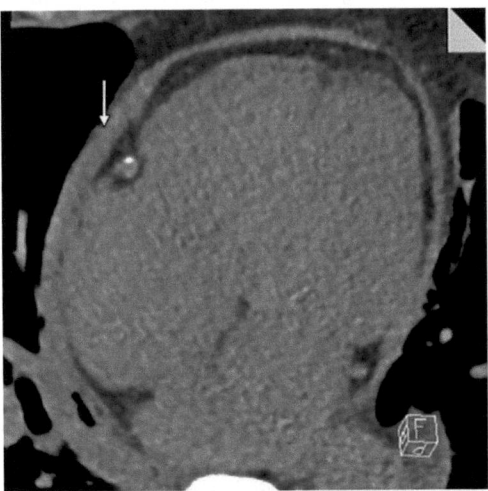

FIG. 5: Thickened pericardium (arrow) without calcification in a noncontrast computed tomography acquisition of a patient with constrictive pericarditis

The calcification has a tendency to be thick, irregular and amorphous, appearing mostly in the AV grooves (Fig. 6). This can be rivaled with the eggshell calcification seen in viral or uremic pericarditis. Calcification is a crucial sign of pericardial constriction, but is not pathognomonic. Pericardial calcification may be present in the absence of any physiologic insult to the heart.[14,19]

Neither pericardial thickening nor calcification in isolation necessarily indicates CP unless accompanied by typical clinical signs. Also, pericardial thickness may be normal in up to 20% of patients with surgically confirmed CP.[20,21]

Tamponade is a frequent complication of TB CP, but patients do well with appropriate therapy; abscess formation is a rare complication.

Limitations of MDCT include the use of ionizing radiation and potentially nephrotoxic contrast media. Also, MDCT offers inadequate functional information and limited tissue characterization.[19] Cardiac MR imaging is better for addressing these issues.

Cardiac Magnetic Resonance Imaging

Constrictive pericarditis is probably the most frequent indication for MR imaging of the pericardium.

Cardiac magnetic resonance includes multitude of imaging sequences done in standard cardiac planes for detailed pericardial and myocardial assessment.

Black-blood sequences comprising of T1 and T2-weighted turbo spin echo and/or fluid-sensitive (double or triple inversion recovery) imaging are used for measurement of pericardial thickness and tissue characterization. Bright-blood cine images are acquired for evaluation of chamber dimensions and functional analysis, diastolic restriction, septal bounce, tubular/conical deformity of the ventricles and myocardial tethering.[18]

Myocardial tagging is used to evaluate epicardial/pericardial tethering and real-time cine imaging is done for evaluation of ventricular interdependence.[18,22,23]

Late gadolinium enhancement (LGE) phase sensitive inversion recovery images are used

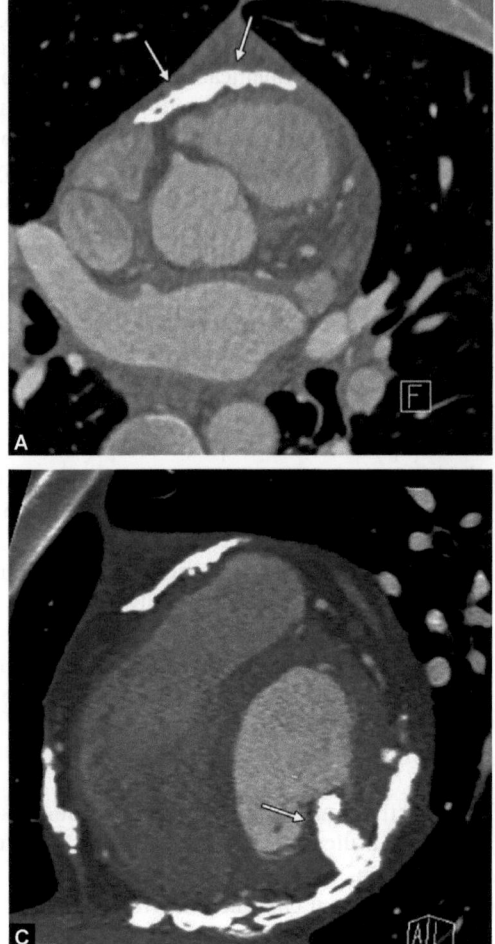
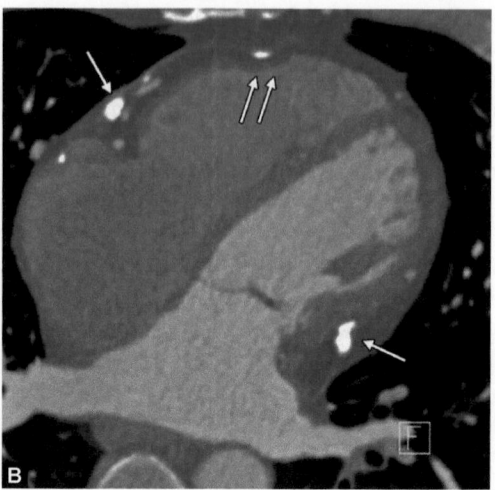

FIG. 6: Pericardial calcification. **A,** Axial computed tomography (CT) section at the level of aortic root showing amorphous pericardial calcification; **B,** axial CT section four-chamber view, discrete pericardial calcification in both right and left atrioventricular groove (single arrow) with impression of the left ventricle (double arrows), indicating the hemodynamic effects of the calcification; **C,** computed tomography scan short-axis view of heart, amorphous irregular pericardial calcification with infiltration of myocardium (arrow)

to evaluate for myocardial fibrosis and inflammation, as well as pericardial inflammation.[18]

Magnetic resonance findings of pericarditis include pericardial thickening greater than 4 mm and an associated effusion that may be simple or complex.[9]

Thickened pericardium has intermediate signal intensity on proton density-weighted spin echo and double inversion sequences. Multiplanar evaluation allows the detection of subtle focal areas of thickening. In CP, thickening may be focal or diffuse. When focal, the right heart border is frequently involved.

Characterization of pericardial effusions is inadequate in patients with normal cardiac function and small effusions. Movement of pericardial fluid during the cardiac cycle may cause signal loss, and therefore simple effusions can appear as a signal void on proton density-weighted and T2-weighted images.[9]

Septations and debris may be seen on any sequence, indicating a complex effusion. Hemorrhagic and proteinaceous or exudative effusions tend to show increased signal intensity on T1-weighted sequences.

Pericardial thickening may be seen without constrictive physiology, and rarely patients with CP show no pericardial thickening.[21] Thus, it is imperative to look out for abnormal cardiac morphology—tubular-shaped ventricles, enlarged atria, focal contour deformities of the ventricles.

Other noncardiac signs of constriction comprise inferior vena cava (IVC) dilatation

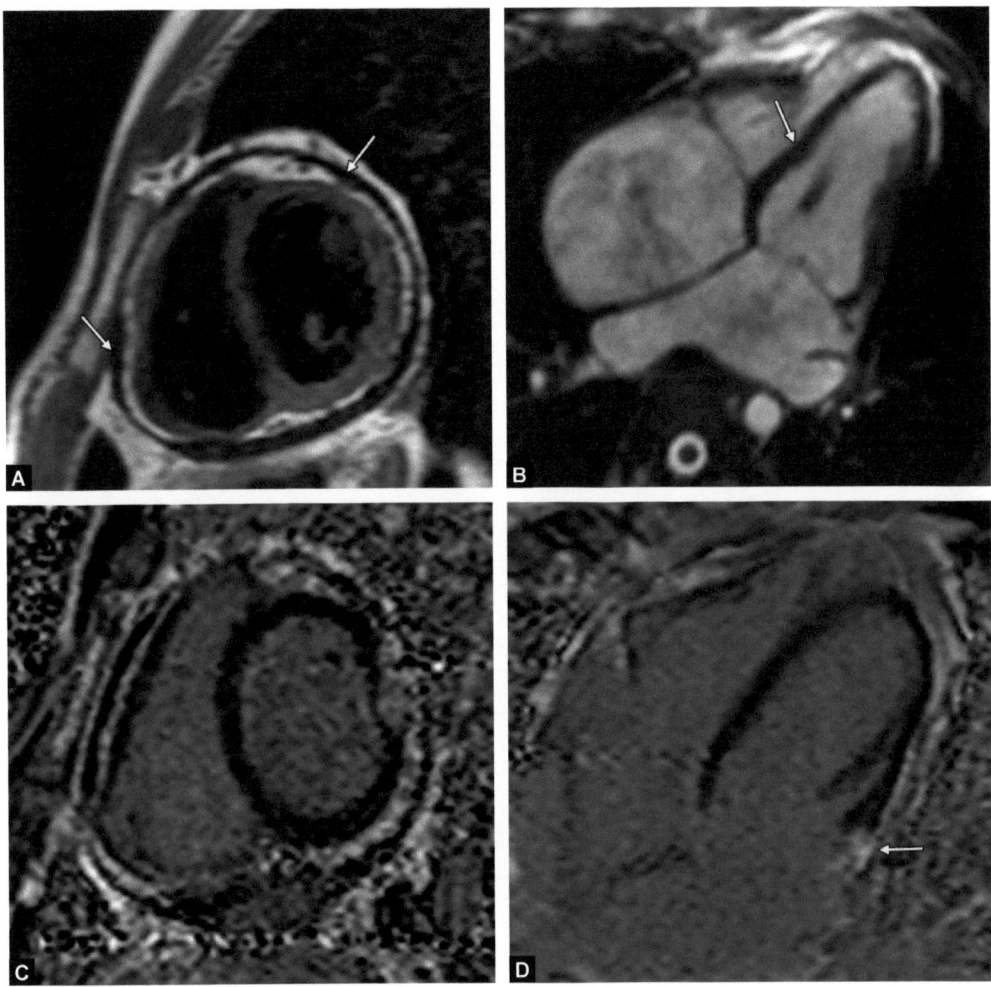

FIG. 7: Magnetic resonance imaging images. **A,** Short axis T1-weighted image showing diffusely thickened hypointense pericardium (arrow); **B,** four-chamber view static cine image shows biatrial dilatation with tubular ventricles along with straightening of interventricular septum (arrow); **C** and **D,** delayed enhancement phase-sensitive inversion recovery sequence short axis and four-chamber view showing delayed enhancement of pericardium and myocardial enhancement near left atrioventricular groove region (straight arrow)

with subsequent hepatic venous congestion. Ascites and pleural effusions are other indirect and nonspecific findings that can occur (Fig. 7).

Dynamic Cine Magnetic Resonance Imaging

There is frequent loss of normal rightward septal convexity in CP. Deviant configuration of the interventricular septum to the left is commonly observed in the initial diastolic phase. Cine imaging in constrictive physiology can reveal this abnormal ventricular interdependence as septal "bounce" or shivering septum, indicating the abnormal ventricular filling dynamics caused by limitation of right ventricular filling secondary to the inelastic pericardium (Fig. 8).

Real-time cine imaging during a deep inspiration is helpful in distinguishing RCM from CP. In CP, septal flattening or inversion is usually observed, whereas this finding is mostly absent in patients with RCM. This is indicative of the reduced compliance of the pericardium such that any increase in right ventricular filling (such as that caused by a deep inspiration) results in shift of the septum to the left.[24]

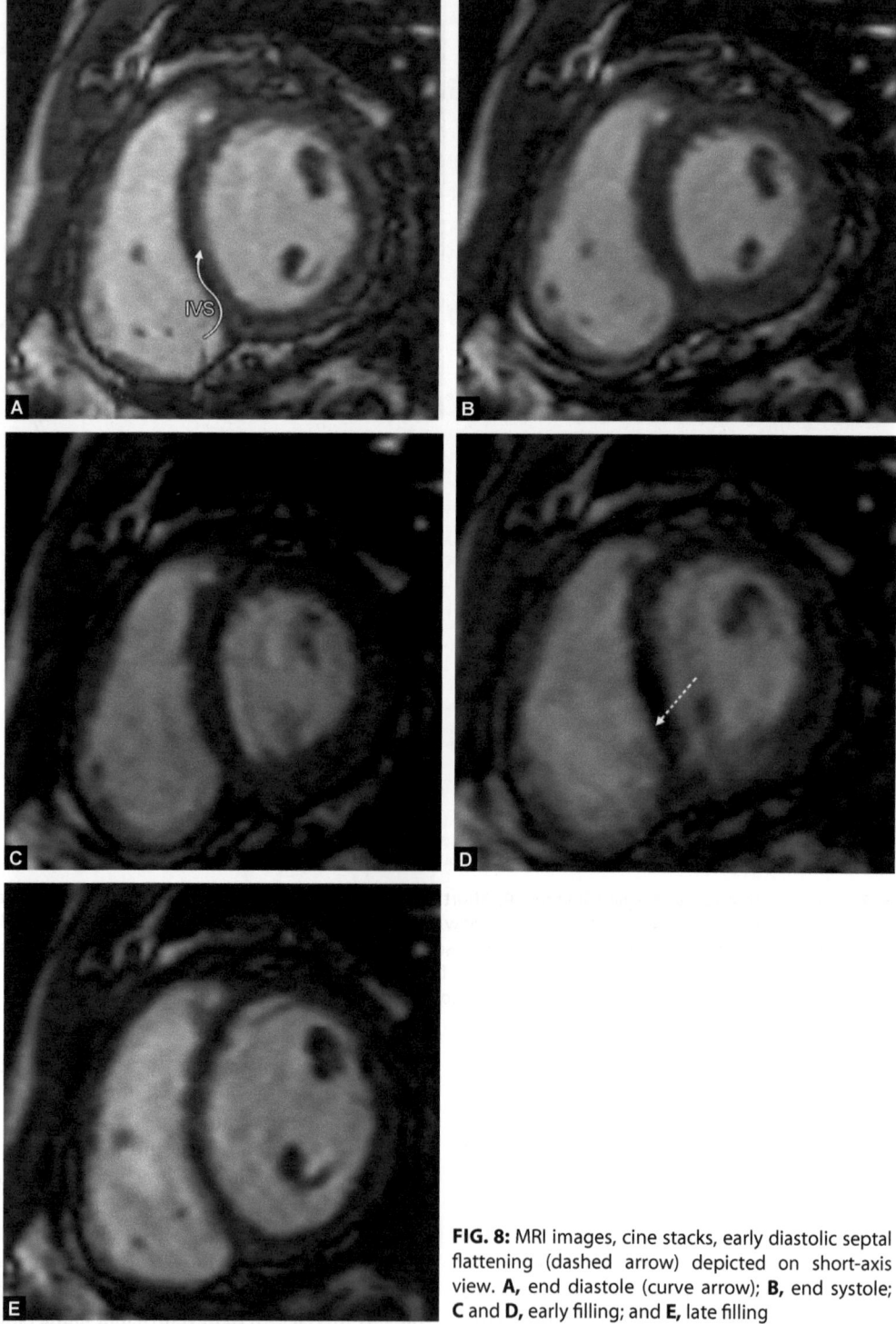

FIG. 8: MRI images, cine stacks, early diastolic septal flattening (dashed arrow) depicted on short-axis view. **A,** end diastole (curve arrow); **B,** end systole; **C** and **D,** early filling; and **E,** late filling

Myocardial tagging: Myocardial tagging is performed most commonly in the four-chamber plane, optimal for evaluation of the pericardium along the right ventricular free wall. Tag lines are seen as dark saturation bands 4–5 mm thick and typically spaced at intervals of approximately 1 cm over the entire image. In normal patients, these lines lose continuity at the parietal and visceral pericardium during the cardiac cycle, which indicates a normal sliding motion between the pericardial layers. In patients with pericardial constriction and adhesions between these layers, the bands bend but remain unbroken, indicating abnormal tethering of the pericardium.[25]

Effusive-constrictive Pericarditis

It is a condition in which there is tamponade caused by tense effusion and constriction caused by inflamed and noncompliant visceral pericardium. A visceral pericardiectomy may be needed in this situation.[26]

Imaging depicts pericardial effusion, a thickened pericardium, and hemodynamic evidence of constriction and can be readily demonstrated by MDCT or CMR (Fig. 9). This entity can be considered as a transitional phase in between acute pericarditis/pericardial tamponade and CP.[11] Features of constriction persist even after removal or resolution of pericardial fluid.[18]

Pericardial Abscess

This is an uncommon complication, usually seen with tubercular CP. Multidetector CT demonstrates a localized biconvex pericardial collection with hypodense core and enhancing walls, causing compression of an adjoining cardiac chamber. On CMR, a rim enhancing lesion is seen with typically hyperintense core on both T1 and T2-weighted images (Fig. 10). Enhancing septae may be seen. Presence of hypointensity on T2-weighted images may suggest tubercular etiology.[27]

MYOCARDIAL TUBERCULOSIS

It occurs most commonly by contiguous involvement from pericardial TB, mediastinal lymph nodes, or retrograde lymphatic and hematogenous spread.

Three patterns of myocardial involvement seen pathologically are:
1. Miliary tuberculosis
2. Diffuse infiltrating interstitial disease
3. Caseating nodular disease (tuberculoma).

The miliary form is by far the most common; tuberculomas are much rarer. The lesions may involve the atria, the ventricles, or the interventricular septum. The favored sites are the right atrium and left ventricle.[28]

Myocardial TB can present with rhythm disturbances, congestive heart failure, ventricular aneurysms, right ventricular outflow obstruction or left ventricular obstruction, coronary involvement, caval obstruction and aortic insufficiency.[29] It is important to recognize TB as a cause of myocarditis because it has the potential of presenting as sudden death, particularly with miliary TB.[30,31]

Though being clinically silent, it is possible that with the increased clinical use and the high resolution of magnetic resonance imaging (MRI), more patients with either nodular or miliary forms of tuberculous myocarditis will be recognized antemortem.

Imaging features of miliary or diffusely infiltrative interstitial myocardial TB are non-

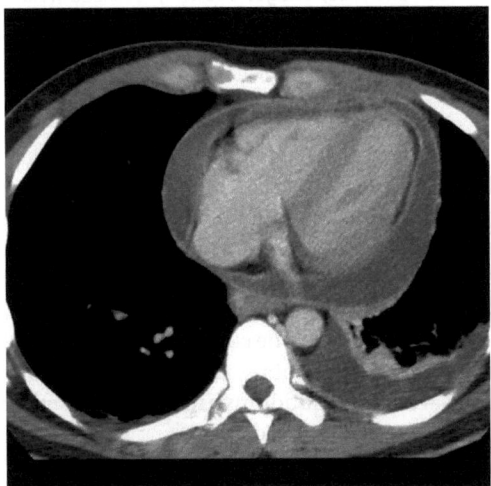

FIG. 9: Axial contrast-enhanced computed tomography image showing pericardial effusion with thick and enhancing pericardium and ventricular constriction significant of effusive constrictive pericarditis. Associated left-sided pleural effusion

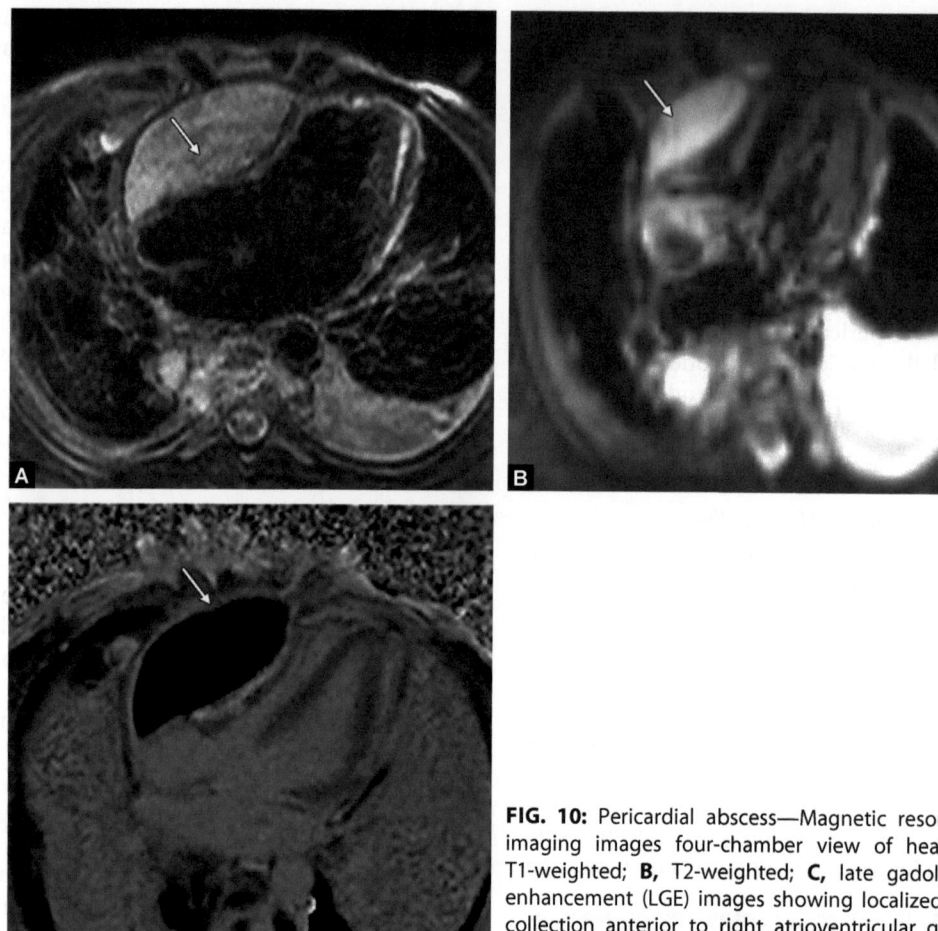

FIG. 10: Pericardial abscess—Magnetic resonance imaging images four-chamber view of heart. **A,** T1-weighted; **B,** T2-weighted; **C,** late gadolinium enhancement (LGE) images showing localized fluid collection anterior to right atrioventricular groove (arrow) causing indentation of heart and showing rim enhancement on LGE (arrow)

specific, similar to other forms of myocarditis with altered hyperintense signal on black blood T2/T2 fat-suppressed sequences suggesting edema and multifocal ill-defined heterogeneous areas of LGE not conforming to vascular territory.

Cardiac Tuberculoma/Mass

Isolated cardiac tuberculomas are exceedingly rare, especially in immunocompetent persons.

These are mostly solitary, well-defined, and distinct from the adjoining tissue. The mass can penetrate the myocardium, causing surface ulceration and thus initiating the thrombus formation with consequent thromboembolism. This occurrence may lead to hematogenous spread and disseminated TB.

All four cardiac chambers can be involved. The right heart chambers, mainly the free wall of right atrium, are frequently affected, maybe because of the frequent involvement of the right mediastinal lymphatic drainage with subsequent spread to the pericardium and myocardium. Other differentials to be considered in right atrial mass include thrombus, myxoma, lymphoma, myosarcoma, rhabdomyosarcoma, vascular tumor, and secondary deposit.[32]

Imaging

Echocardiography

This may show heterogeneously hypoechoic/ echogenic immobile mass adjacent to or within the affected myocardium in case of a noncalcified/calcified myocardial tuberculoma respectively.

Cardiac Magnetic Resonance Imaging

Cardiac MRI may show tuberculoma as a heterogeneous mass, iso to hypointense to muscle on both T1W and T2W. On gadolinium-enhanced MRI, mass may show heterogenous and thick peripheral enhancement, and central irregular nonenhancing areas.[33]

When tuberculomas present as infiltrative cardiac masses these may show iso to mildly hyperintense lesions on T1 and T2-weighted spin echo images, indistinct pericardium and contrast enhancement with mild heterogeneity (Fig. 11). These imaging features help to differentiate the lesion from metastasis (usually quite hyperintense on T2-weighted images with pericardial effusion and prominent enhancement), sarcoma (similar to metastasis with prominent heterogeneity due to hemorrhage and necrosis, and intramyocardial involvement) and lymphoma (which usually enhance homogenously).[34]

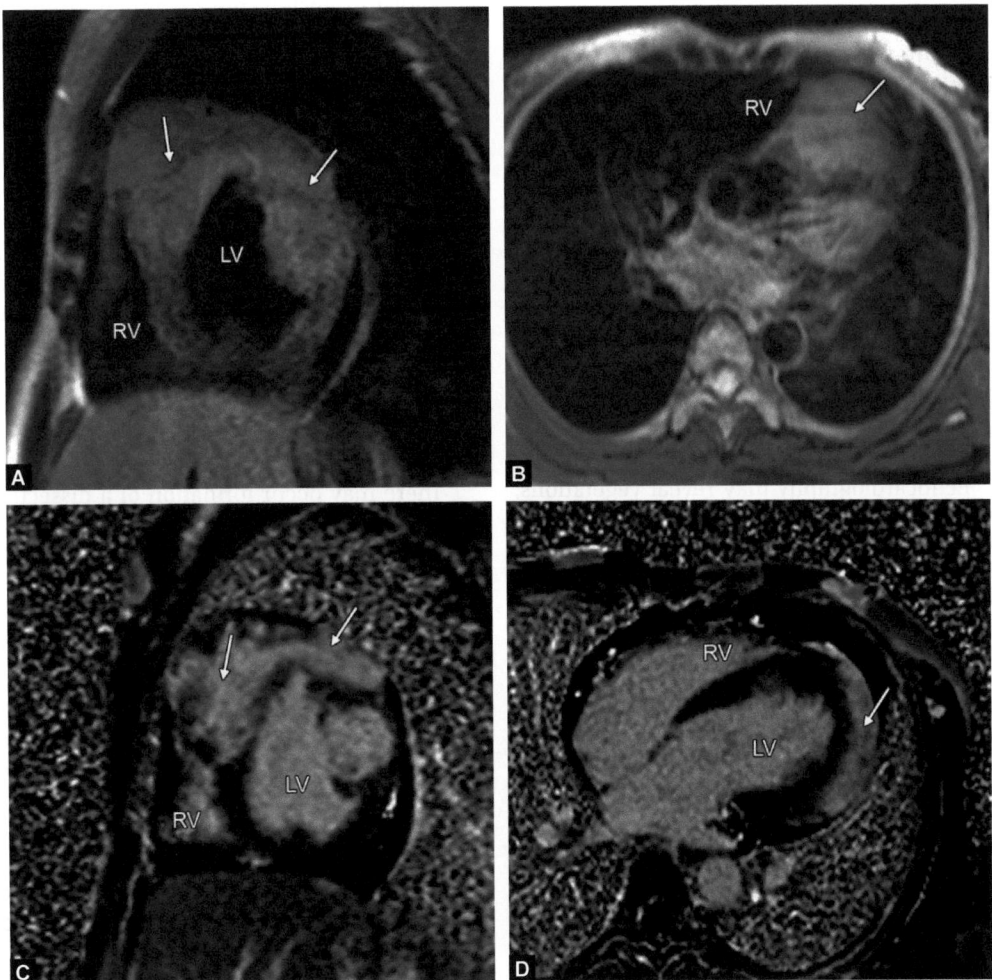

FIG. 11: Cardiac tuberculoma/mass—MRI images. **A,** T1 short axis; **B,** T2 four chamber; **C** and **D,** late gadolinium enhancement (LGE) images showing heterogeneous sheet-like mass diffusely infiltrating left ventricle myocardium and right ventricle outflow tract (arrow) with heterogeneous enhancement on LGE images (arrow)

Cardiac TB may lead to RCM and differentiating from CP is very difficult at times.[35]

The differential diagnoses of cardiac TB include granulomatous disorders like sarcoidosis, giant cell myocarditis, fungal infections, rheumatic fever, abscesses, and metastatic tumors containing giant cells.[36]

TUBERCULOUS ENDOCARDITIS

The endocardial involvement can be either miliary with multiple small tuberculomas (<3 mm in diameter), or nodular, formed by confluent foci of tuberculomas.

Endocardial involvement by tuberculous infection may affect the valvular surfaces presenting as valvular infective endocarditis,[37] or it can involve the endothelial surfaces of the cardiac chambers or great vessels.

Valvular involvement is usually seen in immunocompromised patients with disseminated TB.

This may manifest as formation of subvalvular left ventricular aneurysms, tuberculoma extension into the left ventricular free wall with pseudoaneurysm formation, pulmonary vein obstruction from left atrial tuberculoma, right ventricular outflow tract obstruction and superior vena cava (SVC) obstruction.[38-40]

Echocardiography may reveal vegetations, regurgitant lesions and subvalvular aneurysms. Rarely, a large tuberculoma mimicking a cardiac tumor is formed in one of the cardiac chambers or great vessels. Cardiac MRI may provide additional information about the nature of the cardiac mass.

VASCULAR TUBERCULOSIS

Tuberculous aneurysms are somewhat rare but there has been a recent resurgence with coexisting human immunodeficiency virus (HIV). These aneurysms carry a high mortality rate due to perforation or rupture, with massive hemorrhage and shock.

Different locations of tubercular pseudoaneurysm have distinct names, e.g., pulmonary pseudoaneurysm is called Rasmussen aneurysm,[41] and aortic pseudoaneurysm is called Pott's disease.[42]

Takayasu arteritis, affecting aorta and its branches has also been associated with mycobacterial infection, though the exact cause and effect relationship remains unproven.[43]

Pathogenesis

Tubercle bacilli reach the vessel wall in the following ways:
- Direct implantation on the intimal surface in miliary TB
- Carried to the adventitia or media by the vasa vasorum
- Through lymphatics
- Direct extension (most common) from the adjacent infected lymph node, abscess, or bone.

Once the focus of infection becomes established, subsequent complications depend upon the extent and speed with which the inflammation progresses.

Full thickness involvement of the aortic wall may end in perforation, either causing massive hemorrhage, or forming a perivascular hematoma. The latter may encapsulate and communicate with the lumen leading to false aneurysm. Longitudinal extension of the inflammatory process within the aortic wall favors the development of a true aneurysm (Flowchart 1).

There may occur formation of a dissecting aneurysm, or infection may extend into the lumen resulting in hematogenous dissemination of tubercle bacilli.[44]

Most common site of involvement is abdominal aorta, followed by descending thoracic aorta (DTA), ascending aorta, and arch. Aortic root involvement is very rare. Aneurysms may also involve vertebral, intracranial, visceral (thoracic and abdominal), iliofemoral, and popliteal arteries. Single site involvement is common although multifocal disease can also be seen.

Tubercular aneurysms are mostly pseudoaneurysm (87%) and rarely true (9%) or dissecting (4%). Most commonly, the aneurysms are saccular in shape. These usually rupture into adjacent viscera. With early diagnoses, incidence of rupture has decreased in recent decades.

Rarely, a stenosing type of tubercular aortoarteritis is seen in young patients secondary to

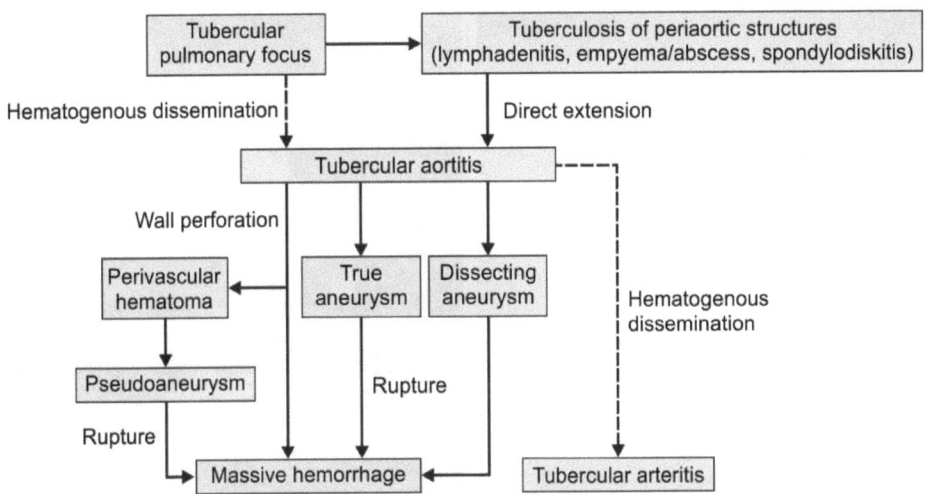

FLOWCHART 1: Modified diagram depicting pathogenesis and complications of vascular involvement in aortic tuberculosis.

a tubercular focus elsewhere in the body.[45,46] It is postulated to be immune-mediated secondary to recurrent exposure to infections from childhood with development of natural immunity.[47] This stenosing type of aortic tubercular involvement has been sometimes linked to Takayasu aortoarteritis with conflicting evidences in the medical literature.

Imaging

Radiograph

Radiographs may demonstrate an aneurysm, which may have calcific wall, periaortic tuberculous disease, such as spondylitis, paravertebral abscesses, and empyema and concurrent pulmonary TB (Fig. 12).[44]

Cross-sectional and Multi-planar Imaging

Multidetector CT and MRI scans can precisely define disease extension and help planning surgical or endovascular intervention.

Computed Tomography Angiography and Contrast-enhanced Computed Tomography

Computed tomography angiography (CTA) provides excellent vessel to background distinction to enable complete assessment of both luminal and mural anatomy. Delayed CECT should be acquired to assess wall enhancement and organ/visceral enhancement depicting complications secondary to aortitis and vasculitis.

Computed tomography angiography with delayed CECT is the imaging modality of choice, demonstrating aortic diameter, aortic wall thickening and regularity, mural calcification, branch vessel involvement, periaortic fluid or soft-tissue accumulation, rapidly progressing saccular aneurysm or pseudoaneurysm or any associated aortic dissection (Fig. 13).

Computed tomography imaging characterizes mural thickening (i.e., >2–3 mm is considered diagnostic for aortitis) and inflammatory periaortic soft tissue changes, such as fat stranding (Fig. 14). Computed tomography allows identification of hazardous mimics of aortitis, such as intramural hematoma and penetrating atheromatous ulcer, which appear as eccentric crescent-shaped or circumferential thickening with potential intimal or subintimal disruption on contrast imaging (Fig. 15). A positron emission tomography (PET)-CT can be useful in these cases to identify the diagnosis.

Computed tomography angiography (CTA) has also been used to identify complications of advanced aortitis, such as saccular aneurysm, pseudoaneurysm and thrombosis. Computed tomography angiography is useful in guiding

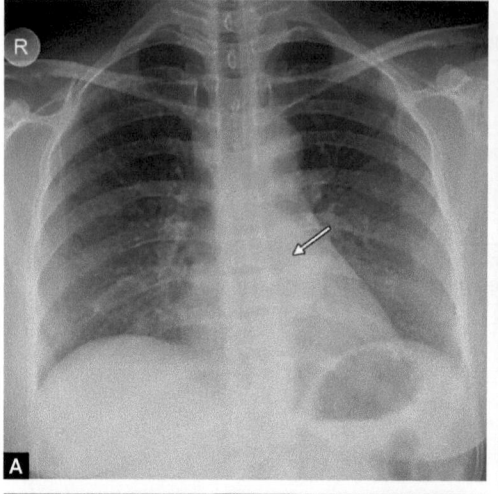
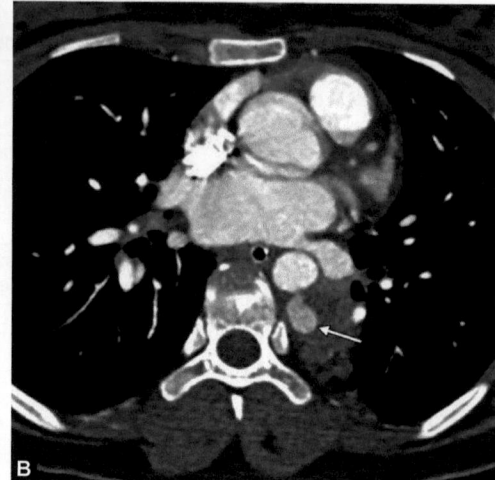
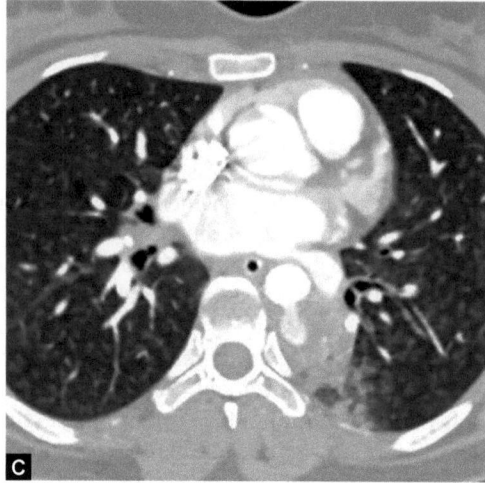

FIG. 12: Mycotic aneurysm of descending thoracic aorta. **A,** Chest X-ray posteroanterior view showing added opacity in left paravertebral region (arrow) obscuring the descending thoracic aortic outline along with ill-defined miliary infiltrates in bilateral lung parenchyma; **B,** corresponding computed tomography images mediastinal window; **C,** lung window showing descending thoracic aortic pseudoaneurysm (curved arrow) with miliary nodules in lung, confirming the findings

revascularization in those with arterial insufficiency of branch vessels causing claudication, cerebrovascular ischemia, intestinal angina, renal failure, or refractory hypertension. Besides, endovascular stent graft reconstruction is best planned using CTA.[48]

Electrocardiogram-gated CTA may be useful for characterizing aortic root and anatomic aortic valvular abnormalities. It readily identifies aortitis-associated ostial and proximal coronary stenosis and may be used as a guide for revascularization.[49]

Computed tomography angiography can also be used as a follow-up tool to assess the treatment response and/or activity of the disease.[50]

Magnetic Resonance Imaging Studies

Magnetic resonance imaging with gadolinium contrast enhancement is becoming an imaging modality of choice for aortitis. It provides imaging of the entire aorta with excellent resolution and without radiation exposure. Areas of aortitis may be seen as vessel wall edema, enhancement, or wall thickening.

Cardiovascular Magnetic Resonance

Magnetic resonance imaging detects mural thickening and depicts mural edema on T2 "edema-weighted" sequences. Gadolinium contrast-enhanced MR identifies mural fibrosis; like PET, both potentially provide essential

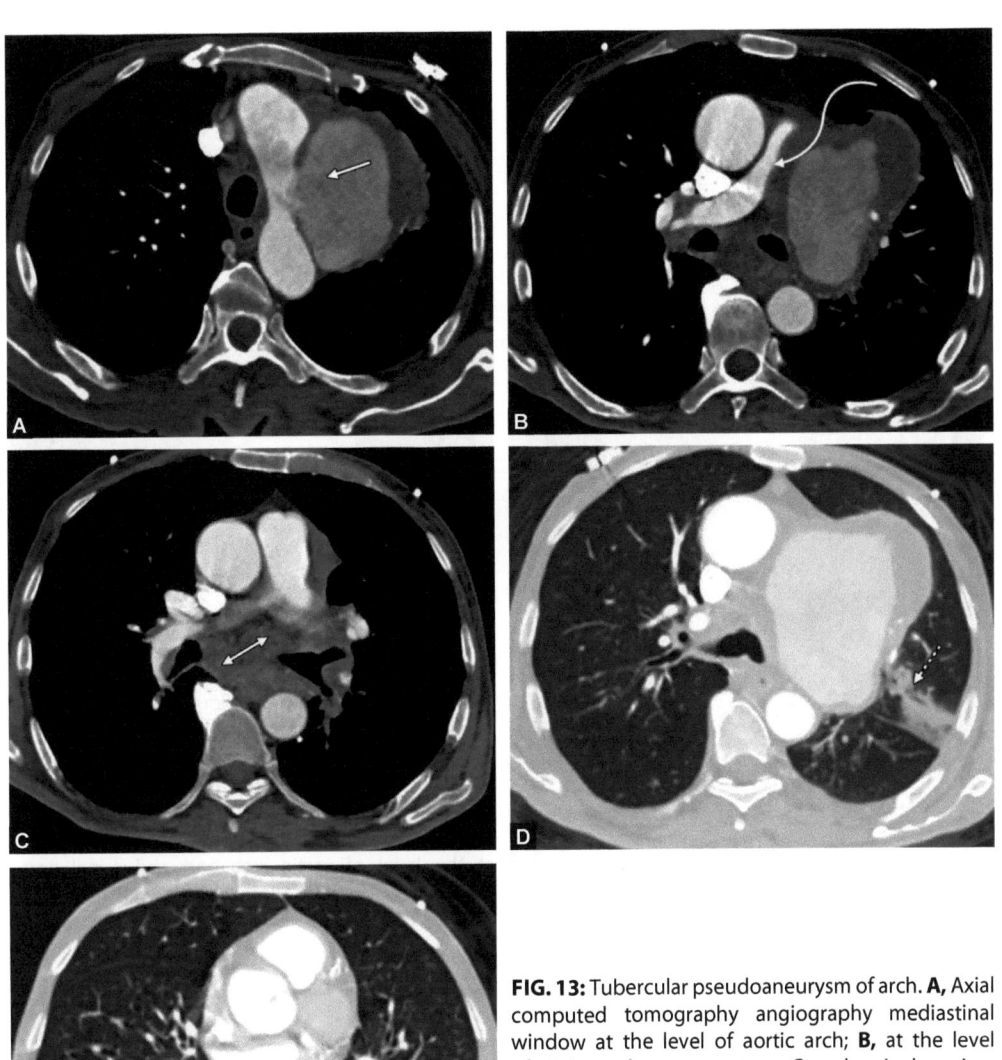

FIG. 13: Tubercular pseudoaneurysm of arch. **A,** Axial computed tomography angiography mediastinal window at the level of aortic arch; **B,** at the level of right pulmonary artery; **C,** subcarinal region; and **D** and **E,** lung window showing large, wide neck pseudoaneurysm (arrow), arising from arch with eccentric thrombus causing compression of pulmonary artery (curved arrow) and associated with significant mediastinal lymph nodes (double arrow) in addition to patchy consolidation and ill-defined centrilobular nodules in left lower lobe

information regarding disease activity before development of luminal changes (Fig. 16).[51]

Magnetic resonance angiography (MRA) extracts luminal details, including arterial stenosis, dilatation and thrombosis, comparable to that of CTA but without the need for iodinated contrast or ionizing radiation. Both contrast and noncontrast angiography protocols are available, relieving concerns in those with renal impairment. Coronary MRA may be useful in identifying ostioproximal coronary involvement in aortitis.[52]

Magnetic resonance is the modality of choice for screening of aneurysm development and routine monitoring of established aneurysms, and it is useful in guiding revascularization.[49]

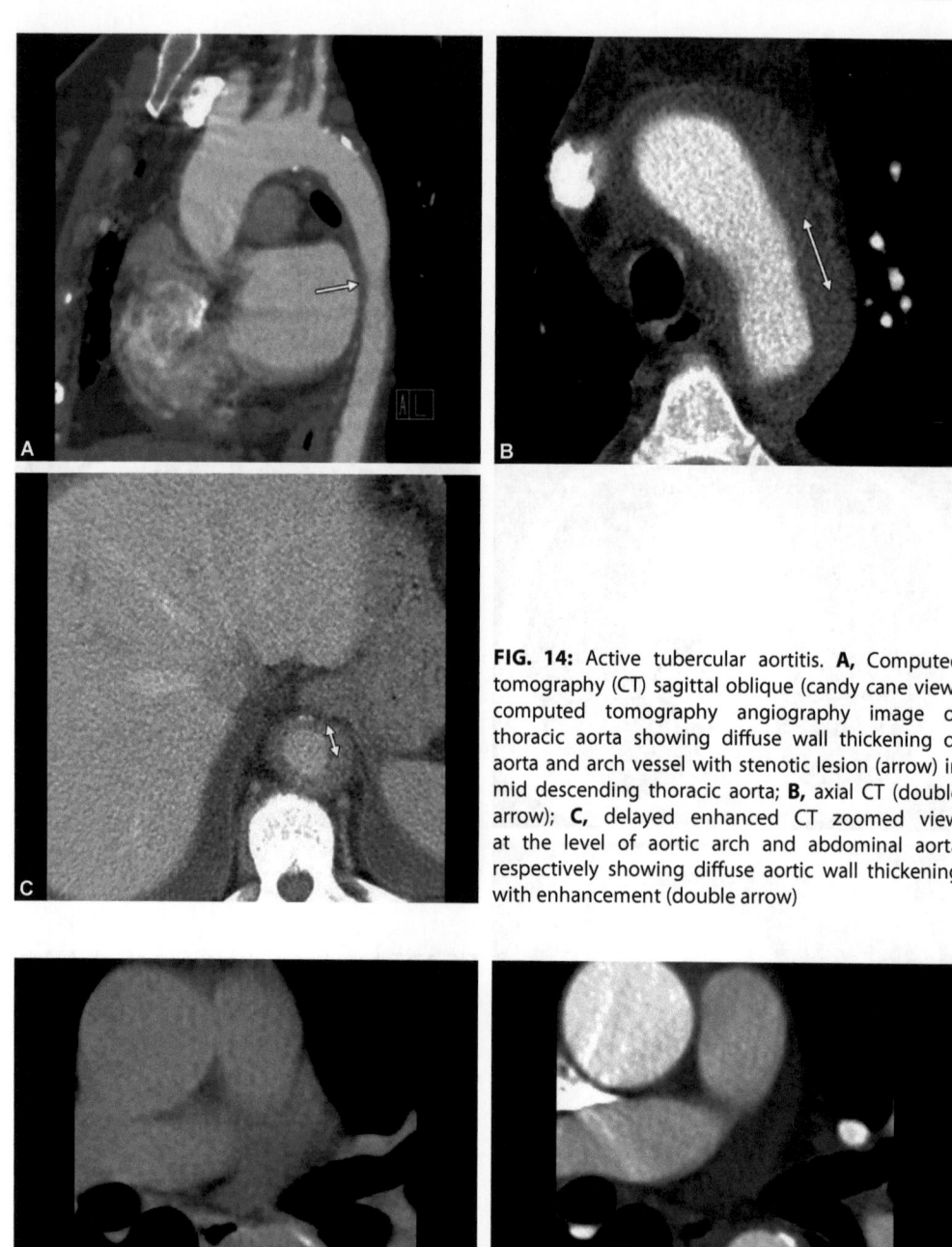

FIG. 14: Active tubercular aortitis. **A,** Computed tomography (CT) sagittal oblique (candy cane view) computed tomography angiography image of thoracic aorta showing diffuse wall thickening of aorta and arch vessel with stenotic lesion (arrow) in mid descending thoracic aorta; **B,** axial CT (double arrow); **C,** delayed enhanced CT zoomed view at the level of aortic arch and abdominal aorta respectively showing diffuse aortic wall thickening with enhancement (double arrow)

FIG. 15: Variants of aortitis—Intramural hematoma. **A,** Axial computed tomography images noncontrast image showing hyperdense eccentric fluid collection (asterisk) with displaced intimal calcification (white arrow head); **B,** contrast-enhanced image showing nonenhancing eccentric hypodense fluid collection (white arrow head) with smooth interface with aortic lumen (black arrow head) as opposed to enhancing and irregular interface in aortitis

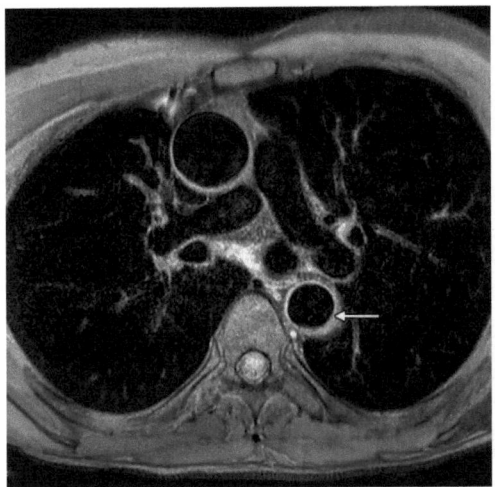

FIG. 16: Wall edema in acute aortitis: T2-weighted axial image showing wall thickness and hyperintense signal intensity in descending thoracic aortic wall (arrow)

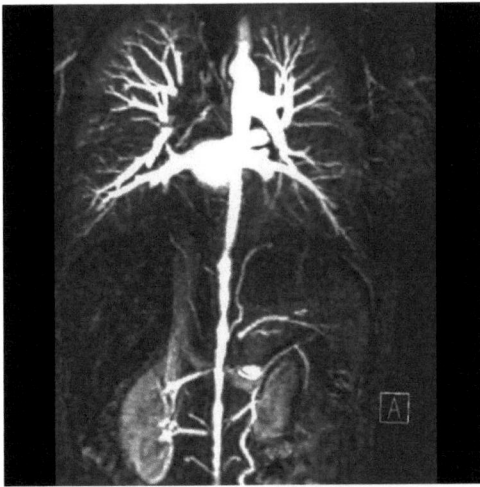

FIG. 17: Coronal magnetic resonance angiogram of aorta showing diffuse narrowing of thoracoabdominal aorta along with significant abdominal visceral branch artery stenosis

The limitations of MR are lower spatial resolution than CT, lengthy scan times demanding multiple breath holds, artifacts and safety concerns associated with implanted cardiovascular devices, overestimation of branch point stenosis, poor evaluation of distal branches and suboptimal imaging of calcium (Fig. 17).[49]

Magnetic resonance/MRA and CT/CTA are equally good in the structural characterization of inflammatory and infectious aortitis. An added benefit of MR is the choice to perform cardiac sequences revealing endocardial, myocardial and pericardial complications related to aortitis. Aortic root and valve morphology are well assessed with MR. Cine and phase-contrast MR is the gold standard for evaluation of cardiac function and aortic regurgitation. This is particularly relevant, as aortic root inflammation and dilation, valvulitis and aortic valve insufficiency may occur in tubercular aortitis.[49]

Nuclear Imaging

18-fluorodeoxyglucose (18-FDG)-PET-CT has a growing role in evaluating inflammatory changes such as vasculitis. FDG does not accumulate in normal vessel wall. Thus, any uptake of 18-FDG in the aortic wall is abnormal because of inflammatory or infectious processes. Although inflammatory activity is well appreciated demonstrated on nuclear imaging, morphological assessment is limited because of the relatively low special resolution; thus, nuclear scans are beneficial when acquired in fusion with either CT or MRI, increasing the sensitivity and specificity of this test.[49,50]

TUBERCULAR MYCOTIC ANEURYSMS INVOLVING AORTIC BRANCHES

Tubercular involvement of carotids, vertebral, systemic (subclavian, iliac, femoral, and popliteal) and visceral (mesenteric, celiac, hepatic, splenic, and renal arteries) has been described in the literature. Pathophysiology and imaging findings are similar to mycotic aneurysms involving aorta with clinical symptomatology varying as per the body region involved. Treatment options are available in the form of surgery and radiologic intervention procedures as per the suitability and morbidity of patient along with antitubercular medical therapy (Fig. 18).[53,54]

MYCOTIC ANEURYSMS AS THE CAUSE OF HEMOPTYSIS IN PULMONARY TUBERCULOSIS

Pulmonary TB is complicated with vascular lesions including pulmonary or bronchial arteritis

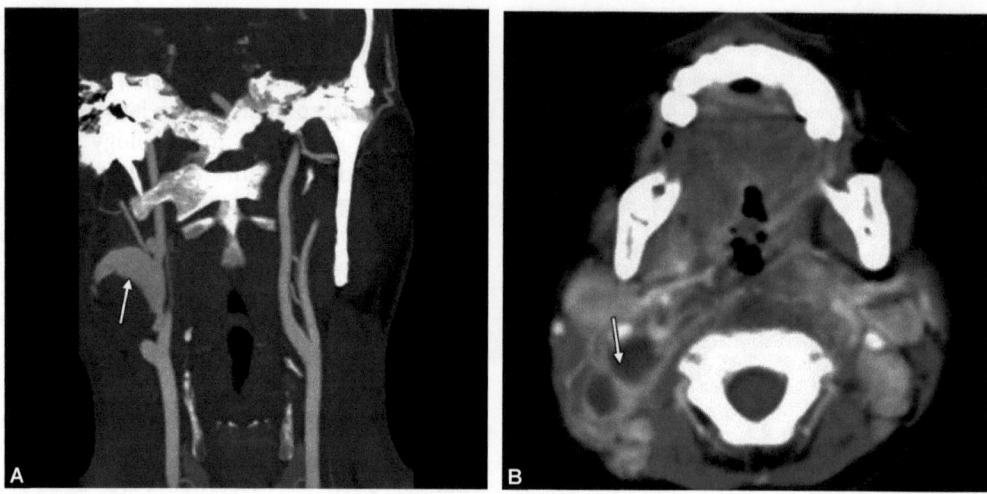

FIG. 18: Tubercular carotid artery pseudoaneurysm. **A,** Computed tomography (CT) neck coronal image showing large contrast filled outpouching with eccentric thrombus (curved arrow) in right carotid fossa arising from internal carotid artery; **B,** axial CT neck showing multiple necrotic lymph nodes in right carotid fossa (arrow)

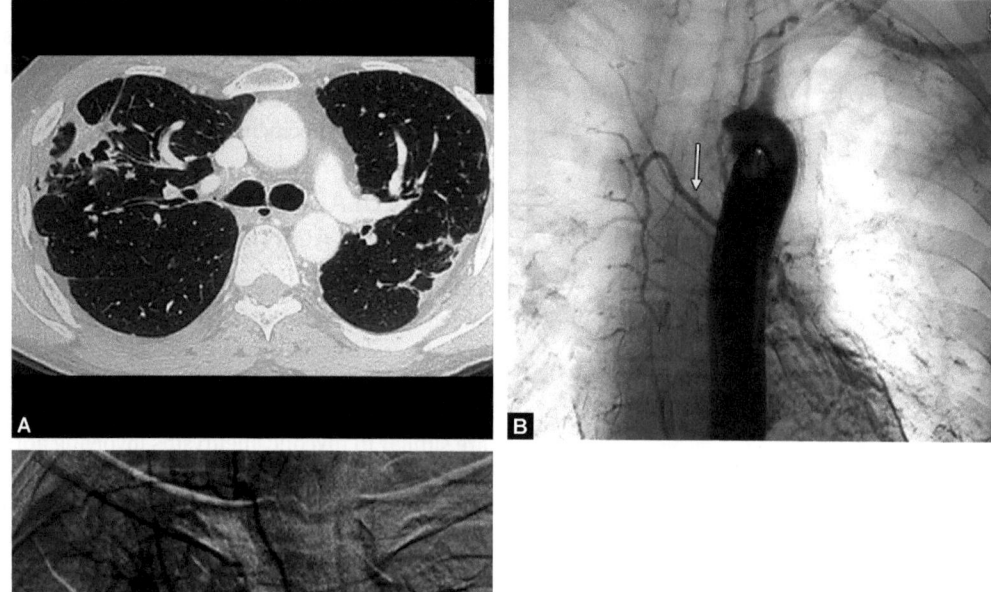

FIG. 19: A, Computed tomography axial image lung window in a patient who presented with moderate hemoptysis, shows cavitary fibrotic lesion in the anterior segment of right upper lobe. Fibrotic lesions are also seen in left upper lobe; **B,** flush aortogram in the same patient showing hypertrophied right intercostobronchial trunk (arrow); **C,** selective cannulation of intercostobronchial trunk shows hypertrophied common bronchial trunk supplying both lungs. Abnormal vascular blush in right upper zone

and thrombosis, bronchial artery hypertrophy/dilatation, and pulmonary artery aneurysms.

Angiographic findings in TB patients presenting with massive hemoptysis include hypervascularity, hypertrophy of systemic arteries, aneurysms, systemic to pulmonary anastomosis and rarely, contrast extravasation. Bronchial arteries are the source of hemorrhage in majority of these cases with nonbronchial systemic or pulmonary arteries being less common as the source (Fig. 19).

BRONCHIAL ARTERY ANEURYSM

It is a rare complication of tubercular infection, which may lead to life-threatening hemoptysis. Bronchial artery aneurysms are effectively depicted with MDCT. The term pseudoaneurysm is often used interchangeably with the aneurysm.

These aneurysms arise either within the mediastinum or from the intrapulmonary portion of the artery. Rupture of bronchial artery aneurysms located in mediastinum may cause hemothorax and mediastinal hemorrhage whereas rupture of the intrapulmonary aneurysm can give rise to massive hemoptysis.

Bronchial artery aneurysm has also been associated with congenital causes such as pulmonary sequestration or pulmonary agenesis, or acquired causes like atherosclerosis, inflammatory lung disease, bronchiectasis, sarcoidosis, Osler-Weber-Rendu disease and trauma.

Most of the intrapulmonary bronchial artery aneurysms are successfully treated with transcatheter embolization; however, large aneurysms and those located in mediastinum may require surgery or aortic stent graft. As bronchial artery embolization only treats the hemoptysis, the underlying disease process needs to be properly addressed to prevent recurrent hemoptysis.[55,56]

PULMONARY ARTERY ANEURYSM

Inflammatory pulmonary artery aneurysms are an extremely uncommon cause of hemoptysis in pulmonary TB.

On CECT imaging, there is focal dilatation of one of the segmental pulmonary arteries adjacent to tuberculous parenchymal alteration or chronic tuberculous cavity. Multidetector CT angiography provides the anatomic and morphological information including the source of the aneurysm, the pathway to bleeding places and orthotopic bronchial arteries. The three-dimensional (3D) reconstruction achieves the conventional angiogram-like images showing a clear-cut road map for the interventional radiologist in performing an endovascular treatment for hemoptysis. In addition, CT is good at depicting an anterior spinal artery that could help prevent spinal cord ischemia.[57]

Endovascular occlusion of the neck of the pulmonary aneurysm is usually successful in treating the hemoptysis. Steel coils are the occlusive material of choice although thrombin and cyanoacrylate injection percutaneously under fluoroscopic and ultrasound guidance has been used where vascular access is not possible (Fig. 20).

VASCULAR INVOLVEMENT SECONDARY TO ABDOMINAL TUBERCULOSIS

Local extension of a tubercular mass may result in involvement of adjacent vascular structures. Involvement of the adjacent mesentery and major mesenteric vessels can be seen with intestinal TB. When present, granulomas in or near the vessel wall, subintimal fibrosis, intraluminal thrombi and perivascular cuffing may be seen.[58]

Tubercular lymph nodal mass can cause encasement and stenosis of the portal vein, resulting in portal hypertension. Local extension of a TB mass can result in stenosis and occlusion of splenic vessels with subsequent splenic infarction. Both arterial as well as venous involvement can be seen in patients with pancreatic TB (Fig. 21).[59]

TUBERCULOSIS AND VENOUS THROMBOEMBOLISM

Tuberculosis is an independent risk factor for venous thromboembolism (VTE). Active pulmonary TB may be complicated by deep vein

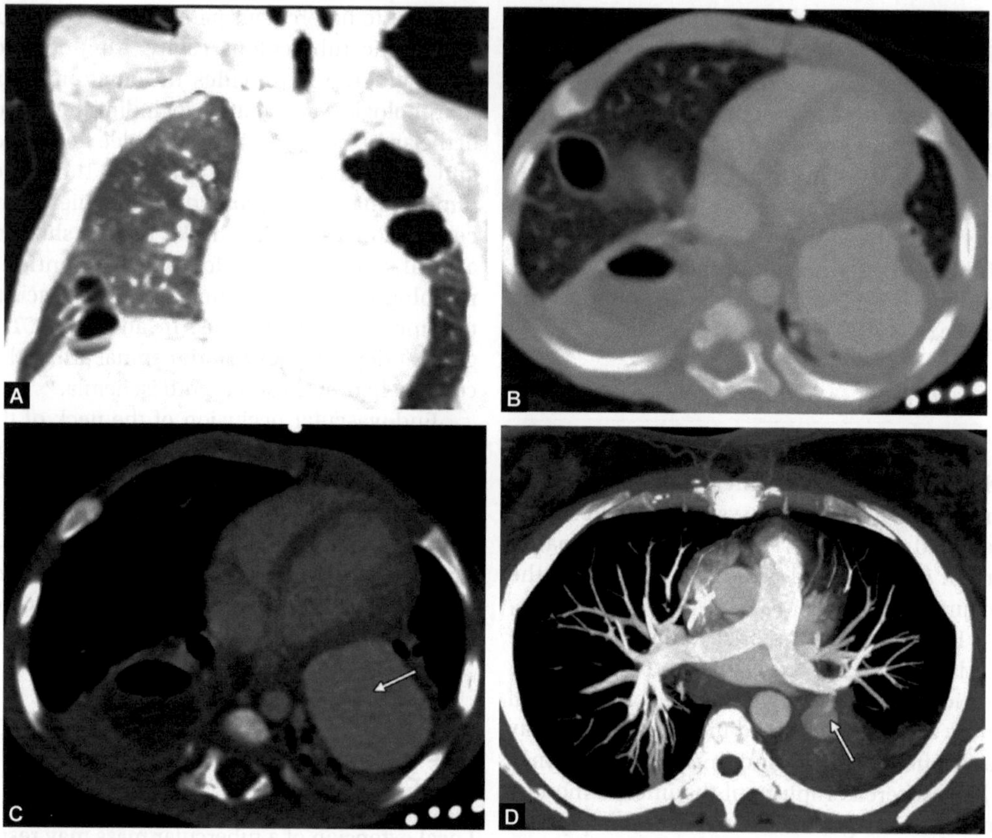

FIG. 20: Tubercular pulmonary pseudoaneurysm—Computed tomography (CT) images. **A** and **B,** Coronal and axial lung window showing multiple cavitary lung lesions; **C,** axial image mediastinal window show large pseudoaneurysm (broken arrow) form left lower lobe pulmonary artery branch; **D,** another patient, multiplanar reconstruction CT image of pulmonary artery showing pseudoaneurysm from left main pulmonary artery (arrow)

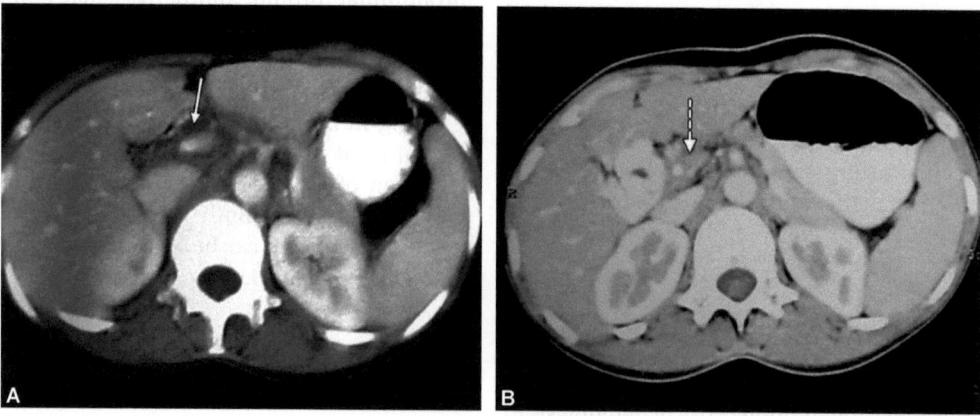

FIG. 21: A, Computed tomography abdomen in a patient with tuberculosis shows hypodense lymph nodes at porta hepatis, encasing the main portal vein (arrow); **B,** following antitubercular treatment for 1 year there is complete resolution of nodes at porta. The portal vein is replaced by multiple collateral channels (broken arrow)

inflammation; however, it requires CT or MRI for anatomic localization.

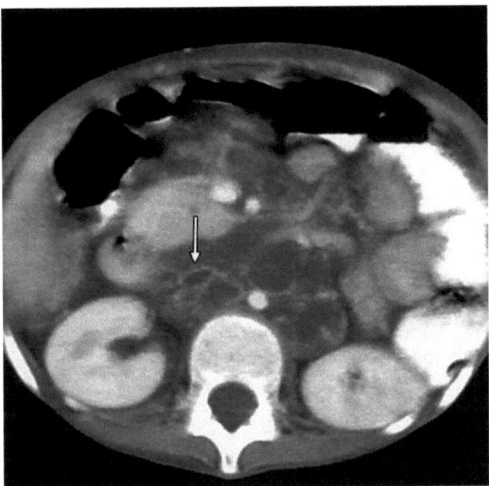

FIG. 22: Computed tomography abdomen in a patient with abdominal tuberculosis shows multiple necrotic lymph nodes encasing aorta and inferior vena cava with thrombus within inferior vena cava (arrow)

thrombosis associated with a hypercoagulable state secondary to the inflammatory state.

Risks of hypercoagulability are increased by the immobility and bed rest; because of the morbidity caused by the disease.

Local factors may also induce the thrombosis of pulmonary arteries. Organ infection can trigger local thrombosis possibly due to endothelial cell alteration and adhesion molecule expression.

Thrombosis of IVC can also result from venous compression by retroperitoneal lymph nodes in abdominal TB, in the absence of any hemostatic abnormalities (Fig. 22).[60,61]

CONCLUSION

Cardiovascular TB may present with myriad manifestations and a multimodality imaging approach is required for diagnosis. Conventional radiography has limited role in the evaluation of cardiovascular TB. Echocardiography and ultrasonography remain the initial diagnostic imaging modalities for evaluation of a clinically suspected case. On the other hand, both CT and MRI with the added advantage of performing 3D angiography, are preferred for holistic evaluation of the morphologic and functional features of cardiovascular TB. Positron emission tomography is a sensitive test for early vessel

REFERENCES

1. Fowler NO. Tuberculous pericarditis. JAMA. 1991;266(1): 99-103.
2. Bashi VV, John S, Ravikumar E, et al. Early and late results of pericardiectomy in 118 cases of constrictive pericarditis. Thorax. 1988;43(8):637-41.
3. Rose AG. Cardiac tuberculosis. A study of 19 patients. Arch Pathol Lab Med. 1987;111(5):422-6.
4. Fairley CK, Ryan M, Wall PG, et al. The organisms reported to cause infective myocarditis and pericarditis in England and Wales. J Infect. 1996;32(3):223-5.
5. Kannangara DW, Salem FA, Rao BS, Thadepalli H. Cardiac tuberculosis: TB of the endocardium. Am J Med Sci. 1984;287(3):45-7.
6. Brar R, Prasada A, Kumara A, et al. Myocardial tuberculosis presenting with congestive heart failure and pulmonary venous occlusion. Eur J Radiol. 2010;74(3):e47-50.
7. Rajesh S, Sricharan KN, Jayaprakash K, et al. Cardiac involvement in patients with pulmonary tuberculosis. J Clin Diagn Res. 2011;5(3):440-2.
8. Pawsat DE, Lee JY. Inflammatory disorders of the heart. Pericarditis, myocarditis, and endocarditis. Emerg Med Clin North Am. 1998;16(3):665-81.
9. Glockner JF. Imaging of pericardial disease. Magn Reson Imaging Clin N Am. 2003;11(1):149-62.
10. Manheimer E. Chest roentgenography for cardiovascular evaluation. In: Walker HK, Hall WD, Hurst JW (Eds). Clinical Methods: The History, Physical, and Laboratory Examinations, 3rd edition. Boston: Butterworths; 1990.
11. Yared K, Baggish AL, Picard MH, et al. Multimodality imaging of pericardial diseases. JACC Cardiovasc Imaging. 2010;3(6):650-60.
12. Jung HO. Pericardial effusion and pericardiocentesis: role of echocardiography. Korean Circ J. 2012;42(11):725-34.
13. Napolitano G, Pressacco J, Paquet E. Imaging features of constrictive pericarditis: beyond pericardial thickening. Can Assoc Radiol J. 2009;60(1):40-6.
14. Gowda RM, Boxt LM. Calcifications of the heart. Radiol Clin North Am. 2004;42(3):603-17.
15. Verhaert D, Gabriel RS, Johnston D, et al. The role of multimodality imaging in the management of pericardial disease. Circ Cardiovasc Imaging. 2010;3(3):333-43.
16. Shammas NW, Padaria RF, Coyne EP. Pericarditis, myocarditis, and other cardiomyopathies. Prim Care. 2013;40(1):213-36.
17. Garcia MJ. Constrictive Pericarditis Versus Restrictive Cardiomyopathy? J Am Coll Cardiol. 2016;67(17):2061-76.
18. Rajiah P. Cardiac MRI: Part 2, pericardial diseases. AJR Am J Roentgenol. 2011;197(4):W621-34.
19. O'Leary SM, Williams PL, Williams MP, et al. Imaging the pericardium: appearances on ECG-gated 64-detector row cardiac computed tomography. Br J Radiol. 2010;83(987):194-205.
20. Nishimura RA. Constrictive pericarditis in the modern era: a diagnostic dilemma. Heart. 2001;86(6):619-23.

21. Khandaker MH, Espinosa RE, Nishimura RA, et al. Pericardial disease: diagnosis and management. Mayo Clin Proc. 2010;85(6):572-93.
22. Kojima S, Yamada N, Goto Y. Diagnosis of constrictive pericarditis by tagged cine magnetic resonance imaging. N Engl J Med. 1999;341(5):373-4.
23. Francone M, Dymarkowski S, Kalantzi M, et al. Assessment of ventricular coupling with real-time cine MRI and its value to differentiate constrictive pericarditis from restrictive cardiomyopathy. Eur Radiol. 2006;16(4):944-51.
24. Grizzard JD. Magnetic resonance imaging of pericardial disease and intracardiac thrombus. Heart Fail Clin. 2009;5(3):401-19.
25. Groves R, Chan D, Zagurovskaya M, et al. MR imaging evaluation of pericardial constriction. Magn Reson Imaging Clin N Am. 2015;23(1):81-7.
26. Hancock EW. A clearer view of effusive-constrictive pericarditis. N Engl J Med. 2004;350(5):435-7.
27. Gulati GS, Sharma S. Pericardial abscess occurring after tuberculous pericarditis: image morphology on computed tomography and magnetic resonance imaging. Clin Radiol. 2004;59(6):514-9.
28. Horn H, Saphir O. The involvement of the myocardium in tuberculosis: a review of the literature and report of three cases. Am Rev Tuberc. 1935;32(1):492-506.
29. Njovane X. Intramyocardial tuberculosis--a rare under-diagnosed entity. S Afr Med J. 2009;99(3):152-3.
30. Alkhuja S, Miller A. Tuberculosis and sudden death: a case report and review. Heart Lung. 2001;30(5):388-91.
31. Chan AC, Dickens P. Tuberculous myocarditis presenting as sudden cardiac death. Forensic Sci Int. 1992;57(1):45-50.
32. Ngow HA, Khairina WM. Right atrial tuberculoma: a diagnosis too late. Cardiol J. 2011;18(5):560-3.
33. Jagia P, Gulati GS, Sharma S, et al. MRI features of tuberculoma of the right atrial myocardium. Pediatr Radiol. 2004;34(11):904-7.
34. Gulati GS, Kothari SS. Diffuse infiltrative cardiac tuberculosis. Ann Pediatr Cardiol. 2011;4(1):87-9.
35. Bali HK, Wahi S, Sharma BK, et al. Myocardial tuberculosis presenting as restrictive cardiomyopathy. Am Heart J. 1990;120(3):703-6.
36. Ozer N, Aytemir K, Sade E, et al. Cardiac tuberculosis with multiple intracardiac masses: a case report. J Am Soc Echocardiogr. 2002;15(7):756-8.
37. Shaikh Q, Mahmood F. Triple valve endocarditis by mycobacterium tuberculosis: a case report. BMC Infect Dis. 2012;12:231.
38. Chang BC, Ha JW, Kim JT, et al. Intracardiac tuberculoma. Ann Thorac Surg. 1999;67(1):226-8.
39. Halim MA, Mercer EN, Guinn GA. Myocardial tuberculoma with rupture and pseudoaneurysm formation--successful surgical treatment. Br Heart J. 1985;54(6):603-4.
40. Deshpande J, Vaideeswar P, Sivaraman A. Subvalvular left ventricular aneurysms. Cardiovasc Pathol. 2000;9(5):267-71.
41. Keeling AN, Costello R, Lee MJ. Rasmussen's aneurysm: a forgotten entity? Cardiovasc Intervent Radiol. 2008;31(1):196-200.
42. Li FP, Wang XF, Xiao YB. Endovascular stent graft placement in the treatment of a ruptured tuberculous pseudoaneurysm of the descending thoracic aorta secondary to Pott's disease of the spine. J Card Surg. 2012;27(1):75-7.
43. Aggarwal A, Chag M, Sinha N, et al. Takayasu's arteritis: role of Mycobacterium tuberculosis and its 65 kDa heat shock protein. Int J Cardiol. 1996;55(1):49-55.
44. Volini FI, Olfield RC, Thompson JR, et al. Tuberculosis of the aorta. JAMA. 1962;181:78-83.
45. Choudhary SK, Bhan A, Talwar S, et al. Tubercular pseudo-aneurysms of aorta. Ann Thorac Surg. 2001;72(4):1239-44.
46. Kolhari VB, Bhairappa S, Prasad NM, et al. Tuberculosis: still an enigma. Presenting as mycotic aneurysm of aorta. BMJ Case Rep. 2013;2013.
47. Gajaraj A, Victor S. Tuberculous aortoarteritis. Clin Radiol. 1981;32(4):461-6.
48. Kicska G, Litt H. Preprocedural planning for endovascular stent-graft placement. Semin Intervent Radiol. 2009;26(1):44-55.
49. Hartlage GR, Palios J, Barron BJ, et al. Multimodality imaging of aortitis. JACC Cardiovasc Imaging. 2014;7(6):605-19.
50. Litmanovich DE, Yıldırım A, Bankier AA. Insights into imaging of aortitis. Insights Imaging. 2012;3(6):545-60.
51. Raman SV, Aneja A, Jarjour WN. CMR in inflammatory vasculitis. J Cardiovasc Magn Reson. 2012;14:82.
52. Greil GF, Stuber M, Botnar RM, et al. Coronary magnetic resonance angiography in adolescents and young adults with kawasaki disease. Circulation. 2002;105(8):908-11.
53. Forbes TL, Harris JR, Nie RG, et al. Tuberculous aneurysm of the supraceliac aorta--a case report. Vasc Endovascular Surg. 2004;38(1):93-7.
54. Oran I, Parildar M, Memis A. Mesenteric artery aneurysms in intestinal tuberculosis as a cause of lower gastrointestinal bleeding. Abdom Imaging. 2001;26(2):131-3.
55. Karmakar S, Nath A, Neyaz Z, et al. Bronchial Artery Aneurysm due to Pulmonary Tuberculosis: Detection with Multidetector Computed Tomographic Angiography. J Clin Imaging Sci. 2011;1:26.
56. Cheng YS, Lu ZW. Bronchial aneurysm secondary to tuberculosis presenting with fatal hemoptysis: a case report and review of the literature. J Thorac Dis. 2014;6(6):E70-2.
57. Wang W, Gao L, Wang X. Rasmussen's aneurysm with aspergilloma in old, healed pulmonary tuberculosis. Clin Imaging. 2012;37(3):580-2.
58. De Backer AI, Mortelé KJ, De Keulenaer BL, et al. Vascular involvement secondary to tuberculosis of the abdomen. Abdom Imaging. 2005;30(6):714-8.
59. Rana SS, Sharma V, Sampath S, et al. Vascular invasion does not discriminate between pancreatic tuberculosis and pancreatic malignancy: a case series. Ann Gastroenterol. 2014;27(4):395-8.
60. El Fekih L, Oueslati I, Hassene H, et al. Association deep veinous thrombosis with pulmonary tuberculosis. Tunis Med. 2009;87(5):328-9.
61. Dentan C, Epaulard O, Seynaeve D, et al. Active tuberculosis and venous thromboembolism: association according to international classification of diseases, ninth revision hospital discharge diagnosis codes. Clin Infect Dis. 2014;58(4):495-501.

CHAPTER 16

Whole Body Imaging in Tuberculosis

Mudit Gupta, Rakesh K Gupta

INTRODUCTION

Tuberculosis (TB) has emerged as a potentially serious infectious disease especially after human immunodeficiency virus (HIV) and it continues to be an important cause of morbidity and mortality in the developing world. *Mycobacterium tuberculosis* usually spreads by droplets, leading to primary disease focus in the lung, and disseminates via the hematogenous route to extrapulmonary sites. When the immune system weakens, the bacilli start multiplying rapidly, manifesting as clinical tubercular disease.

Virtually all organ systems may be affected by TB, and simultaneous involvement of multiple organ systems is not unusual.[1,2] Lung is the most commonly affected organ, however extrapulmonary involvement can be seen in up to a third of patients, of which lymph node (LN), pleural, and bone and joint diseases are more common, whereas pericardial, meningeal and miliary forms are more likely to result in fatal outcome.[3] It is known that extrapulmonary TB potentially spreads through hematogenous route; there is likelihood that it may affect multiple organs concurrently even when the patient presents with symptoms limited to single-organ/site involvement.[4] For optimum management, disease mapping in various body organs is important. Treatment duration is long, and can be prolonged for extrapulmonary sites of infection, such as neuro TB including meningitis and musculoskeletal disease.[5] Imaging has an important role to play in assessing treatment response and in deciding the therapeutic end point.[6]

Positron emission tomography-computed tomography (PET-CT) is the whole body (WB) imaging modality used in the diagnosis and management of oncology patients. A number of studies have shown the false positivity of fluorodeoxyglucose (FDG)-PET studies in the diagnosis of neoplastic lesions. This is due to the fact that FDG is utilized by the active inflammatory cells as well as the neoplastic cells and confounds the diagnosis.

Magnetic resonance imaging (MRI) is another modality which has the potential for WB imaging. Takahara et al. demonstrated that respiratory motion does not affect diffusion-weighted contrast.[7] These insights led to the development of a new diffusion-weighted MR imaging technique with free breathing, which allowed for thin-section acquisitions in a reasonable time frame and was referred to as WB diffusion-weighted imaging with background body signal suppression, (DWIBS).[8]

Diffusion-weighted imaging with background body signal suppression is being routinely used to assess the disease burden in WB oncology imaging on routine clinical scanners.[9] Recently, it has been shown to have a complementary role to PET-CT.[10,11] There are isolated reports on the use of WB imaging which includes PET-CT and MRI.[12,13] Recently, WB-DW-MRI appears to have found a comparable diagnostic value to ^{18}F-FDG-PET/CT in staging patients with gastrointestinal lymphoma.[14] However, DWIBS, in isolation, suffers from poor spatial resolution, inability to differentiate malignant from nonmalignant lesions, and visibility of highly cellular physiological structures such as ovaries, testes, prostate, endometrium, tonsils, spleen, spinal cord, and peripheral nerves.[10]

WHOLE BODY MAGNETIC RESONANCE IMAGING

Since MRI is free of ionizing radiation hazards it is ideally suited for WB imaging. There are many different ways of achieving this like DWIBS, WB short T1 inversion recovery (STIR) and of late contrast-enhanced Dixon based technique has been added to this list.

Dixon water-fat separation entails a spectroscopic technique for fat suppression that is based on chemical shift properties instead of T1 relaxation characteristics such as STIR. The original two-point Dixon technique acquired two images using a modified spin-echo pulse sequence so that fat and water are in-phase and 180° out-of-phase.[15] One image is a conventional spin-echo image with water and fat in-phase, the second is acquired with the read out gradient shifted to produce an image with 180° water-fat phase difference. These images then undergo complex addition or subtraction to produce water only and fat only images, respectively, from which a fat-water ratio image can be calculated. However, the technique was marred by a number of inherent limitations. For example, B0 inhomogeneity-induced phase errors resulted in incorrect fat-water separation, and limitations were imposed on the pulse sequences because the echo time (TE) had to be exactly in-phase and 180° out-of-phase. Therefore, the two-point Dixon technique was noted to be more susceptible to motion artifacts.[16]

The three-point Dixon technique was developed to reduce sensitivity to magnetic field inhomogeneities and, therefore, phase errors associated with two-point Dixon by utilizing a combination of multipoint acquisition and image processing techniques.[17] Recent developments in image processing techniques, such as iterative decomposition of water and fat with echo asymmetry and least-squares estimation (IDEAL) have further helped to separate fat and water signals in inhomogeneous magnetic field regions.[18,19]

Volumetric imaging has been possible by applying DIXON with unrestricted TE approach.[20] The technique utilizes a gradient echo sequence with low flip angles to minimize T1 bias, and acquires multiple echoes at TEs at which fat and water signals are nominally in-phase or out-of-phase relative to each other. This technique helps to reduce acquisition time, minimizes spatial misregistration or ghosting artifact due to motion and allows a higher signal-to-noise ratio by use of multiple echoes. Use of multi-echo Dixon fat-water separation also allows partial k-space acquisitions and, because the sequences extend easily to multi-coil reconstruction, they can be used with parallel imaging to further decrease acquisition time. Multi-echo two-point Dixon coupled with SENSE parallel imaging technique is bundled as "m-DIXON" (modified DIXON). Dixon imaging techniques have been widely used in the literature for fat quantification in hepatic steatosis, cardiac and abdominal imaging, and MR angiography.[21-23]

To overcome the shortcomings of DWIBS, recently high-resolution contrast-enhanced three-dimensional m-DIXON (WB HR-CE-3D m-DIXON) has been successfully added to the whole body magnetic resonance (WB-MRI) protocol to provide robust WB dataset with good spatial and temporal resolution in a practically feasible short duration.[9,24] Whole body-MRI comprising these two sequences have been used to image patients who were clinically suspected to have single site/organ extrapulmonary TB.[25,26]

Recently the role of WB HR-CE-3D m-DIXON versus DWIBS to assess for multifocal tubercular infection and to decide on an easily accessible site for biopsy/aspiration for histopathological confirmation has been shown.[24] Dedicated MR imaging of clinically symptomatic organ/site was followed by WB HR-CE-3D m-DIXON first and then DWIBS (at five stations to cover the WB from the skull to the mid-thigh) using a b-value of 1500 s/mm^2. This was done with an aim to use the same contrast that was being given for the symptomatic site with no extra contrast injection. The mean additional time for WB-MRI was 25-30 minutes. This helps to avoid using any extra dose of contrast which may have issues with cost, toxicity, deposition in the tissue and in patients with renal impairment.[27]

In a study of 18 patients imaged on WB-MRI with clinically suspected single site extrapulmonary TB and tested negative for HIV, 14 patients had concurrent asymptomatic involvement of other organs/sites (78%). Three

(33%) had incidental brain tuberculoma, four patients (44%) had concurrent lung disease and three patients (33%) had LN involvement (Figs 1 to 3). In five of the earlier 14 patients, the information was helpful in choosing an easily accessible site for biopsy/aspiration for

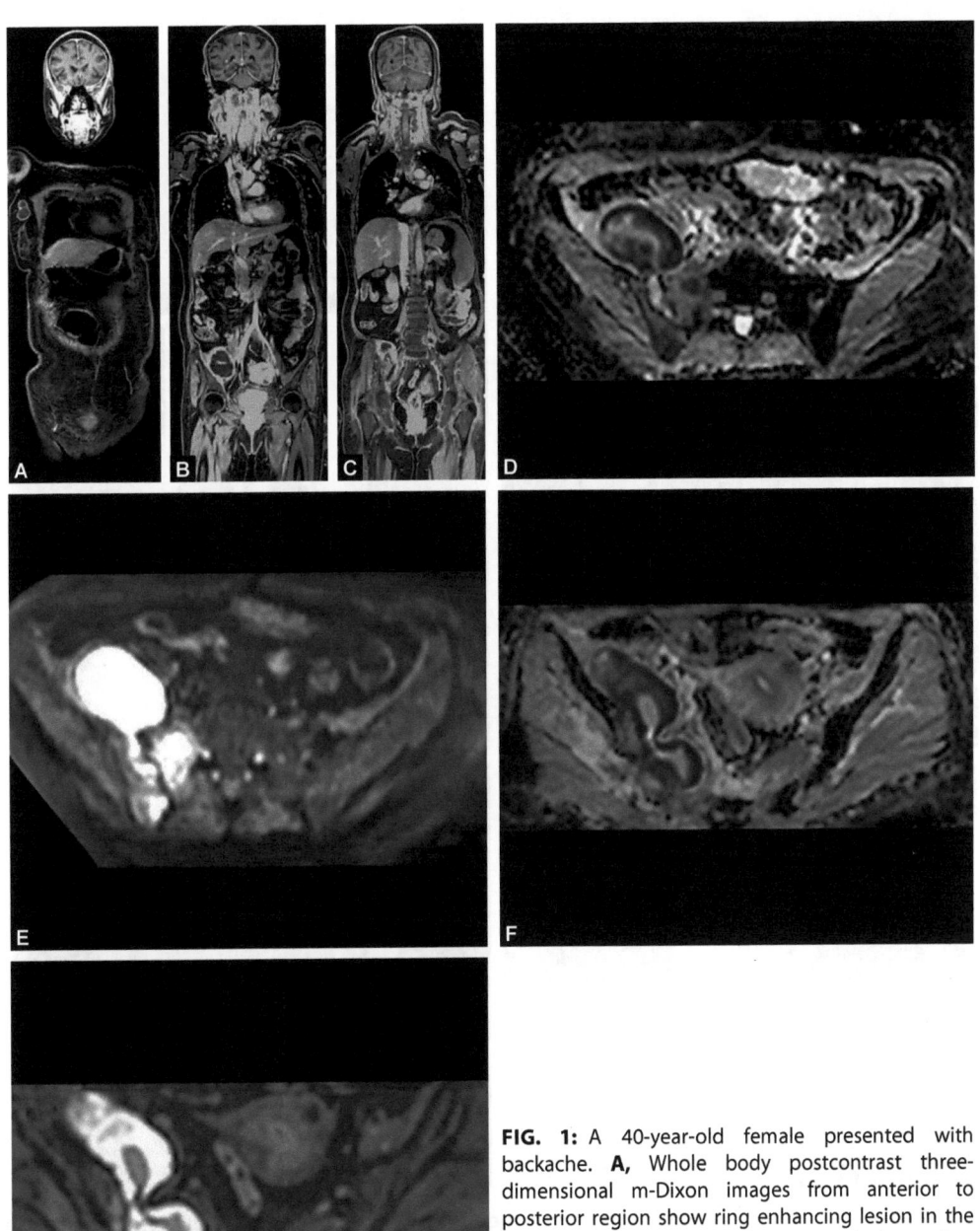

FIG. 1: A 40-year-old female presented with backache. **A,** Whole body postcontrast three-dimensional m-Dixon images from anterior to posterior region show ring enhancing lesion in the right chest, and in the right periventricular region; **B** and **C,** Multiple necrotic and nonnecrotic enlarged lymph nodes in the neck and mediastinum; **D** to **G,** Large abscess in the right sacroiliac region showing restricted diffusion with low apparent diffusion coefficient. Aspiration of pus from the chest wall showed M. tuberculosis bacilli

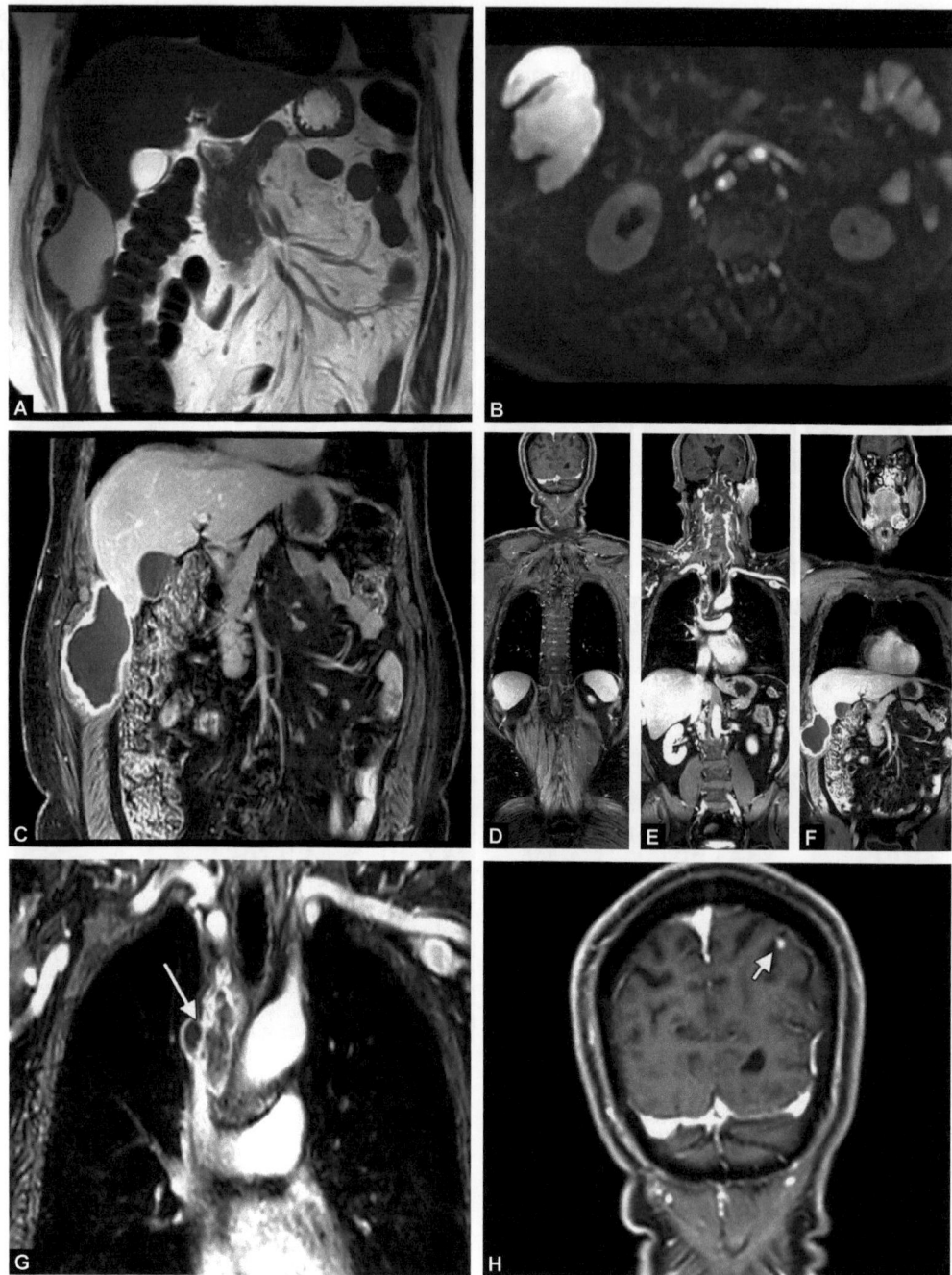

FIG. 2: A 60-year-old man presented with swelling in the right hypochondrium. **A,** magnetic resonance imaging showed a T2 hyperintense lesion in the right subcapsular region of the liver pushing the margin of the liver medially; **B,** on diffusion-weighted imaging, it shows restricted diffusion; **C,** on postcontrast study there is rim enhancement; **D** to **H,** whole body three-dimensional m-Dixon imaging showed multiple rim enhancing lymph nodes in the mediastinum (G, arrow) and disk enhancing lesion (H, small arrow) in the left frontal region. Aspiration revealed about 800 mL pus, the culture of which grew M. tuberculosis bacilli, sensitive to all the first-line drugs. The lesions showed complete resolution after 9 months of treatment

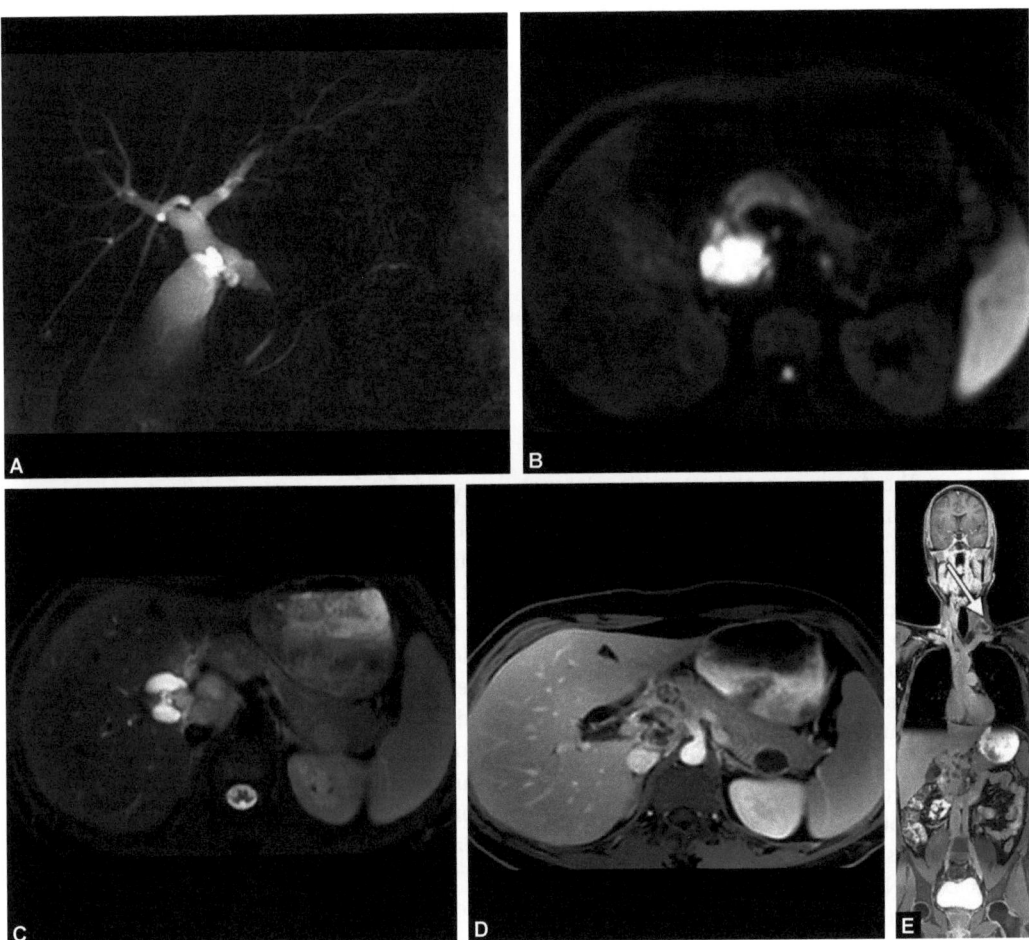

FIG. 3: A 38-year-old man underwent executive health check up and was advised magnetic resonance cholangiopancreatography for deranged liver functions. **A,** Single shot breath-hold MRCP revealed dilatation of the common bile duct (CBD) with narrowing of the distal CBD due to an extrinsic mass; **B,** diffusion-weighted; **C,** Fat suppressed T2-weighted; **D,** Postcontrast T1-weighted axial images revealed necrotic lymph node mass in the peripancreatic and celiac axis region with restricted diffusion and rim enhancement; **E,** Whole body imaging revealed a left supraclavicular lymph node (arrow). Biopsy from the mass showed necrotic tubercular lymphadenopathy. Incidental cyst in the tail of the pancreas was also noted with no restricted diffusion and rim enhancement. Patient showed complete regression of biliary dilatation at the end of 1 year following antitubercular treatment

histopathological confirmation. In addition, WB-MRI was also useful in differentiating necrotic from solid nodes. This is important while choosing which node to biopsy because diagnostic yield from solid LNs is better than from necrotic nodes.

Lesions showing impeded diffusion on DWIBS and ring or disk enhancement on postcontrast m-DIXON images were considered pathological. Lesions were grouped into abscesses, and that of bone, LN, brain, spinal cord, and other soft tissues. Lymph nodes were further categorized into necrotic and solid upon comparison of apparent diffusion coefficient (ADC) values.

One patient who presented with pituitary tumor had clinical symptoms not explained by the tumor alone; WB-MRI was performed to evaluate for any occult pathology, and multifocal extrapulmonary TB was found.

Clinically, asymptomatic brain lesions were detected in three of 10 patients (30%), who presented with spinal TB. These patients with brain lesions need longer duration of antitubercular drugs.

Diffusion-weighted imaging with background body signal suppression demonstrated a superior role in detecting vertebral lesions not evident on postcontrast 3D m-DIXON because these lesions did not show any enhancement. These lesions were detected only on DWIBS owing to impeded diffusion. However, DWIBS had poor sensitivity for brain lesions (69%) and LN lesions (51%). All these lesions were conspicuous on postcontrast 3D m-DIXON sequence. There were two patients with primary brain involvement and had extracranial disease (Figs 4 and 5).

There was 100% concordance of routine chest radiograph with WB-MRI in the five patients who demonstrated pulmonary parenchymal lesions. Chest radiograph was suggestive of enlarged hilar LNs in one patient. Rest of the patients had normal findings on chest radiograph and WB-MRI.

Breast, renal and splenic lesions were evident on both the sequences. In one patient, a single lung lesion was seen only on postcontrast 3D m-DIXON and did not show any impeded diffusion. Remaining lung lesions were seen well on both the sequences. The ADC value of these soft tissue lesions varied widely, with mean [standard deviation (SD)] being $1.26 (0.50) \pm 10^{-3}$ mm^2/s.

All the patients were under regular clinical follow-up. The WB-MRI follow-up was also obtained in all the patients after 3–4 months of antitubercular therapy (ATT). Since it yielded an excellent assessment of TB in various body organs, it helped in choosing the optimum drug regimen and duration of antitubercular treatment.

A WB MR study comprises anatomical and functional data from postcontrast m-DIXON and DWIBS sequence. The authors found the former sequence was highly sensitive and latter sequence was mildly sensitive to detect lymph nodal and cerebral lesions. Both the sequences were complementary to characterize abscesses which demonstrated well-defined peripheral enhancement on postcontrast study and impeded diffusion in the core on DWI (Figs 1 and 2). Similar, results were obtained to characterize necrotic and solid LNs. Few nonenhancing vertebral lesions were conspicuous only on DWIBS, owing to impeded diffusion in the bone marrow.

The high incidence of multifocal lesions in immunocompetent individuals is contrary to literature. The discrepancy may be explained by high sensitivity of DWIBS for pathology as compared with previous studies that were based on clinical data and imaging limited to the clinically symptomatic organs.

Whole body MRI characterized LN disease well. As documented in literature, the necrotic nodes had significantly lower ADC value than that of the solid enhancing nodes.

The authors have pioneered the application of WB-MRI in multisystem infective disease. Extracranial TB is well-known to lead to development of intracranial tuberculomas, despite patients showing good clinical response to the primary disease on appropriate antitubercular drugs. This has been termed as "paradoxical response" and has been discussed extensively. The authors note that the primary diagnosis was made on basis of clinical symptoms and imaging was limited to symptomatic organs, likely underprognosticating the disease spread.

The fact that, in the only available MRI based WB imaging study, clinically asymptomatic brain tuberculomas were detected in three of nine patients presenting with vertebral TB raises a doubt that many cases labeled as paradoxical response previously may be due to undiagnosed clinically silent brain lesions that became symptomatic later on, while the patient is on therapy. Presence of asymptomatic brain tuberculomas has been shown previously in patients with miliary pulmonary TB. The WB-MRI has the potential of providing true estimate of total disease burden in known patients of TB.

Though combining WB postcontrast 3D m-Dixon with DWIBS looks promising in the

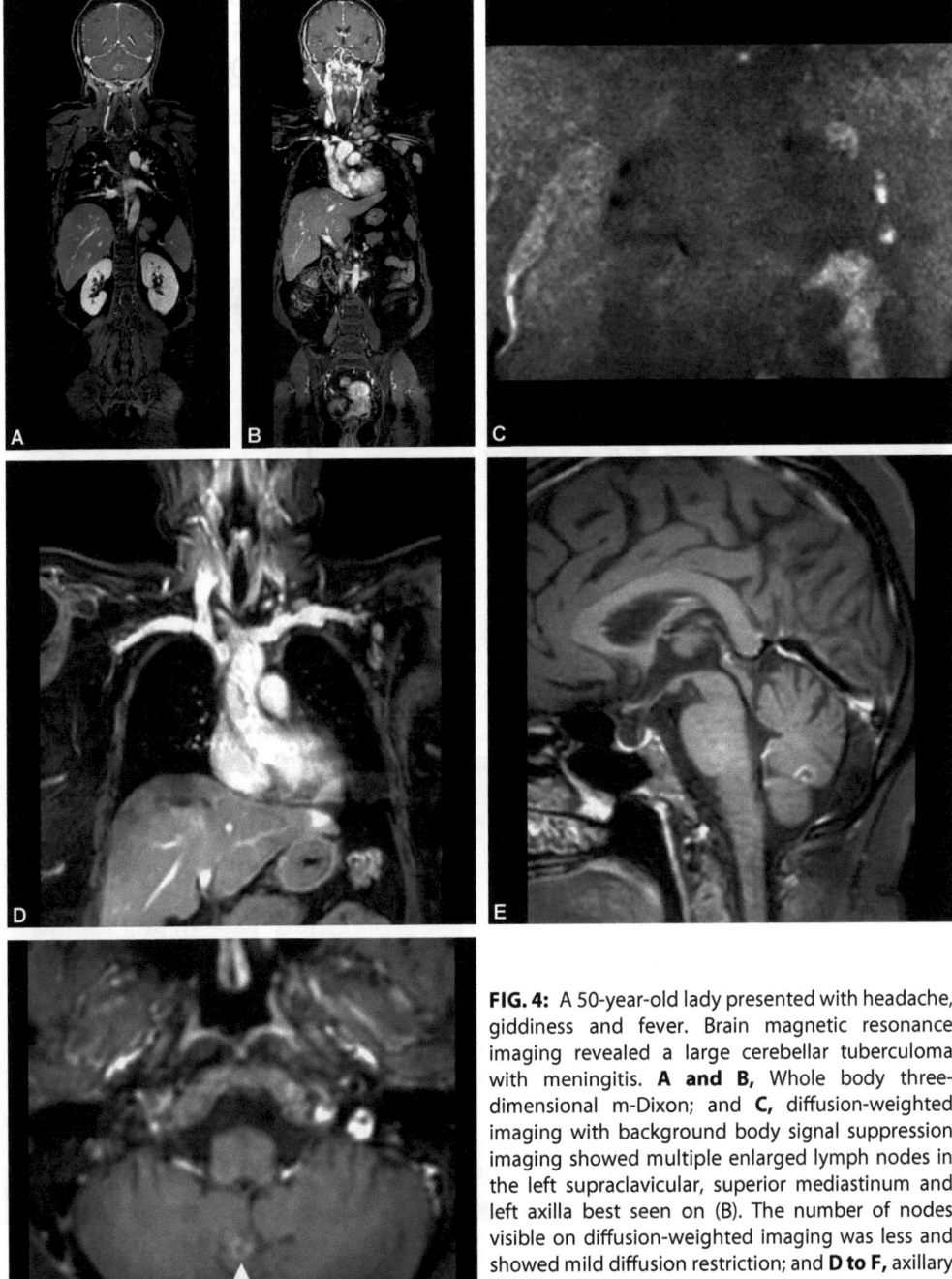

FIG. 4: A 50-year-old lady presented with headache, giddiness and fever. Brain magnetic resonance imaging revealed a large cerebellar tuberculoma with meningitis. **A and B,** Whole body three-dimensional m-Dixon; and **C,** diffusion-weighted imaging with background body signal suppression imaging showed multiple enlarged lymph nodes in the left supraclavicular, superior mediastinum and left axilla best seen on (B). The number of nodes visible on diffusion-weighted imaging was less and showed mild diffusion restriction; and **D to F,** axillary lymph node was biopsied and showed tuberculous lymphadenopathy. She was put on antitubercular therapy and showed complete resolution of lymphadenopathy with visible small residual cerebellar tuberculoma (arrow, E and F) at the end of 1 year

assessment of disease burden in TB. Currently it suffers from some limitations. The need for breath holding for about 15 seconds per station especially in sick patients and children make it difficult in these groups of patients and is a major limitation of the technique. In future free breathing WB imaging using fat-suppressed T2 Dixon and m-Dixon will help in overcoming the limitations.

WHOLE BODY POSITRON EMISSION TOMOGRAPHY-COMPUTED TOMOGRAPHY

Pilot studies have demonstrated the diagnostic value of dual time-point ^{18}F-FDG-PET/CT in imaging for detecting infective lesions in patients with extrapulmonary TB and monitoring response to therapy (Fig. 5).[28-30] During ATT,

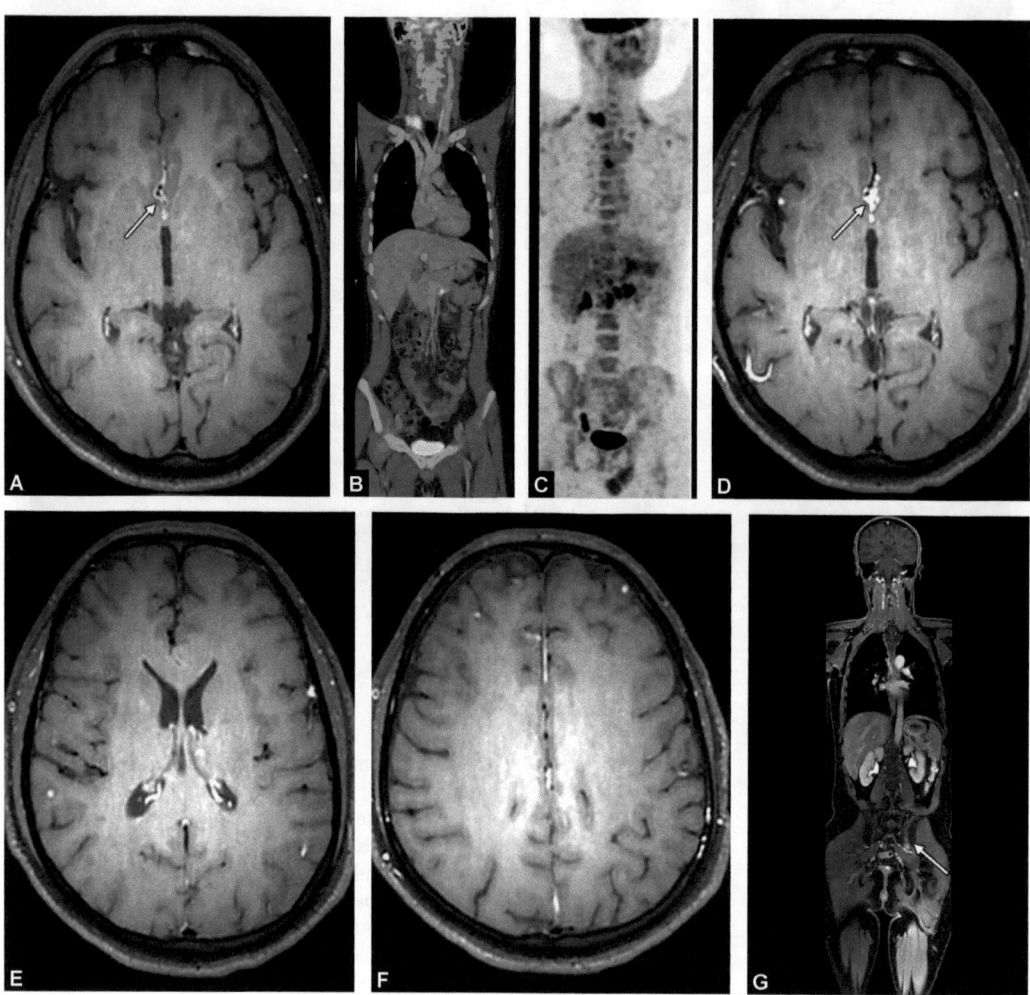

FIG. 5: A 29-year-old man presented with fever and headache. **A,** Postcontrast T1-weighted image shows focal meningeal enhancement in the midline (arrow); **B and C,** fluorodeoxyglucose-positron emission tomography study shows fluorodeoxyglucose avid right supraclavicular and abdominal lymphadenopathy. Biopsy from the supraclavicular lymph node was consistent with tubercular adenitis; **D to F,** Patient was put on antitubercular therapy and a repeat postcontrast magnetic resonance imaging after 2 months shows increase in focal meningeal enhancement and tiny nodular cortical enhancement in bilateral frontal and right parietal regions to suggest appearance of tuberculomas; and **G,** The whole body postcontrast three-dimensional m-Dixon imaging shows regression of supraclavicular and abdominal lymphadenopathy and appearance of left sacroiliitis (arrow). Patient showed complete clinical recovery after antitubercular therapy

some bacillus-negative tuberculomas do not decrease in size and may even increase, making it difficult for the physician to decide whether or not to modify treatment. In these cases, ^{18}F-FDG-PET/CT imaging may help, as the changes in glycolytic activity of the inflammatory lesion, measured by ^{18}F-FDG uptake, correlate well with the clinical markers of response.[31] Ongoing trials hypothesize that a decrease in the uptake of FDG in the foci of TB during treatment permit a noninvasive monitoring of therapeutic response.[32] However, high uptake of FDG by PET may represent ongoing active disease, or simply the host immune system activity.[33] The imaging features of 18F-FDG-PET/CT in TB frequently mimic those of many malignancies.[34,35] Also, TB symptoms could be masked by the concurrent malignancy.[36]

CONCLUSION

Whole body MRI using postcontrast 3D m-DIXON and DWIBS are complementary sequences that provide an excellent tool for WB imaging, yielding both morphological and functional data that can be used for assessing the disease load and involvement of multiple body organs in patients with extrapulmonary TB. The WB-PET-CT using macrophage-specific agents as well as other TB specific agents will certainly help to improve the specificity of the disease and therapeutic response assessment in future. It is likely to help in optimizing the duration of treatment and will have significant bearing on disease management in future.

REFERENCES

1. Ozvaran MK, Baran R, Tor M, et al. Extrapulmonary tuberculosis in non-human immunodeficiency virus-infected adults in an endemic region. Ann Thorac Med. 2007;2(3):118-21.
2. Gupta RK, Kohli A, Gaur V, et al. MRI of the brain in patients with miliary pulmonary tuberculosis without symptoms or signs of central nervous system involvement. Neuroradiology. 1997;39(10):699-704.
3. World Health Organization (WHO). (2010). Treatment of Tuberculosis: Guidelines. [online] Available from: www.apps.who.int/iris/bitstream/10665/44165/1/9789241547833_eng.pdf?ua=1&ua=1. [Accessed June, 2017].
4. Getahun H, Matteelli A, Chaisson RE, et al. Latent Mycobacterium tuberculosis infection. N Engl J Med. 2015;372(22):2127-35.
5. Blumberg HM, Burman WJ, Chaisson RE, et al. American Thoracic Society/Centers for Disease Control and Prevention/Infectious Diseases Society of America: treatment of tuberculosis. Am J Respir Crit Care Med. 2003;167(4):603-62.
6. API Consensus Expert Committee. API TB Consensus Guidelines 2006: Management of pulmonary tuberculosis, extra-pulmonary tuberculosis and tuberculosis in special situations. J Assoc Physicians India. 2006;54:219-34.
7. Takahara T, Imai Y, Yamashita T, et al. Diffusion weighted whole body imaging with background body signal suppression (DWIBS): technical improvement using free breathing, STIR and high resolution 3D display. Radiat Med. 2004;22(4):275-82.
8. Kwee TC, Takahara T, Ochiai R, et al. Whole-body diffusion-weighted magnetic resonance imaging. Eur J Radiol. 2009;70(3):409-17.
9. Costelloe CM, Kundra V, Ma J, et al. Fast Dixon whole-body MRI for detecting distant cancer metastasis: a preliminary clinical study. J Magn Reson Imaging. 2012;35(2): 399-408.
10. Kwee TC, Takahara T, Ochiai R, et al. Complementary roles of whole-body diffusion-weighted MRI and 18F-FDG PET: the state of the art and potential applications. J Nucl Med. 2010;51(10):1549-58.
11. Cafagna D, Rubini G, Iuele F, et al. Whole-body MR-DWIBS vs. [18F]-FDG-PET/CT in the study of malignant tumors: a retrospective study. Radiol Med. 2012;117(2):293-311.
12. Schmidt GP, Haug A, Reiser MF, et al. Whole-body MRI and FDG-PET/CT imaging diagnostics in oncology. Radiologe. 2010;50(4):329-38.
13. Xu GZ, Li CY, Zhao L, et al. Comparison of FDG whole-body PET/CT and gadolinium-enhanced whole-body MRI for distant malignancies in patients with malignant tumors: a meta-analysis. Ann Oncol. 2013;24(1):96-101.
14. Stecco A, Buemi F, Quagliozzi M, et al. Staging of Primary Abdominal Lymphomas: Comparison of Whole-Body MRI with Diffusion-Weighted Imaging and (18)F-FDG-PET/CT. Gastroenterol Res Pract. 2015;2015:104794.
15. Dixon WT. Simple proton spectroscopic imaging. Radiology. 1984;153(1):189-94.
16. Ma J. Dixon techniques for water and fat imaging. J Magn Reson Imaging. 2008;28(3):543-58.
17. Glover GH, Schneider E. Three-point Dixon technique for true water/fat decomposition with B0 inhomogeneity correction. Magn Reson Med. 1991;18(2):371-83.
18. Reeder SB, Pineda AR, Wen Z, et al. Iterative decomposition of water and fat with echo asymmetry and least-squares estimation (IDEAL): application with fast spin-echo imaging. Magn Reson Med. 2005;54(3):636-44.
19. Reeder SB, McKenzie CA, Pineda AR, et al. Water-fat separation with IDEAL gradient-echo imaging., J Magn Reson Imaging. 2007;25(3):644-52.
20. Yu H, McKenzie CA, Shimakawa A, et al. Multiecho reconstruction for simultaneous water-fat decomposition and T2* estimation. J Magn Reson Imaging. 2007;26(4):1153-61.
21. Ishizaka K, Oyama N, Mito S, et al. Comparison of 1H MR spectroscopy, 3-point DIXON, and multi-echo gradient echo for measuring hepatic fat fraction. Magn Reson Med Sci. 2011;10(1):41-8.

22. Eggers H, Börnert P. Chemical shift encoding-based water-fat separation methods. J Magn Reson Imaging. 2014;40(2):251-68.
23. Farrelly C, Shah S, Davarpanah A, et al. ECG-gated multiecho Dixon fat-water separation in cardiac MRI: advantages over conventional fat-saturated imaging. AJR Am J Roentgenol. 2012;199(1):W74-83.
24. Pandey AK, Gupta RK, Jain KK, et al. Role of whole-body magnetic resonance imaging in the evaluation of extrapulmonary tuberculosis in immunocompetent patients. J Comput Assist Tomogr. 2014;38(3):415-23.
25. Costelloe CM, Madewell JE, Kundra V, et al. Conspicuity of bone metastases on fast Dixon-based multisequence whole-body MRI: clinical utility per sequence. Magn Reson Imaging. 2013;31(5):669-75.
26. Blackledge MD, Brown D, Wallace T, et al. Improved morphological information using the Dixon technique in conjunction with DWI for detection of bone metastases. Proc Intl Soc Mag Reson Med. 2011.
27. Perazella MA. Gadolinium-contrast toxicity in patients with kidney disease: nephrotoxicity and nephrogenic systemic fibrosis. Curr Drug Saf. 2008;3(1):67-75.
28. Razak HR, Geso M, Abdul Rahim N, et al. Imaging characteristics of extrapulmonary tuberculosis lesions on dual time point imaging (DTPI) of FDG PET/CT. J Med Imaging Radiat Oncol. 2011;55(6):556-62.
29. Martinez V, Castilla-Lievre MA, Guillet-Caruba C, et al. (18)F-FDG PET/CT in tuberculosis: an early non-invasive marker of therapeutic response. Int J Tuberc Lung Dis. 2012;16(9):1180-5.
30. Vorster M, Sathekge MM, Bomanji J. Advances in imaging of tuberculosis: the role of ^{18}F-FDG PET and PET/CT. Curr Opin Pulm Med. 2014;20(3):287-93.
31. Park IN, Ryu JS, Shim TS. Evaluation of therapeutic response of tuberculoma using F-18 FDG positron emission tomography. Clin Nucl Med. 2008;33(1):1-3.
32. Dureja S, Sen IB, Acharya S. Potential role of F18 FDG PET-CT as an imaging biomarker for the noninvasive evaluation in uncomplicated skeletal tuberculosis: a prospective clinical observational study. Eur Spine J. 2014;23(11):2449-54.
33. Jalil AJ, Rossetti C, Abdul Rahim N, et al. Potential false positive active extra pulmonary tuberculosis lesions on FDG PET/CT imaging in malignancy. Dicle Med J. 2010;37:42-7.
34. Ito K, Morooka M, Minamimoto R, et al. Imaging spectrum and pitfalls of 18fluorodeoxyglucose positron emission tomography/computed tomography in patients with tuberculosis. Jpn J Radiol. 2013;31(8):511-20.
35. Li Y, Su M, Li F, et al. The value of 18F-FDG-PET/CT in the differential diagnosis of solitary pulmonary nodules in areas with a high incidence of tuberculosis. Ann Nucl Med. 2011;25(10):804-11.
36. Bhattacharya A, Agarwal KL, Kashyap R, et al. Coexisting Tuberculosis and Non-Hodgkin's Lymphoma on 18F-Fluorodeoxyglucose PET-CT. J Postgrad Med Edu Res. 2012; 46(1):49-50.

17 CHAPTER

Tuberculosis in the Pediatric Patient

Manisha Jana, Arun K Gupta

INTRODUCTION

Tuberculosis (TB) is an infectious disease caused by *Mycobacterium tuberculosis* and is a significant cause of morbidity and mortality especially in childhood. The annual risk of tuberculosis infection (ARTI) is a reflector of the prevalence of disease in the younger population.[1] The ARTI in India in 2002–2003 was between 1% and 2.5%; and in 2009–2010, in spite of the ongoing National Tuberculosis Control Programs, it was still about 1% in most zones of India.[2,3] Owing to the high prevalence of disease in the society, the children are at risk to contract disease from the infected adults. Although precise epidemiological data is scarce, pulmonary TB in the age group 5–14 year is uncommon compared to adults and is even rarer among those below the age of 5 years.[4]

ROLE OF IMAGING

The proposed algorithm to diagnose pulmonary TB in children by the Working Group on Tuberculosis, Indian Academy of Pediatrics (2012)[4] states that fever and/or cough for longer than 2 weeks with loss of weight and recent history of contact should arouse suspicion of TB. Although detailed description of the algorithm is beyond the scope of this chapter, the radiologist should be aware of the features highly suggestive of TB on chest radiography, i.e., hilar or right paratracheal adenopathy with or without parenchymal disease, miliary lesion and/or fibrocavitary pneumonia. Computed tomography (CT) plays only a limited role in the diagnostic workup of pediatric pulmonary TB[4] (chest radiographic features not suggestive and tuberculin test positive, for example).

IMAGING MODALITIES

Pulmonary Tuberculosis

- As a diagnostic workup of pulmonary TB, chest radiograph is the most commonly utilized imaging modality
- Ultrasound may be used in evaluation of persistent or unusual peripheral lung opacities, pleural pathologies and mediastinal widening
- Computed tomography thorax is uncommonly used in diagnosis, but it remains the most useful imaging tool in detecting complications
- Magnetic resonance imaging (MRI) is not routinely used in evaluation of the lungs but can be used for assessing treatment response in cases of mediastinal nodal involvement.

Extrapulmonary Tuberculosis

- Plain radiograph is the first investigation in musculoskeletal TB, providing a wealth of information
- Ultrasound of abdomen is a useful tool in the diagnostic algorithm of abdominopelvic TB, although the diagnostic criteria on ultrasound is not precise. The suggestive findings are discussed later in this chapter.
- Contrast-enhanced CT (CECT) of abdomen is the most useful investigation in the evaluation of abdominal TB [gastrointestinal (GI), genitourinary or peritoneal]

- Magnetic resonance imaging is of immense diagnostic importance in musculoskeletal and central nervous system (CNS) tuberculosis in pediatric age group.

IMAGING MANIFESTATIONS

Pulmonary Tuberculosis

Primary TB is more common than postprimary lesion in children. Pulmonary TB in younger children and infants shows some differences, with higher chances of miliary TB.[5,6] Except for primary pulmonary complex (PPC), all other forms (progressive primary disease, miliary disease and fibrocavitary disease) are categorized as severe pulmonary TB.[4]

Pulmonary Primary Complex

Primary pulmonary TB starts with a pulmonary focus of infection (a localized area of consolidation), enlarged lymphatics draining this area of consolidation and enlarged draining lymph nodes. The primary focus is termed Ghon's focus and the PPC is known as "Ranke's complex" (Fig. 1). Cavitation and endobronchial spread of disease is rare in children with uncomplicated primary TB.[7-9] There is no specific lobar predominance and, primary TB can cause consolidation of any lobe. Persistent mass-like lesion or tuberculoma is uncommon in children.[10]

Lymph Node Involvement

Lymphadenopathy is a common feature of primary TB and is the radiologic hallmark of disease in children. Enlarged lymph nodes are usually in the hila, the right paratracheal and less commonly, the subcarinal region. The lymphadenopathy can be ipsilateral to the parenchymal lesion; or bilateral in approximately 30% of patients.[10]

Tubercular adenopathy (Figs 2A to D) can show central areas of low attenuation with rim enhancement of thick irregular wall. Less commonly they can be homogenously enhancing or ghost-like ring enhancement in a group of matted nodes. On MRI, the central necrosis of tubercular nodes is seen as hyperintense area on T2-weighted (T2W) images.

Airway Involvement

Tubercular endobronchial disease can cause atelectasis. In primary TB, atelectasis can be seen in the anterior segment of upper lobe or medial segment of middle lobe due to compression by lymph node enlargement.

Pleural Involvement

Pleural effusion is uncommon in primary TB. If present, usually it is free and small in amount. Large pleural effusion or empyema is rare in primary TB.[7]

Primary TB can heal to give rise to postprimary lesion (PPL) or can show progression or reactivation to manifest as progressive primary disease (PPD) (Flowchart 1).

Progressive Primary Disease

Parenchymal Involvement

Consolidation (Figs 3 and 4) in PPD commonly involves apical or posterior segments of upper lobe or superior segment of lower lobe, often involving more than one pulmonary segment. Segmental consolidation can have cavitation or lead to collapse. One of the most striking features of pediatric pulmonary TB is the absence of proliferative apical TB before onset of adolescence.[11]

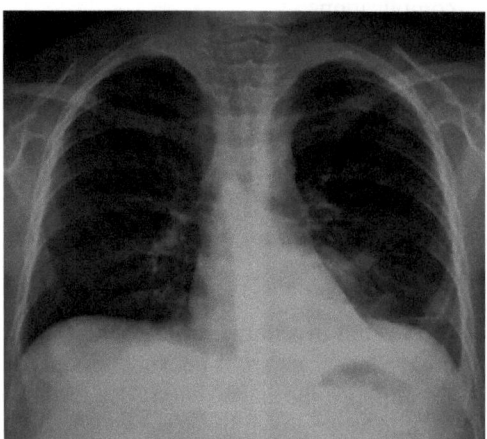

FIG. 1: Chest radiograph in primary pulmonary complex. Chest radiograph reveals left lower zone consolidation, left hilar lymphadenopathy, and mild left pleural effusion

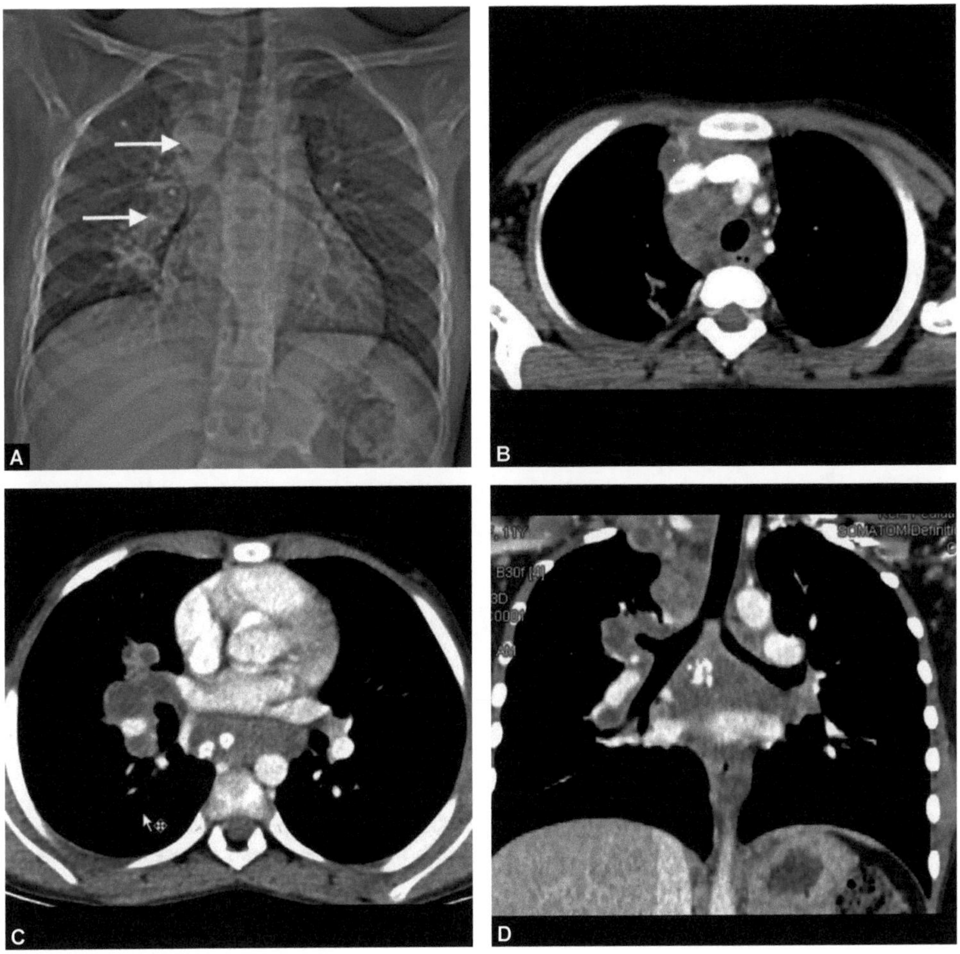

ns in the Pediatric Patient

FIG. 2: Primary tuberculosis, lymph nodal disease. **A,** Chest radiograph shows right paratracheal and right hilar adenopathy (arrows); **B** and **C,** on contrast-enhanced computed tomography axial; **D,** coronal reformatted images, the nodes show central nonenhancing necrotic area and peripheral rim enhancement

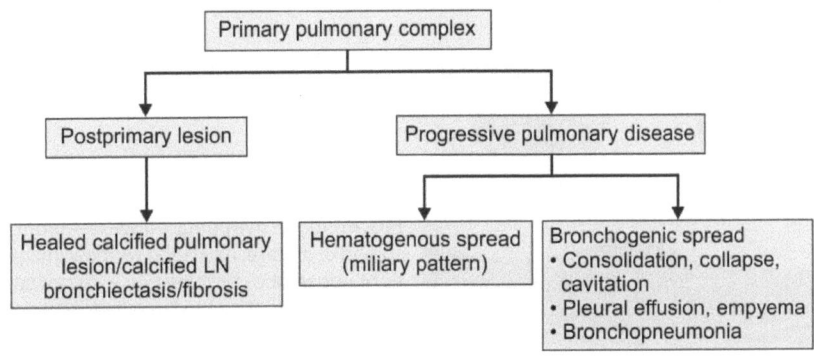

FLOWCHART 1: Course of pulmonary TB in children

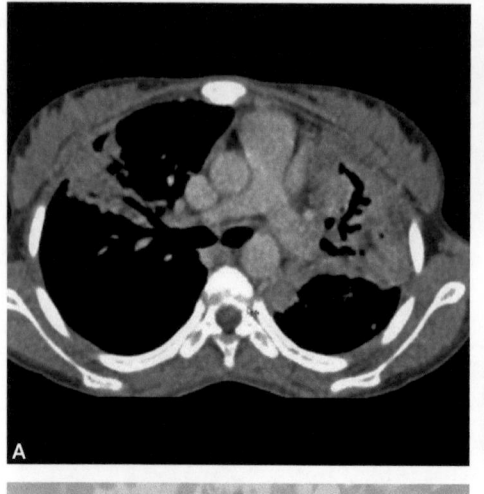
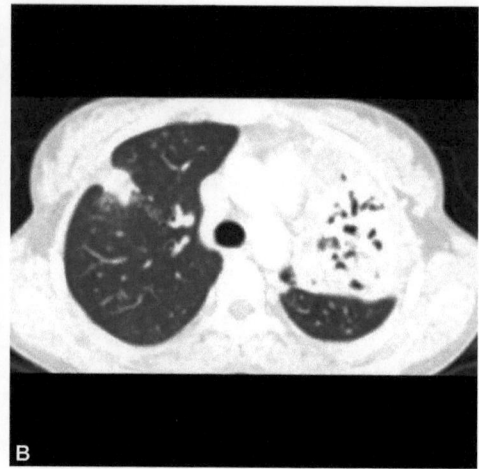
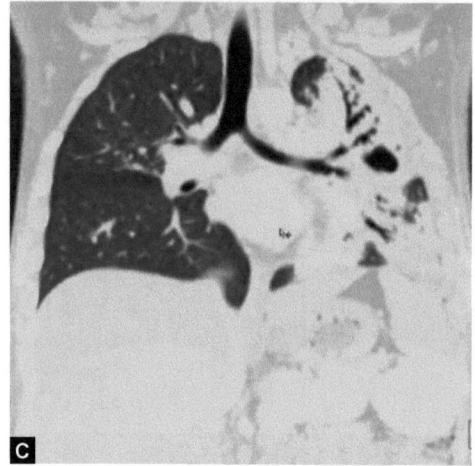

FIG. 3: Progressive primary disease in a 12-year-old girl, bronchogenic spread of disease. **A,** Axial soft tissue; **B,** lung window images; and **C,** coronal reformatted image reveal bilateral extensive consolidation with cavitation involving both upper lobes

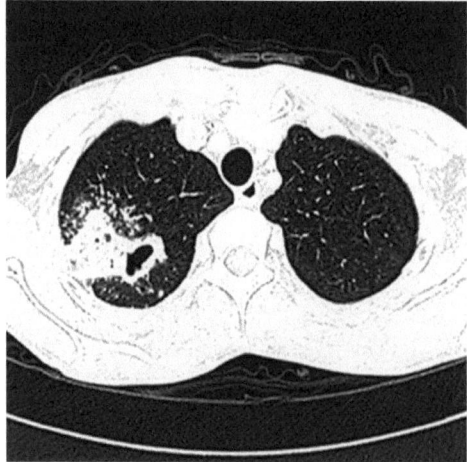

FIG. 4: Progressive primary disease—bronchogenic spread of disease. Axial lung window image reveals right upper lobe consolidation with cavitation, and acinar nodules showing "tree-in-bud" appearance, involving right upper lobe

Cavitation within a consolidation is a typical imaging feature of PPD. The consolidated lung shows areas of breakdown and gives rise to irregular thick-walled cavities. With healing, the cavities become thin and smooth walled.

Pleural Involvement

Pleural effusion in PPD is usually moderate to large in amount; unlike that in PPC. Usually it is unilateral, free, and with or without an ipsilateral lung lesion. The effusion may get complicated to form empyema (Fig. 5), pleural thickening, pyopneumothorax, or fibrothorax after healing.

Tuberculous Bronchopneumonia

Endobronchial spread of tubercular parenchymal lesion can occur when the lesion causes local erosion into the bronchial lumen. After bronchial communication, infection spreads through the bronchial tree to ipsilateral or bilateral lung parenchyma. It results in multiple acinar nodules (ill-defined with fluffy margins), show branching (tree-in-bud appearance).

Miliary Tuberculosis

Hematogenous dissemination of primary TB (Fig. 6) occurs when primary lesion erodes into a vascular channel, causing miliary dissemination into the lungs and many organs. The miliary lesions in lung (Fig. 7) are tiny, discrete pinpoint opacities evenly distributed throughout both lungs with some basal predominance. High-resolution CT (HRCT) is sensitive to detect these miliary nodules (seen as pinpoint well-defined nodules about 1–3 mm in diameter).

Postprimary Lesion

The PPL results from healing of primary pulmonary TB, and results in parenchymal (Fig. 8) or nodal calcification and/or fibrotic lesions.

Extrapulmonary Tuberculosis

Extrapulmonary TB can be divided into severe and nonsevere groups [Revised National Tuberculosis Control Programme (RNTCP) classification]. Central nervous system TB, tubercular pericarditis, tubercular peritonitis and intestinal TB, spinal TB with neurological symptoms, bilateral and extensive pleurisy, disseminated TB are considered severe form; whereas unilateral pleural effusion, lymph node TB, peripheral bone and joint involvement (excluding spine) are considered nonsevere forms.[12-14]

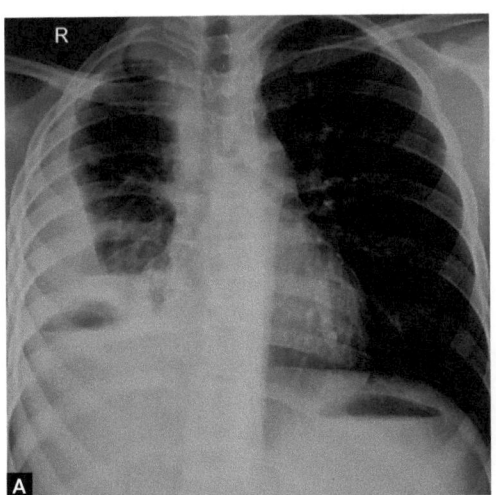 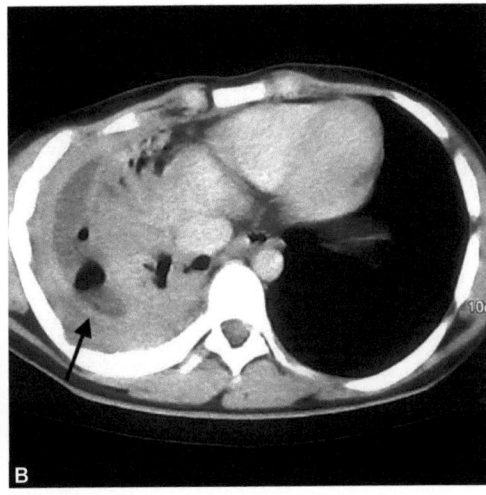

FIG. 5: Empyema. **A,** Chest radiograph reveals homogeneous opacity occupying right lower hemithorax having air loculations and a concave upper margin; **B,** contrast-enhanced computed tomography (CECT) chest axial image reveals volume loss, rib crowding on right side and gross pleural thickening with pleural enhancement (split pleura sign, arrow) and adjacent pulmonary collapse

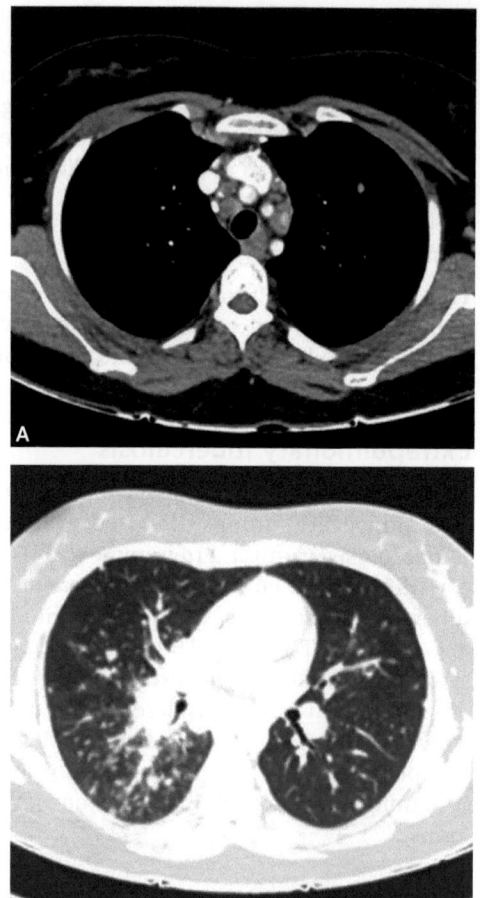
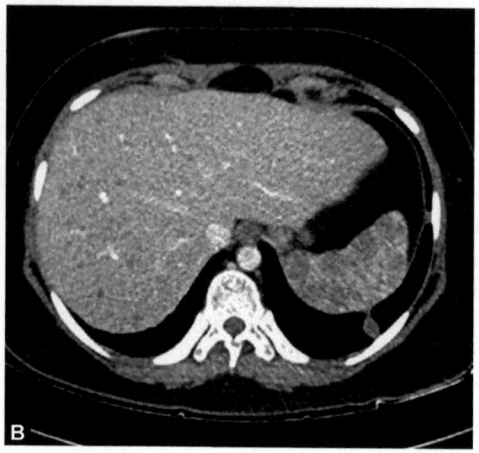

FIG. 6: Disseminated tuberculosis in a 16-year-old girl. **A** and **B,** axial soft tissue window images reveal necrotic mediastinal adenopathy and small focal hypodense lesions in the liver; **C,** axial lung window image shows extensive centriacinar nodules in both the lungs

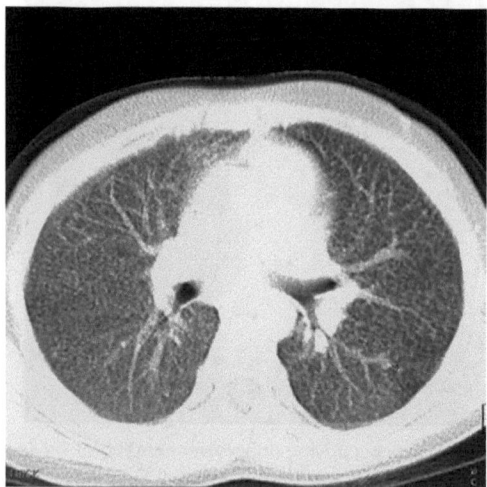
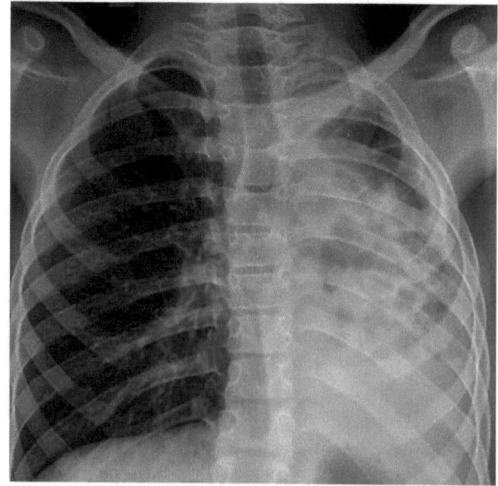

FIG. 7: Miliary tuberculosis. Axial lung window image reveals fine miliary nodules spread over both the lungs

FIG. 8: Tubercular bronchiectasis with destroyed left lung. Chest radiograph reveals opaque left hemithorax with ipsilateral mediastinal shift and multiple cystic lucencies within left hemithorax

Intracranial Tuberculosis

Central nervous system TB (Figs 9 to 12) may present either as meningitis or parenchymal TB. Depending on the type, however, it is classified as diffuse meningeal [tuberculous meningitis (TBM)], tuberculomas, tuberculous abscess and focal cerebritis.

Tuberculous Meningitis

The diagnosis of TBM is based on clinical suspicion and cerebrospinal fluid (CSF) examination. Imaging has a role in corroborating the diagnosis, and is useful for assessing complications including hydrocephalus and infarcts.

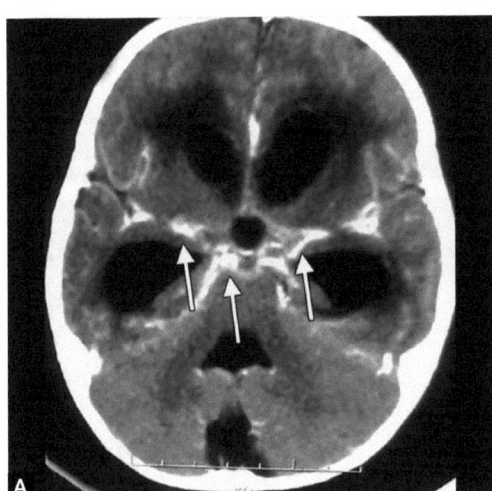
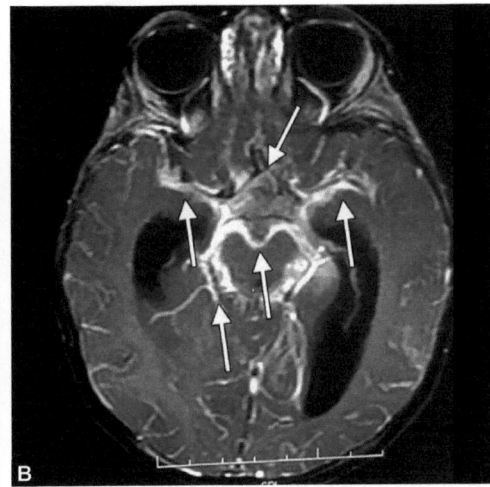

FIG. 9: Enhancing basal exudates in tubercular meningitis in an 11-year-old boy. **A** and **B,** Axial contrast-enhanced computed tomography and contrast-enhanced T1-weighted fat-suppressed magnetic resonance images reveal abnormal meningeal enhancement (arrows) along the sylvian cisterns, prepontine, ambient, and suprasellar cistern

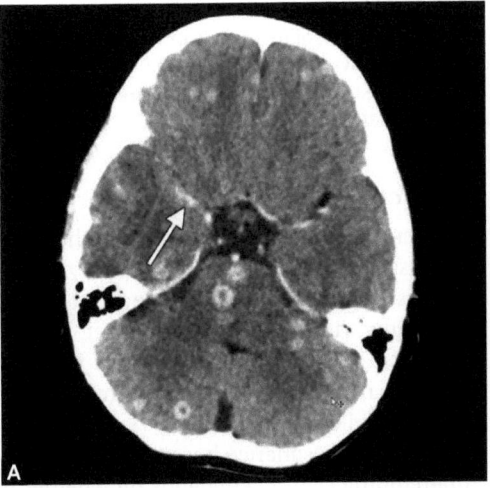
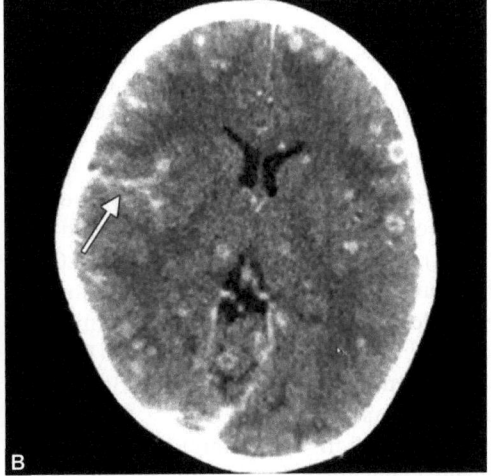

FIG. 10: Central nervous system tuberculosis, tuberculoma with meningitis. Contrast-enhanced computed tomography brain reveals multiple disk and ring enhancing focal lesions and meningeal enhancement in right sylvian fissure cistern (arrow)

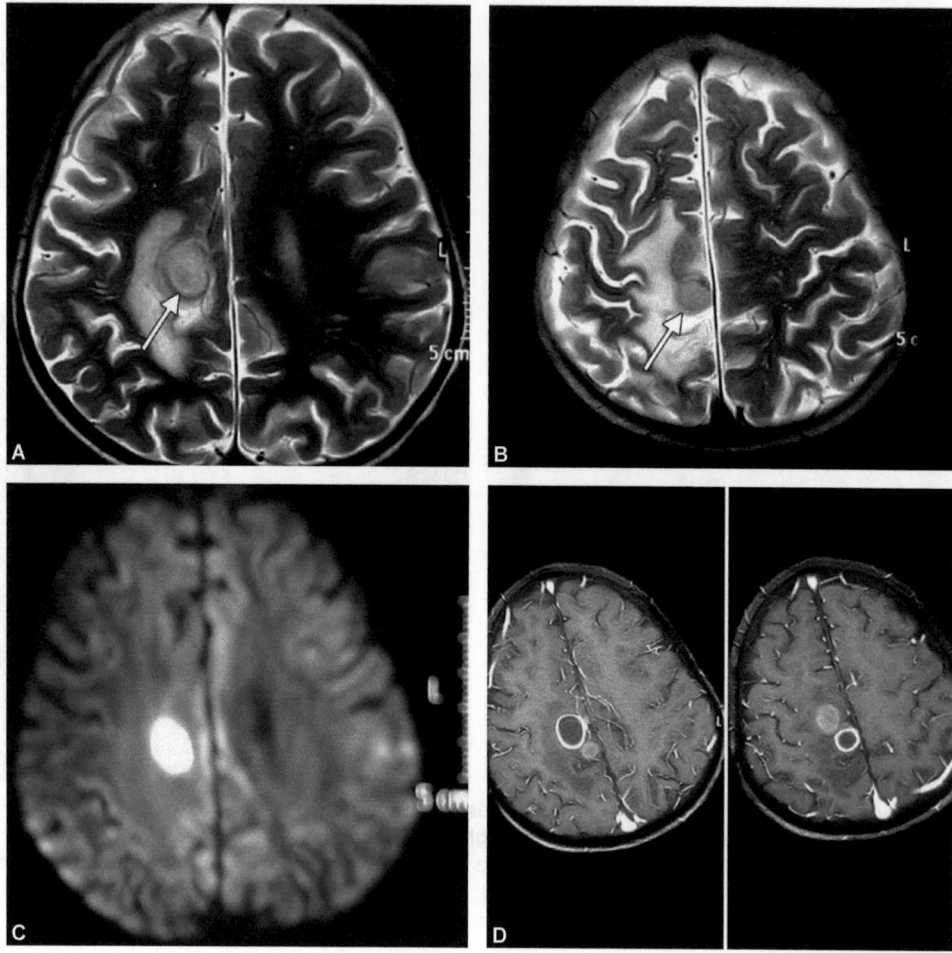

FIG. 11: A and **B,** Magnetic resonance imaging appearance of tubercular abscess and tuberculoma with T2-weighted hypointense core. Axial T2-weighted magnetic resonance imaging image shows two parenchymal lesions, one having a hyperintense core (abscess arrow in figure A) and another with hypointense core (tuberculoma arrow in figure B); **C** and **D,** the former lesion shows restriction of diffusion; whereas both lesions show thin and smooth rim enhancement after gadolinium administration

The exudates in the basal cisterns are iso/hyperdense on noncontrast-enhanced CT (NCCT), and show enhancement on CECT.[15] The meningeal enhancement is usually smooth and thick (Fig. 9A) but can sometimes be nodular.[16,17] Contrast-enhanced MRI (Fig. 9B) is more sensitive than CT for detecting subtle meningeal enhancement.

Complications of tubercular meningeal enhancement are hydrocephalus and infarcts in the basal ganglia. Late sequelae of TBM include atrophy, meningeal calcifications and focal infarcts.

Intracranial Tuberculomas

Tuberculomas (Fig. 10) may occur either alone or in association with TBM. On NCCT, they are seen as hypodense to isodense focal lesions, and show rim enhancement after contrast administration. Tuberculoma can be either single or multiple or conglomerate, and have variable perilesional edema.

Magnetic resonance imaging appearance of tuberculoma (Fig. 11) depends on whether the tuberculoma is noncaseating, caseating with a solid center or caseating with a liquid center.[18] The signal characteristics are shown in table 1.

Tuberculosis in the Pediatric Patient

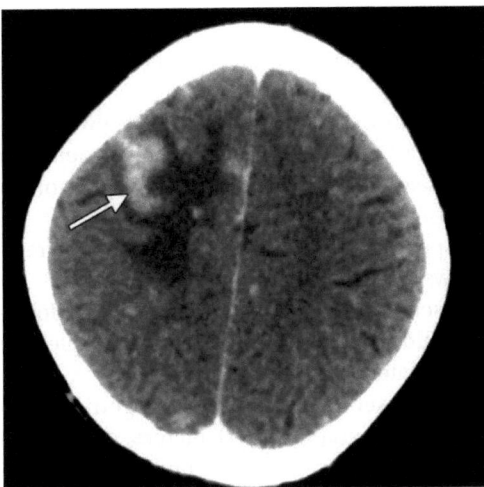

FIG. 12: Tuberculoma with focal cerebritis. Contrast-enhanced computed tomography brain reveals multiple tiny disk enhancing focal lesions and focal gyral enhancement with surrounding edema in right frontal lobe (arrow)

Advanced MR imaging techniques including spectroscopy and magnetization transfer imaging have also been shown to be helpful in differentiating tuberculomas from other lesions. Tuberculomas on MR spectroscopy characteristically show lipid peak with or without raised choline.[19] Magnetization transfer images have been shown to be more sensitive than T2-weighted images (T2WIs) in detecting small tuberculomas.[20]

The differential diagnoses of tuberculoma include neurocysticercosis, pyogenic abscess and fungal abscess. Computed tomography and MR features may help in differentiating tuberculoma from cysticercosis (Table 2).[19,21]

Tubercular abscess and focal cerebritis are rare presentations of intracranial TB. Imaging features of tubercular abscess are similar to pyogenic abscess. A noncaseating tuberculoma with ring enhancement is differentiated from a tuberculous abscess by noting the attenuation values of the center of the lesion which will be similar to normal brain in the former and low in the latter. Magnetic resonance spectroscopy of a tubercular abscess also shows lactate and lipid peaks without any amino acid peak which helps in differentiating it from pyogenic abscess.

Focal cerebritis (Fig. 12) is diagnosed in presence of focal edema with gyral enhancement without an evident abscess or tuberculoma in the same region.

Table 1: Magnetic resonance imaging features of tuberculoma			
	T1-weighted image	T2-weighted image	Contrast enhancement
Noncaseating	Hypointense	Hyperintense	Homogeneous
Caseating with solid center	Hypo to isointense	Iso to hypointense center, hypointense rim	Rim enhancement
Caseating with liquid center	Hypointense center	Centrally hyperintense with hypointense rim	Rim enhancement

Table 2: Differentiating features of tuberculoma and neurocysticercosis		
	Tuberculoma	Neurocysticercosis
Size of lesion	Larger (>2 cm)	Small
Associated meningitis	Favors diagnosis	Unlikely
Enhancement	Irregular thick rim	Smooth thin rim enhancement
Central/eccentric hyperdensity	Central hyperdensity	Eccentric hyperdensity (scolex)
T2W signal of center	Variable, can be T2W hypointense to isointense in solid caseation necrosis	Usually hyperintense
Lipid-lactate peak on magnetic resonance spectroscopy	Present	Absent

T2W, T2-weighted.

Abdominal Tuberculosis

Pediatric abdominal TB may present as localized involvement as in peritoneal disease, intestinal disease or mesenteric lymphadenopathy; or disseminated disease with visceral involvement. Although there are no standard guidelines for sonographic diagnosis of abdominal tuberculosis, suggestive findings include echogenic thickened mesentery with lymph nodes greater than 15 mm in size, dilated and matted bowel loops, thickened omentum and ascites.[22]

Peritoneal Tuberculosis (Figs 13 and 14)

Peritoneal TB in children differs from adult peritoneal TB in the following ways:[23,24]

- The "dry" or "sclerotic" type peritoneal TB is very uncommon in childhood; unlike in adults
- Pediatric peritoneal TB is almost always secondary to intestinal (contiguous extension) disease or lymphadenopathy; or pulmonary disease.

The spectrum of findings in peritoneal TB are as follows:

- Ascitic fluid of high density [25–45 Hounsfield unit (HU) on CT] with multiple fine delicate septations
- Increased mesenteric echogenicity on ultrasonography (USG), increased density of the mesentery on CT and matting of bowel loops

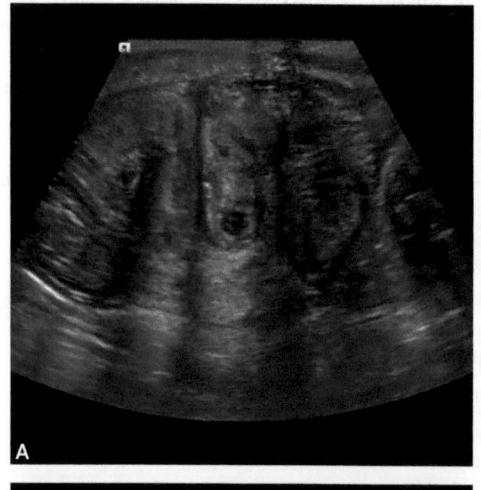
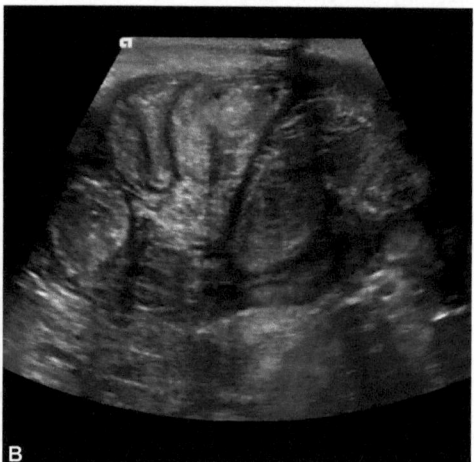
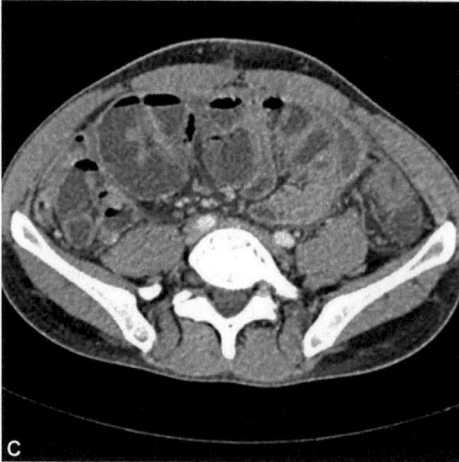

FIG. 13: Peritoneal tuberculosis. **A** and **B,** Ultrasound images reveal increased mesenteric echogenicity and matted bowel loops arranged in a stellate fashion; **C,** contrast-enhanced computed tomography abdomen axial image reveals smooth peritoneal thickening and palisading of small bowel loops

Tuberculosis in the Pediatric Patient

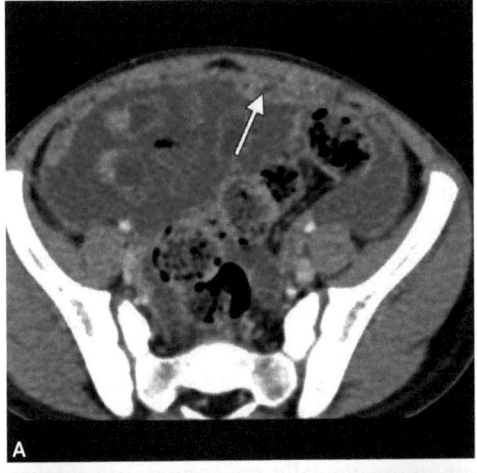
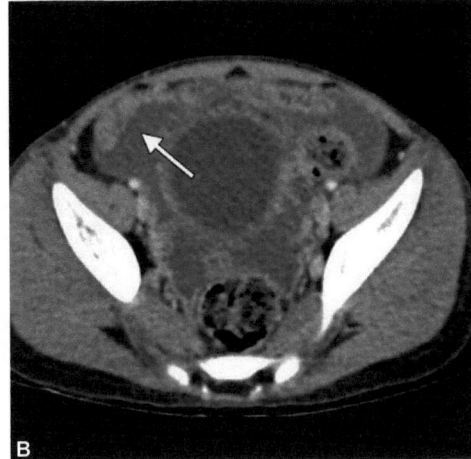
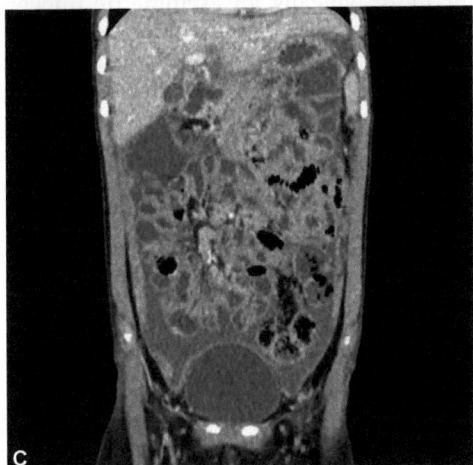

FIG. 14: Peritoneal tuberculosis (wet type) on computed tomography. **A** and **B,** Contrast-enhanced computed tomography axial images; **C,** coronal reformatted image reveal high density ascites, smooth peritoneal thickening and omental thickening (arrow)

- Smooth peritoneal thickening; omental "caking"
- "Sliced bread" appearance on sonography
- Loculated fluid collection in the abdomen with peritoneal thickening
- Associated mesenteric adenopathy, showing rim enhancement and central low attenuation.

Gastrointestinal Tuberculosis

Intestinal TB in children has the following clinical features:[23]
- Primary intestinal TB (caused by ingestion of infected milk; by *M. bovis*) is more common in children
- Primary intestinal TB has a higher association with CNS TB, than secondary intestinal TB has
- Secondary intestinal TB (secondary to a pulmonary pathology; or hematogenous dissemination) usually has TB contacts in the family
- Cause of mortality in primary TB is usually intestinal obstruction; whereas in secondary TB the causes are GI bleeding and obstruction
- In children, the abdominal disease more commonly manifests as peritoneal disease and lymph nodal enlargement. The hyperplastic type of intestinal disease and strictures is rare in children.

Plain radiograph of the abdomen can reveal multiple dilated bowel loops with air-fluid levels in intestinal obstruction (Fig. 15), calcified mesenteric or retroperitoneal nodes and enterolith. Chest radiograph may reveal a primary focus in the lungs.

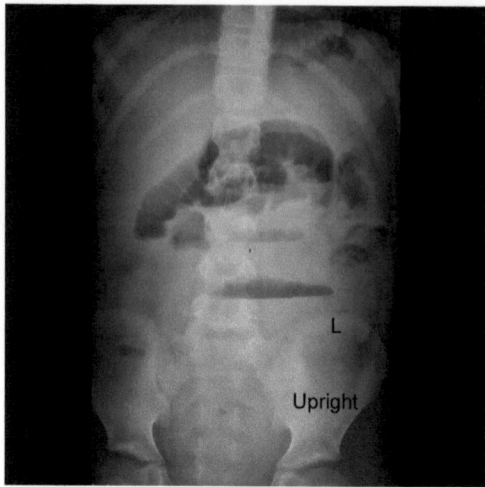

FIG. 15: Abdominal tuberculosis. Plain radiograph of the abdomen reveals multiple dilated air-fluid levels in central abdomen suggestive of intestinal obstruction

Although not a part of the proposed diagnostic protocol, barium studies can show findings suggestive of GI TB. Classically, the ileocecal (IC) area is commonly involved and typical imaging findings include a pulled-up contracted cecum with obtuse angle of the IC junction, narrowing of the terminal ileum and proximal bowel dilation. Ulcerations/strictures in one or more areas of small bowel, sparing the IC area, can also be seen. Crohn's disease is also not uncommon in pediatric age group; and should be considered in the differential diagnosis of terminal ileal strictures.

Contrast-enhanced CT (Fig. 16) demonstrates the circumferential wall thickening or more typically an asymmetric thickening of the IC valve, medial wall of the cecum and terminal ileum along with pericecal regional lymphadenopathy which are highly suggestive

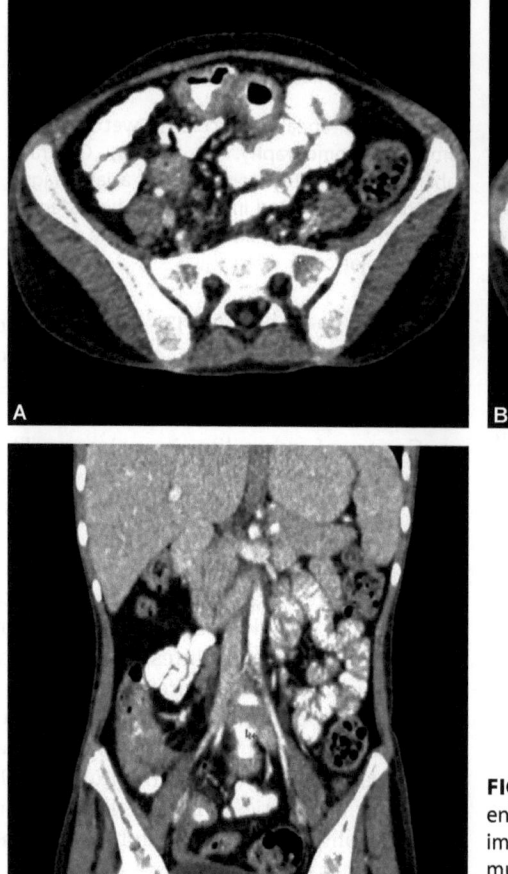

FIG. 16: Intestinal tuberculosis on contrast-enhanced computed tomography. **A** and **B,** Axial images; **C,** coronal reformatted image reveal mural thickening of ileal loops, and multiple small mesenteric lymph nodes

of IC TB on CT. Computed tomography and MR enterography are superior investigations in suspected GI TB because of better luminal distension and demonstration of strictures along with delineation of bowel wall and mesenteric findings.

Abdominal Adenopathy (Fig. 17)
Tubercular adenopathy has a tendency to involve mesenteric and peripancreatic lymph nodes. Tubercular nodes are usually seen in the upper retroperitoneum and are uncommon in the infrarenal location.

Visceral Tuberculosis (Fig. 18)
Liver, spleen, and rarely pancreas may be involved with disseminated disease. There is usually only hepatomegaly or splenomegaly but uncommonly focal hypoechoic masses can be seen on sonography. The possibility of lymphoma should be considered in the differential diagnoses of hepatosplenic TB.

Urinary Tract Tuberculosis
Genitourinary TB (Fig. 19) affects the young adults, in their 20s; and is rare in childhood. This can be explained by the fact that there is a time lag of 2–20 years between the initial pulmonary infection and the diagnosis of secondary genitourinary TB.[24,25] Currently, it is seen in children almost exclusively with miliary disease. The diagnosis of genitourinary TB is most often delayed because of minimal and nonspecific symptoms.

Intravenous urography (IVU) still remains the best imaging modality to document early radiological changes in genitourinary TB. The early findings on IVU would include poor definition of the calyceal outline (moth-eaten calyx); late findings secondary to fibrosis and scarring include infundibular stenosis and focal caliectasis, contracted "hiked-up" pelvis. Advanced disease results in diffuse fibrosis and the kidney becomes nonfunctional, the so-called "autonephrectomy". This stage is usually not seen in children.

Ureteric involvement is associated with ipsilateral renal disease and might show strictures (single or multiple), "pipe-stem ureter" in case of extensive fibrosis, "golf-hole ureter" at the vesicoureteric junction (VUJ) owing to patulous and fibrosed VUJ, small capacity urinary bladder.

Musculoskeletal Tuberculosis
Musculoskeletal TB has an overall incidence of 1–3% among all tubercular infections.[26] Most of them having coexisting pulmonary TB. Tubercular spondylitis accounts for the majority of cases (50%), other manifestations being osteomyelitis, peripheral arthritis, tenosynovitis, and bursitis.[27-34]

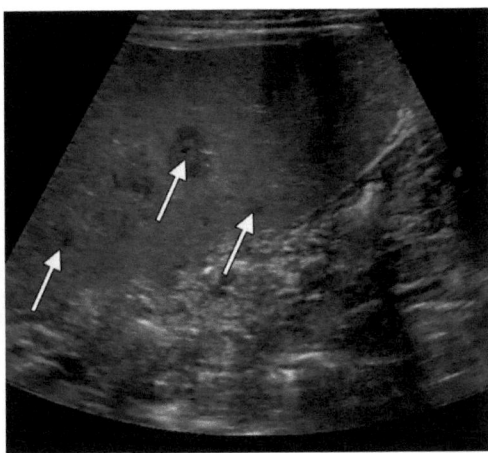

FIG. 18: Visceral tuberculosis. Ultrasound abdomen reveals multiple hypoechoic solid focal lesions (arrows) in the liver

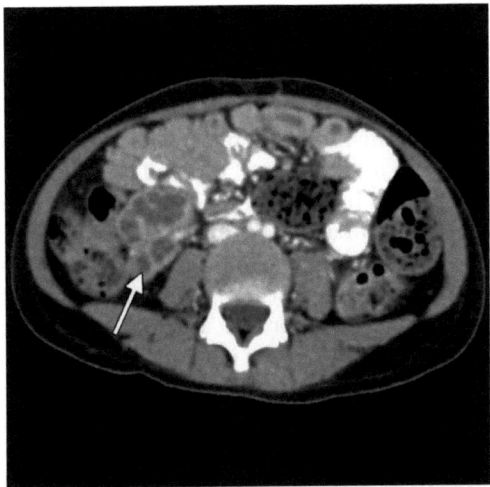

FIG. 17: Abdominal tuberculosis, lymphadenopathy. Contrast-enhanced computed tomography abdomen reveals conglomerate necrotic adenopathy (arrow) in the mesentery

Imaging in Tuberculosis: Clinicopathological Correlation

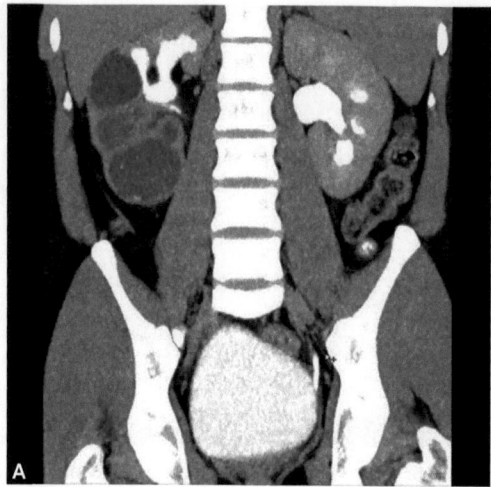 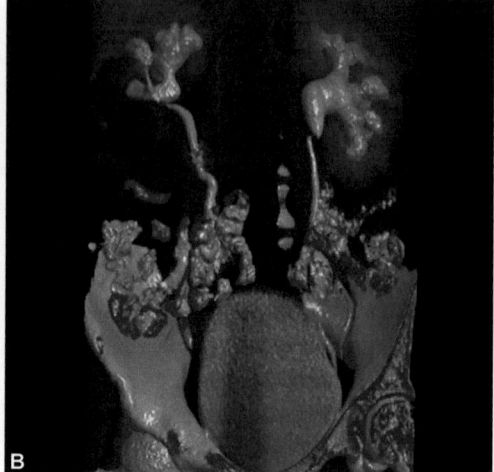

FIG. 19: Genitourinary tuberculosis in an adolescent male. **A,** Coronal maximum intensity projection; **B,** volume rendering technique image reveal focal caliectasis of the mid and lower pole of right kidney, with lack of contrast accumulation (phantom calyces) *(For color version, see Plate 12)*

Tubercular Spondylitis (Figs 20 and 21)

Thoracic vertebrae are most commonly affected in children, unlike the predilection for thoracolumbar junction in the adults.[26-29] Either single or multiple vertebrae can be affected. The patterns of involvement might be classified into paradiskal, anterior subligamentous, central or posterior element TB. Plain radiographic imaging findings include:
- Irregular vertebral endplates and erosions of the vertebral bodies adjacent to the endplates
- Narrowed or obliterated disk spaces
- Collapse of the vertebral bodies, "vertebra plana" appearance
- Calcified paraspinal abscess
- Kyphosis and fused vertebrae.

In the evaluation of tubercular spondylitis, plain radiograph is often not adequate and CT or MRI are needed for complete evaluation of disease extent. On T2WIs, the affected marrow and disk spaces show a relative increase in signal intensity and enhancement after contrast administration. The paraspinal abscesses may show rim enhancement. Spinal cord changes secondary to compression may be seen on T2WI (myelomalacia or atrophy).

Tubercular Arthritis[29-33]

Tubercular arthritis (Figs 22 and 23) typically is a monoarthritis, less than 10% cases having multiple joint involvement. Plain radiographic findings are slow to appear and imaging findings are nonspecific; at an early stage include joint effusion with soft tissue edema with normal appearing bones. The triad of juxtaarticular osteoporosis, marginal bony erosions and gradual narrowing of joint space is termed Phemister's triad and is characteristic of tuberculous arthritis.

Magnetic resonance imaging is the imaging modality of choice for early detection of tubercular arthritis. Synovial hypertrophy is seen as isointense to muscle on T1WI and hyperintense on T2WI. A hypointense signal on T2WI due to fibrosis can also be found. Biphasic pattern of active pannus (enhances postcontrast) and chronic fibrotic nonenhancing pannus is characteristic for TB arthritis. Magnetic resonance imaging also demonstrates the articular surface erosions and soft tissue changes.[31]

Synovial involvement in young patients leads to chronic hyperemia, hypertrophy of epiphyseal centers, and an early epiphyseal fusion with resultant leg-length discrepancy.

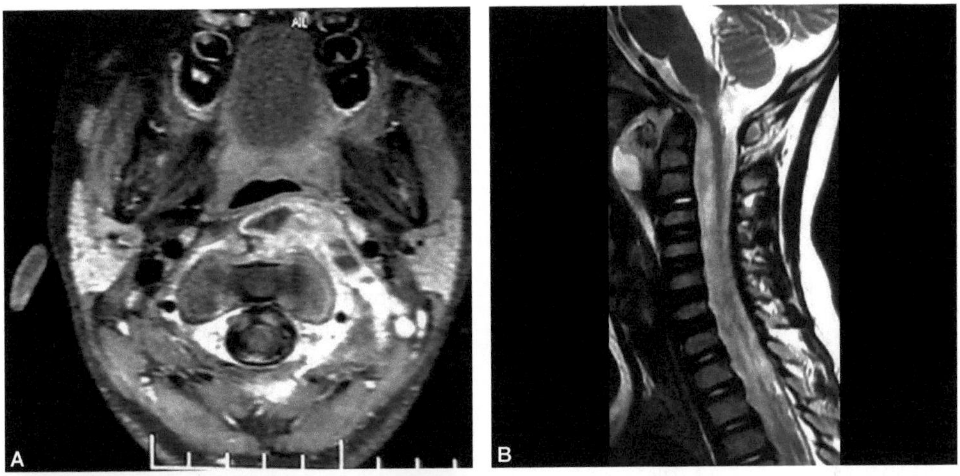

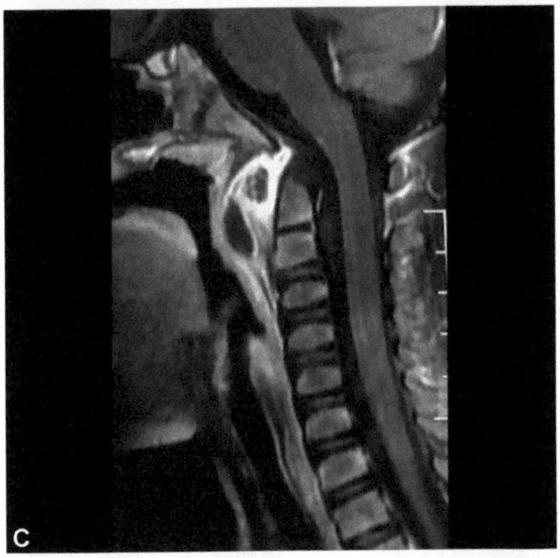

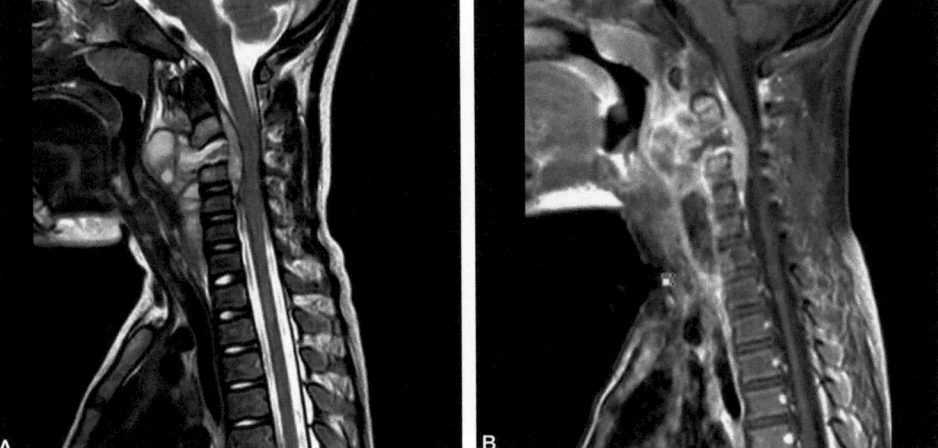

FIG. 20: Cervical spine tuberculosis. **A,** Axial contrast-enhanced T1-weighted (T1W) fat suppressed image; **B,** sagittal T2WI; **C,** sagittal T1W fat suppressed image reveal a large multiloculated collection in the prevertebral space, with enhancement of the adjacent endplates of second and third cervical vertebrae

FIG. 21: Tuberculous spondylodiskitis in a 5-year-old boy. **A,** Sagittal T2-weighted image (T2WI); **B,** sagittal T1W fat suppressed image reveal a large multiloculated collection in the prevertebral space, with collapse of third cervical vertebra and epidural collection (arrow) causing spinal cord compression

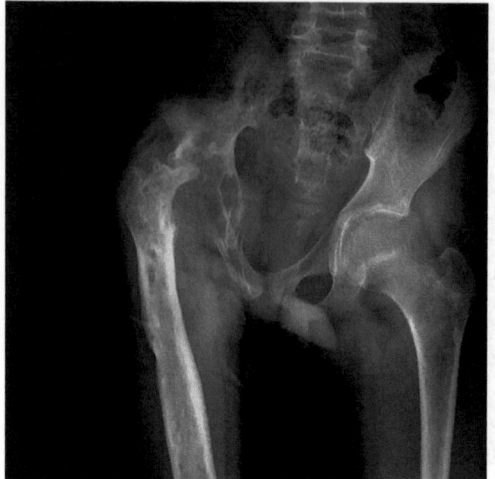

FIG. 22: Tubercular arthritis of the right hip joint, advanced stage. Plain radiograph reveals destruction of the right femoral head with lytic lesions of the right iliac bone and acetabulum, "wandering acetabulum", and chronic osteomyelitis involving right femur

This is similar to that seen in hemophiliacs or juvenile rheumatoid arthritis.

Differentiating features of tubercular and pyogenic arthritis are listed in table 3.

Tuberculous Osteitis/Osteomyelitis (Fig. 24)

Tuberculosis of short bones of hands and feet (tuberculous dactylitis): Involvement of these bones is considered a disease of childhood. It is known by the name of spina ventosa due to the cystic, ballooned out appearance of the involved bone. Radiographically it manifests as soft tissue swelling, expansion of the medullary space of the small bones causing thinning of cortex and periosteal reaction.

Tuberculosis in Primary Immunodeficiency Diseases

Children suffering from primary immunodeficiency (PI) are more prone to mycobacterial

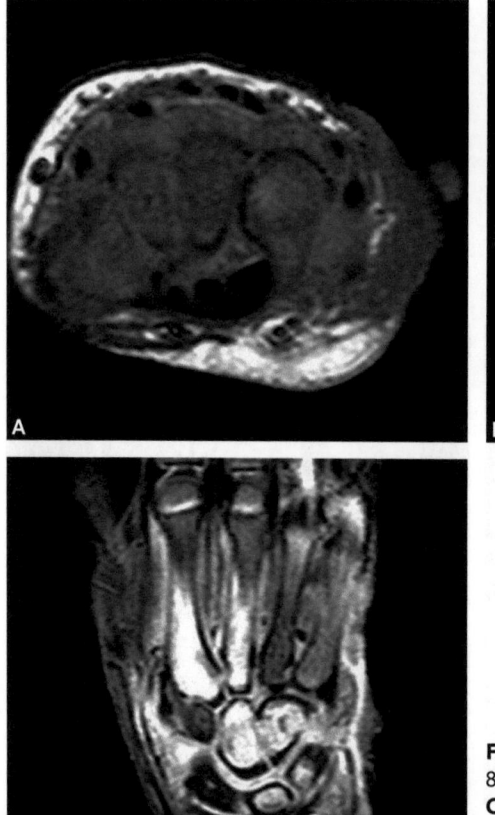

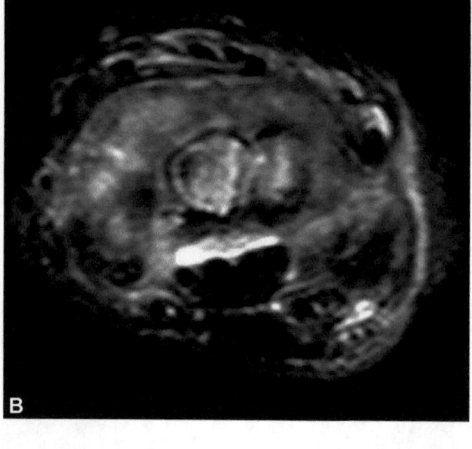

FIG. 23: Tubercular arthritis of the wrist joint in an 8-year-old boy. **A,** Axial T1-weighted (T1W); **B,** T2W; **C,** coronal T2W fat suppressed images reveal T1W hypointense and T2W hyperintense marrow signal intensity involving multiple carpal and metacarpal bones and soft tissues

Table 3: Differentiation of tubercular and pyogenic arthritis[33]

Feature	Tubercular	Pyogenic
Onset of symptoms	Insidious	Acute
Bone destruction	Slow	Rapid
Periosteal reaction	Less common	More common
Appearance of extraarticular extension of infection on magnetic resonance imaging	Smooth outline	Ill-defined
Walls of extraosseous abscess on magnetic resonance imaging	Thin and smooth	Thick and irregular

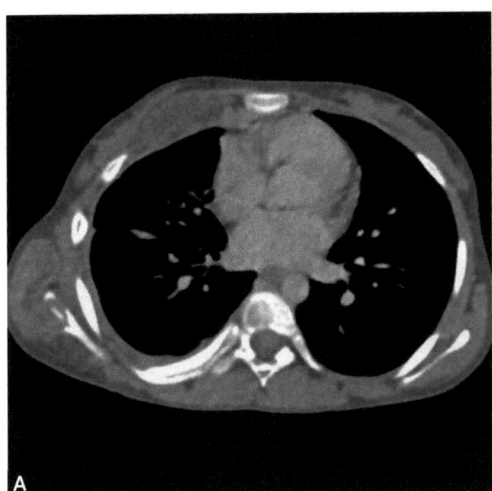
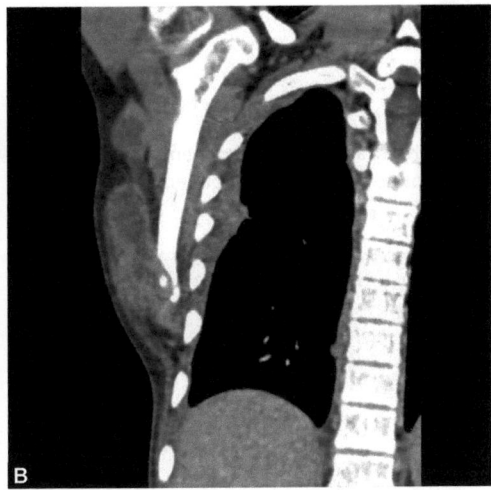

FIG. 24: Tubercular osteomyelitis of scapula in a 13-year-old girl. **A,** Computed tomography (CT) axial bone window image; **B,** coronal soft tissue window image reveal bone destruction and associated soft tissue collection involving angle of right scapula

infections.[34] Subsets of PI including disorders of phagocytosis, combined T and B-cell deficiency are specifically prone to develop extensive fulminant disease. Disseminated TB after Bacillus Calmette-Guerin (BCG) vaccination is also encountered in PI.[35]

Congenital Tuberculosis[36-38]

Congenital TB can occur due to vertical transmission of TB (transplacental transmission through umbilical veins to the fetal liver and lungs); or aspiration and swallowing of infected amniotic fluid in utero or intrapartum (fetal lungs and gut affected). The diagnostic criteria used for congenital TB were described by Beitzke in 1935.[36] Cantwell et al. revised them in 1994[37] as follows: the presence of proven tubercular disease and at least one of the following: (i) lesions in the newborn baby during the 1st week of life, (ii) a primary hepatic complex or caseating hepatic granulomata, (iii) tuberculous infection of the placenta or the maternal genital tract and (iv) exclusion of the possibility of postnatal transmission by investigation of contacts, including hospital staff.

The imaging findings (Figs 25 and 26) in congenital TB[38] are:
- Abnormal chest radiograph and computed tomography: Miliary or interstitial pattern (hematogenous dissemination)
  - Bronchopneumonic pattern (in case of aspirated of infected contents)
  - Multiple nodules, may show cavitation
  - Mediastinal or hilar adenopathy
- Abdominal imaging: Necrotic abdominal adenopathy

- Hepatosplenic enlargement and focal lesions
- Periportal hypodensities
- Ascites.

CONCLUSION

Pediatric TB, especially in infants, is different from adult TB. There is a tendency towards more severe and disseminated disease. Diagnosis of TB in children is a technical challenge; as clinical assessment is often unreliable high degree of clinical suspicion and familiarity with unusual imaging appearances is required. Congenital TB is another unique entity which needs to be kept in mind in cases of unexplained and atypical radiographic findings in a newborn.

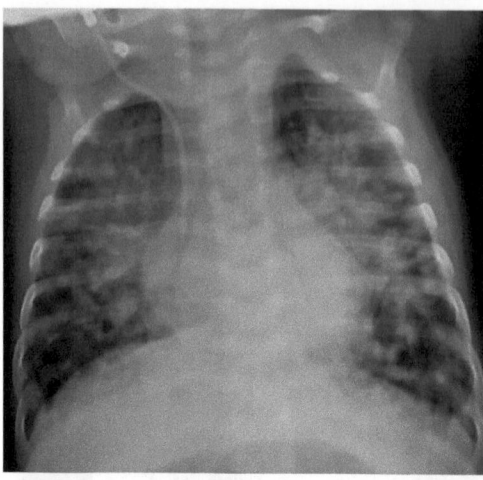

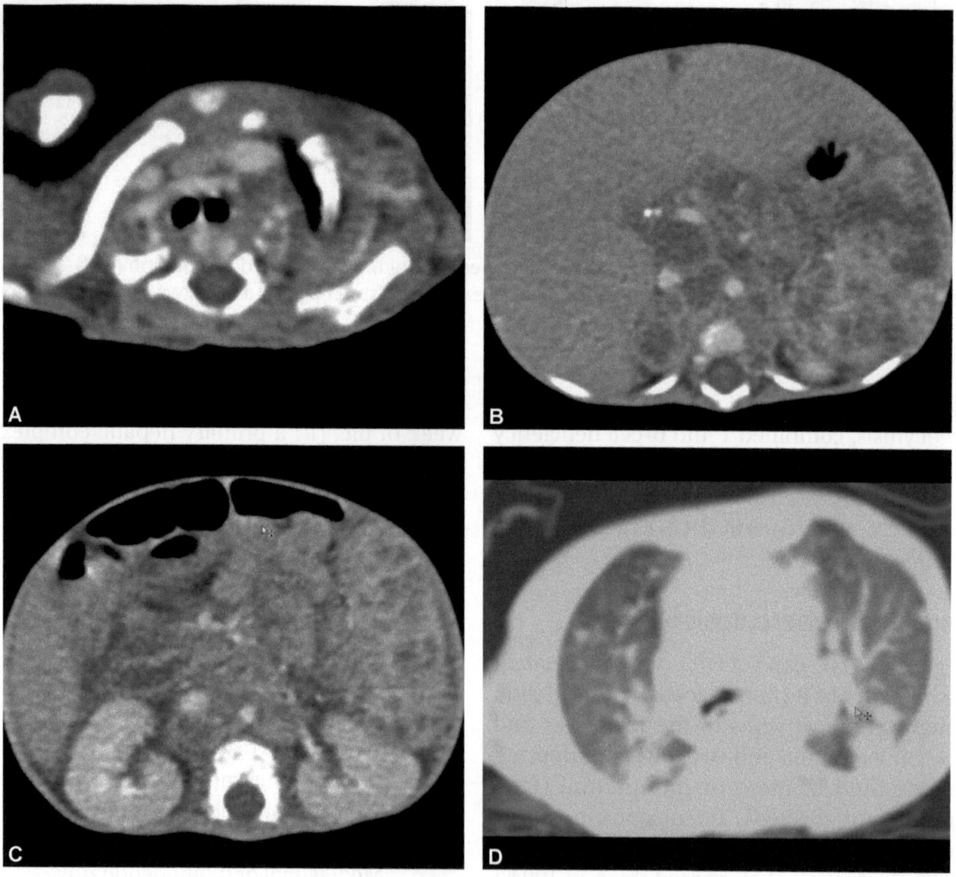

FIG. 25: Chest radiograph in congenital tuberculosis showing coarse reticulonodular pattern

FIG. 26: An 1-day-old girl with congenital tuberculosis. **A** to **C,** Axial soft tissue window images of chest and abdomen reveal necrotic axillary and abdominal adenopathy, and focal splenic lesions with hepatosplenomegaly; **D,** axial lung window image shows multiple pulmonary nodules in both lungs

REFERENCES

1. Chadha VK, Kumar P, Jagannatha PS, et al. Average annual risk of tuberculous infection in India. Int J Tuberc Lung Dis. 2005;9(1):116-8.
2. Chadha VK, Sarin R, Narang P, et al. Trends in the annual risk of tuberculous infection in India. Int J Tuberc Lung Dis. 2013;17(3):312-9.
3. Suryanarayana L, Suryanarayana HV, Jagannatha PS. Prevalence of pulmonary tuberculosis among children in a South Indian Community. Indian J Tuberc. 1999;46(3):171-7.
4. Working Group on Tuberculosis, Indian Academy of Pediatrics (IAP). Consensus statement on childhood tuberculosis. Indian Pediatr. 2010;47(1):41-55.
5. Schaaf HS, Gie RP, Beyers N, et al. Tuberculosis in infants less than 3 months of age. Arch Dis Child. 1993;69(3):371-4.
6. Vallejo JG, Ong LT, Starke JR. Clinical features, diagnosis, and treatment of tuberculosis in infants. Pediatrics. 1994;94(1):1-7.
7. Weber AL, Bird KT, Janower ML. Primary tuberculosis in childhood with particular emphasis on changes affecting the tracheobronchial tree. AJR Am J Roentgenol. 1968;103(1):123-32.
8. Stansberry SD. Tuberculosis in infants and children. J Thorac Imaging. 1990;5(2):17-27.
9. Solomon A, Rabinowitz L. Primary cavitating tuberculosis in childhood. Clin Radiol. 1972;23(4):483-5.
10. Leung AN, Müller NL, Pineda PR, et al. Primary tuberculosis in childhood: radiographic manifestations. Radiology. 1992;182(1):87-91.
11. Kim WS, Moon WK, Kim IO, et al. Pulmonary tuberculosis in children: evaluation with CT. AJR Am J Roentgenol. 1997;168(4):1005-9.
12. Marais BJ. Childhood tuberculosis: epidemiology and natural history of disease. Indian J Pediatr. 2011;78(3):321-7.
13. IAP Working Group. Consensus statement of IAP Working Group: status report on diagnosis of childhood tuberculosis. Indian Pediatr. 2004;41(2):146-55.
14. Management of Pediatric Tuberculosis under the Revised National Tuberculosis Control Program (RNTCP). A joint statement of the Central TB Division, Directorate General of Health Services, Ministry of Health and Family Welfare, and experts from Indian Academy of Pediatrics. Indian Pediatr. 2004;41(1):901-5.
15. Andronikou S, Smith B, Hatherhill M, et al. Definitive neuroradiological diagnostic features of tuberculous meningitis in children. Pediatr Radiol. 2004;34(11):876-85.
16. Bhargava S, Gupta AK, Tandon PN. Tuberculous meningitis—a CT study. Br J Radiol. 1982;55(651):189-96.
17. Jenkins JR. CT of intracranial tuberculosis. Neuroradiology. 1991;33(1):126-35.
18. Gupta RK, Jena A, Sharma A, Guha DK, et al. MR imaging of intracranial tuberculomas. J Comput Assist Tomogr. 1988;12(2):280-5.
19. Gupta RK, Roy R, Dev R, et al. Finger printing of Mycobacterium tuberculosis in patients with intracranial tuberculomas by using in vivo, ex vivo, and in vitro magnetic resonance spectroscopy. Magn Reson Med. 1996;36(6):829-33.
20. Gupta RK, Kathuria MK, Pradhan S. Magnetization transfer MR imaging in CNS tuberculosis. AJNR Am J Neuroradiol. 1999;20(5):867-75.
21. Gupta RK, Prakash M, Mishra AM, et al. Role of diffusion weighted imaging in differentiation of intracranial tuberculoma and tuberculous abscess from cysticercus granulomas-a report of more than 100 lesions. Eur J Radiol. 2005;55(3):384-92.
22. Jain R, Sawhney S, Bhargava DK, et al. Diagnosis of abdominal tuberculosis: sonographic findings in patients with early disease. AJR Am J Roentgenol. 1995;165(6):1391-5.
23. Sharma AK, Agarwal LD, Sharma CS, et al. Abdominal tuberculosis in children: experience over a decade. Indian Pediatr. 1993;30(9):1149-53.
24. Sharma A, Rattan KN, Kumar S. Renal tuberculosis in children. Trop Doct. 2000;30(3):183-4.
25. Engin G, Acunaş B, Acunaş G, et al. Imaging of extra-pulmonary tuberculosis. Radiographics. 2000;20(2):471-88.
26. Jaovisidha S, Chen C, Ryu KN, et al. Tuberculous tenosynovitis and bursitis: imaging findings in 21 cases. Radiology. 1996;201(2):507-13.
27. Andronikou S, Jadwat S, Douis H. Patterns of disease on MRI in 53 children with tuberculous spondylitis and the role of gadolinium. Pediatr Radiol. 2002;32(11):798-805.
28. Dixit R. Tuberculosis of the spine. In: Berry M, Chowdhury V, Mukhopadhyay S, Suri S (Eds). Diagnostic Radiology: Musculoskeletal and Breast Imaging, 2nd edition. New Delhi: Jaypee Brothers Medical Publishers (P) Ltd; 2005. pp. 111-29.
29. Hoffman EB, Crosier JH, Cremin BJ. Imaging in children with spinal tuberculosis. A comparison of radiography, computed tomography and magnetic resonance imaging. J Bone Joint Surg Br. 1993;75(2):233-9.
30. Sawlani V, Chandra T, Mishra RN, et al. MRI features of tuberculosis of peripheral joints. Clin Radiol. 2003;58(10):755-62.
31. Harisinghani MG, McLoud TC, Shepard JA, et al. Tuberculosis from head to toe. Radiographics. 2000;20(2):449-70.
32. Prasad A, Manchanda S, Sachdev N, et al. Imaging features of pediatric musculoskeletal tuberculosis. Pediatr Radiol. 2012;42(10):1235-49.
33. Hong SH, Kim SM, Ahn JM, et al. Tuberculous versus pyogenic arthritis: MR imaging evaluation. Radiology. 2001;218(3):848-53.
34. Galkina E, Kondratenko I, Bologov A. Mycobacterial infections in primary immunodeficiency patients. Adv Exp Med Biol. 2007;601:75-81.
35. Rezai MS, Khotaei G, Mamishi S, et al. Disseminated Bacillus Calmette-Guerin infection after BCG vaccination. J Trop Pediatr. 2008;54(6):413-6.
36. Beitzke H. About congenital Tuberculosis infection. Ergeb Ges Tuberk Forsch. 1935;7:1-30.
37. Cantwell MF, Shehab ZM, Costello AM, et al. Brief report: congenital tuberculosis. N Engl J Med. 1994;330(15):1051-4.
38. Neyaz Z, Gadodia A, Gamanagatti S, et al. Imaging findings of congenital tuberculosis in three infants. Singapore Med J. 2008;49(2):e42-6.

CHAPTER 18

Positron Emission Tomography-Computed Tomography: Does It Have a Role in Tuberculosis?

Rakesh Kumar, Krishan K Agarwal, Abhishek Behera

INTRODUCTION

Tuberculosis (TB) is a contagious and airborne infectious disease. Tuberculosis remains a worldwide concern despite substantial improvement in health service. Patients with sputum-negative pulmonary TB (PTB), and extrapulmonary TB (EPTB) are difficult to diagnose and may be missed at all points of care. Imaging for diagnosis of TB is challenging because it can mimic other diseases such as sarcoidosis or neoplasm.

To improve diagnostic accuracy and facilitate timely diagnosis, the broad imaging spectrum of this disease has to be kept in mind. Positron emission tomography/computed tomography (PET/CT) is a new noninvasive technique that is being used in selected clinical situations for improving the imaging of TB.

POSITRON EMISSION TOMOGRAPHY

Positron emission tomography is a form of molecular imaging utilizing positron emitting radionuclides attached to biological molecules to form radiopharmaceuticals. It can delineate the biological distribution of these radiopharmaceuticals and provide useful pathophysiological data. The raw data acquired via a PET scanner is then processed to form images and is represented as sectional images in the axial, coronal or sagittal planes. Additionally, PET images are very frequently represented as three-dimensional reconstructions such as maximum intensity projections and multiplanar reconstructions.

However, the functional data provided by PET images is incomplete without anatomical correlation. Hence, in the clinical setting, PET images are most commonly fused with sequentially acquired CT images.

Radiotracers

The most commonly used PET radiotracer in the management of TB is ^{18}F-fluorodeoxyglucose (^{18}F-FDG). Fluorodeoxyglucose is a surrogate marker for glucose metabolism and has consistently been shown to have increased concentration in areas of inflammation associated with active TB. Markers of amino acid metabolism such as ^{11}C-methionine and lipid metabolism tracers such as ^{11}C-choline have also been used for this reason.[1-5] Radiotracer concentration in active tubercular lesions has also been noted in somatostatin receptor scintigraphy.[6]

FLUORODEOXYGLUCOSE-POSITRON EMISSION TOMOGRAPHY/COMPUTED TOMOGRAPHY IN TUBERCULOSIS

As noted earlier, accumulation of ^{18}F-FDG occurs in inflammatory cells such as neutrophils, activated macrophages and lymphocytes at the site of inflammation or infection It is also taken up by tumor cells.[7-9] Consequently, ^{18}F-FDG uptake occurs in PTB, in tuberculoma and in other TB-related lesions. Fluorodeoxyglucose uptake can be quantified using standardized uptake values (SUVs).

Potential Areas of Utility

^{18}F-fluorodeoxyglucose-positron emission tomography/computed tomography though unable to differentiate between TB and other diseases may still have a role in TB diagnosis in conjunction with other modalities.

Positron emission tomography/computed tomography scans may suggest the sites of safe high yield biopsies, thus yielding confirmatory histopathology, cultures, or polymerase chain reaction samples.[10,11]

Though investigations such as tuberculin skin test and gamma-interferon release assays are very sensitive for tubercular exposure, they are unable to differentiate between latent and active disease. Positron emission tomography/computed tomography provides additional metabolic information which can help to locate active disease in lesions which look healed on anatomical imaging.[12,12-14]

Using PET/CT, pulmonary and EPTB involvement can be assessed simultaneously, potentially saving time, resources and simplifying imaging. Additionally using serial SUVmax measurement, response to antitubercular therapy may be evaluated.[12,15-21] It has been shown that metabolic changes seen in ^{18}F-FDG-PET/CT precede anatomical imaging findings.[22] This response assessment is potentially very valuable in patients with drug-resistant TB in order to allow early change of the antitubercular regime. Also, in cases of EPTB requiring very long durations of antitubercular therapy, PET/CT evaluation may allow response guided shortening of therapy duration, potentially reducing adverse effects associated with long-term antitubercular therapy.

FLUORODEOXYGLUCOSE-POSITRON EMISION TOMOGRAPHY/COMPUTED TOMOGRAPHY FINDINGS IN TUBERCULOSIS

Pulmonary Tuberculosis

Pulmonary TB can be divided into primary and postprimary pattern, both of them presenting with different radiological features. There are overlapping features between both patterns on radiological imaging.[23]

Primary Tuberculosis

Primary TB manifests as four different patterns: (i) parenchymal diseases, (ii) lymphadenopathy, (iii) pleural effusion and (iv) miliary disease—or any combination.

On PET-CT imaging, two distinct types of patterns are described: (i) the lung pattern and (ii) the lymphatic pattern. Lung pattern depicts restricted infection to lung parenchyma with mildly enlarged mediastinal and hilar lymphadenopathy. ^{18}F-FDG PET-CT shows tracer uptake in areas of lung consolidation ± cavitations surrounded by micronodules and mild uptake within lymph nodes. Lymphatic pattern depicts systemic and intense infection, with more enlarged hilar and mediastinal lymph nodes and increased tracer uptake in ^{18}F-FDG PET-CT scan.[24]

Dual time-point ^{18}F-FDG PET/CT imaging has shown some benefits in differentiation of tubercular and malignant lesions, however, further investigation in larger cohorts of patients is needed.[25,26] In dual time-point FDG-PET/CT imaging is done at 1 hour and 3 hours instead of just the routine 1 hour images. Usually there is a washout of FDG in inflammatory lesions while malignancy shows retention of ^{18}F-FDG.

Postprimary Tuberculosis

Postprimary TB develops under the influence of acquired immunity which is also called secondary or reactivation TB.[23] PET/CT manifestation of postprimary PTB is focal or patchy heterogeneous, poorly defined consolidation, and cavitation with increased FDG uptake (Fig. 1). Cavitation may progress to endobronchial spread that results in a typical "tree-in-bud" distribution of nodules in addition to cavitation (Fig. 2).[27]

Hilar or mediastinal lymphadenopathy is uncommon in postprimary PTB, seen in only 5–10% of patients.[28,29] Pulmonary tuberculomas, i.e., round or oval granuloma, with the wall lined by inflammatory granulomatous tissue or encapsulated by connective tissue showing increased tracer uptake may be seen, however, it is not specific for TB.[30] For differentiation of lung cancer and tuberculoma, ^{11}C-choline PET scan has a potential role, as a tuberculoma shows low

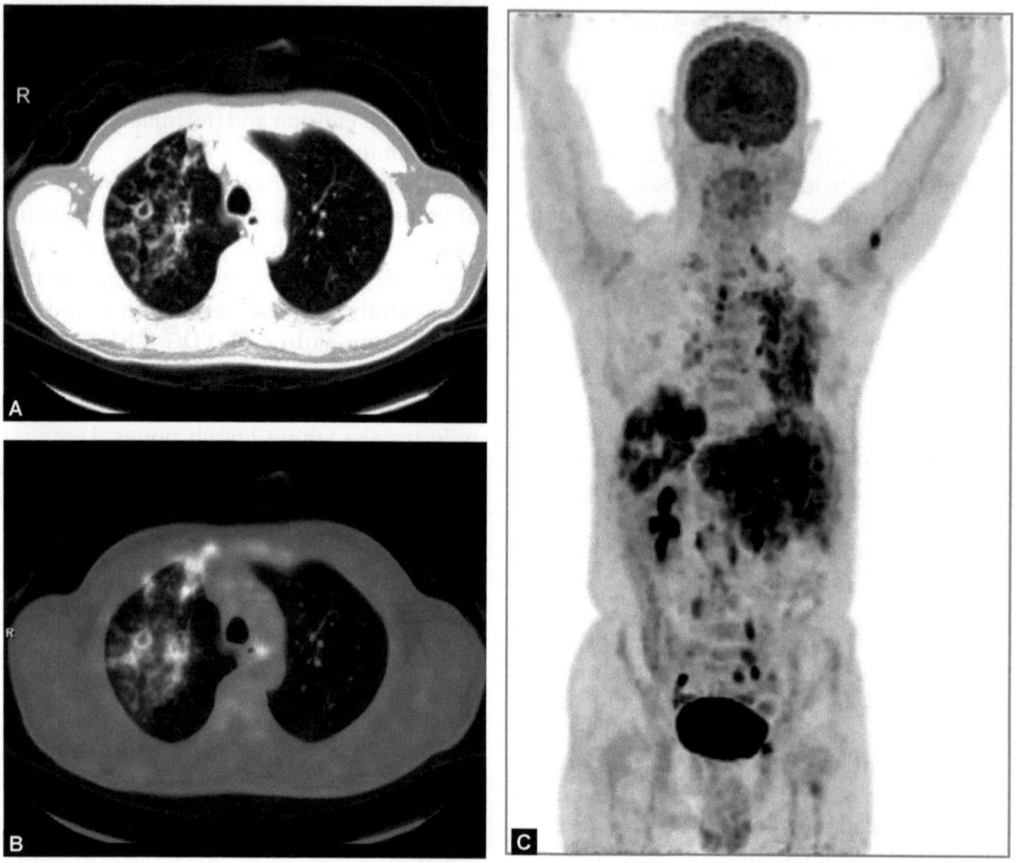

Imaging in Tuberculosis: Clinicopathological Correlation

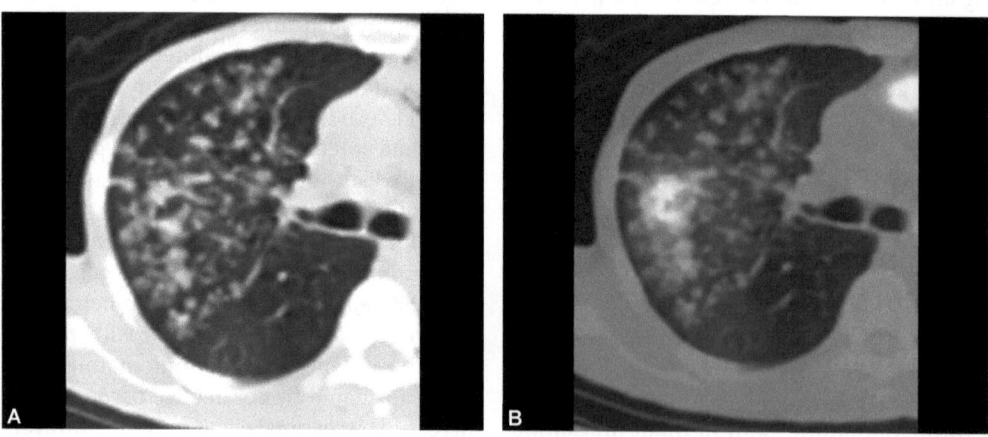

FIG. 1: A 45-year-old male, known case of Type 2 diabetes presented with hemoptysis, positron emission tomography/computed tomography (PET/CT) scan showing lung parenchymal changes, micro and macronodules with cavitations surrounded suggestive of active pulmonary tuberculosis *(For color version, see Plate 13)*

CT, computed tomography; PET, positron emission tomography; TB, tuberculosis.

FIG. 2: A 63-year-old male, known case of pulmonary tuberculosis underwent PET/CT which demonstrated the "tree-in-bud sign" which is reliable marker of active TB *(For color version, see Plate 13)*

tracer uptake on ^{11}C-choline PET scan (choline is a marker of cell membrane synthesis).[1]

Differentiation between Active and Inactive Tuberculosis

Active tubercular lesions have significantly higher SUVmax values (SUV$_{ratio}$ of 1.9 showed a sensitivity of 97% and specificity of 92% in our own study) (unpublished data) compared with inactive disease (Fig. 3).[12,13] ^{18}F-FDG PET/CT has the potential to become a tool for monitoring the treatment response in selected cases of EPTB or multidrug resistance.[31]

Extrapulmonary Tuberculosis

Skeletal Tuberculosis

Skeletal TB usually occurs secondary to hematogenous spread from other lesions.

Spinal TB forms the most common form of skeletal TB forming approximately 50% cases of skeletal TB.[32,33] The lower dorsal and upper lumbar spine are more commonly involved. Spondylodiskitis, also known as Pott's disease (Fig. 4), is the most common form.[34] Skip lesions, large abscesses, epidural extension, and subligamentous spread are seen.[33,35] Serious complications such as vertebral collapse, spinal compression, and spinal deformity may occur.[36]

Schmitz et al. found ^{18}F-FDG PET to be a sensitive imaging tool in the detection of spondylodiskitis.[37,38] ^{18}F-FDG PET correctly identifies the patients with vertebral osteomyelitis. It also differentiates between mild infections and degenerative changes; in addition, extraspinal manifestations are also detected. Changes in the baseline SUV and follow-up studies are helpful to evaluate the treatment response (Fig. 5). This is very relevant in the case of spinal TB as it requires prolonged antitubercular treatment, potentially exposing patients to a high-risk of adverse effects. Thus, FDG-PET response assessment may allow shortening of regimens in selected patients.

Tubercular arthritis most commonly involves the knee and the hip. Initial involvement of the joint begins with synovitis, visible as FDG uptake in the periarticular region.[39] Progression of the disease leads to periarticular osteopenia and involvement of the marginal areas of the joint. Later on, there is significant loss of joint space and destruction of the joint.[40] A cold abscess may be seen in the nearby soft tissue. Subluxation or dislocation of the joint may be seen in the later stages secondary to joint damage. In case of diagnostic dilemma, FDG-PET may be used to guide the site for biopsy. Involvement of the ankle, shoulder, and elbow may also occur, though it is far rarer. Involvement of the small bones of the hands and feet may lead to dactylitis.[41]

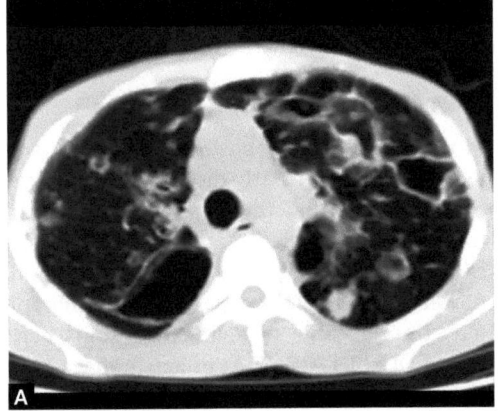
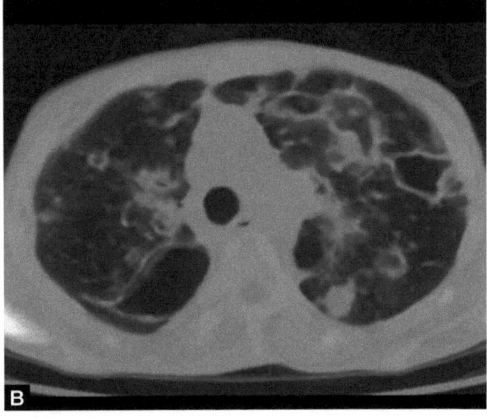

CT, computed tomography; FDG, fluorodeoxyglucose; PET, positron emission tomography.

FIG. 3: A 54-year-old male, known case of pulmonary tuberculosis, treated with antitubercular treatment in 2008. Now presented with chest pain and breathlessness, PET/CT scan was done to see activity of disease which showed multiple fibrocavitary lesions with no significant FDG uptake suggestive of no disease activity *(For color version, see Plate 14)*

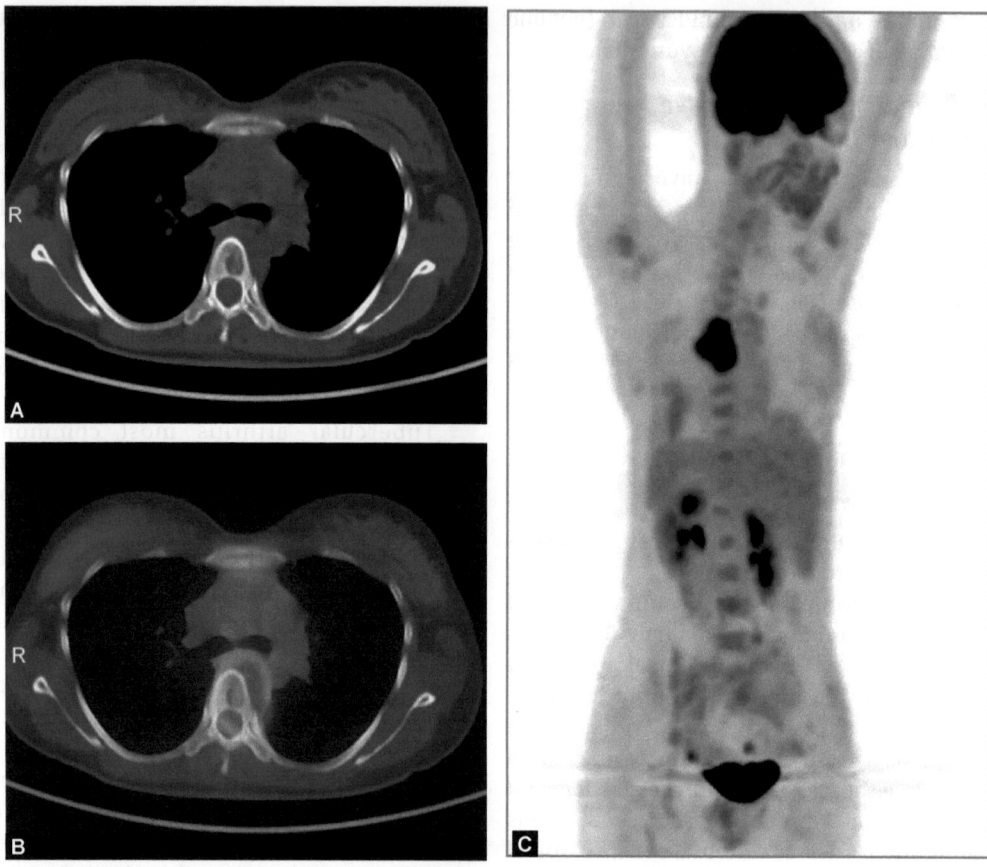

CT, computed tomography; FDG, fluorodeoxyglucose; PET, positron emission tomography.

FIG. 4: A patient with a vertebral lesion consistent with Pott's spine showing FDG uptake indicative of active disease *(For color version, see Plate 14)*

Abdominal Tuberculosis

Abdominal TB may involve the gastrointestinal tract, peritoneum, mesenteric lymph nodes, liver, spleen, or genitourinary tract. Its presentations are nonspecific and diagnosis is frequently elusive.[42,43] Since the presentations of multi-site abdominal TB are even more atypical and insidious, definitive diagnosis requires a high index of suspicion, various laboratory findings, imaging data, and histologic exclusion of malignancy.

^{18}F-fluorodeoxyglucose positron emission tomography/computed tomography image is nonspecific in abdominal TB (including TB of the spleen, lymph nodes, and peritoneum) (Fig. 6).[44] Focal accumulation pattern and a diffuse accumulation pattern of ^{18}F-FDG have been observed in splenic TB.

Bowel Tuberculosis

Most common site of gastrointestinal TB is the ileocecal region.[45] Early disease shows an area of circumferential thickening of cecum and terminal ileum with increased FDG uptake. Ulceration/nodularity may be visible within the bowel loop. PET/CT enteroclysis/enterography may thus be able to delineate lesions better than FDG-PET/CT. Sites of active disease will show increased FDG uptake. Physiological FDG uptake in the gut must be taken into account during any interpretation.[41] Complications such as abscess, perforation, and obstruction may

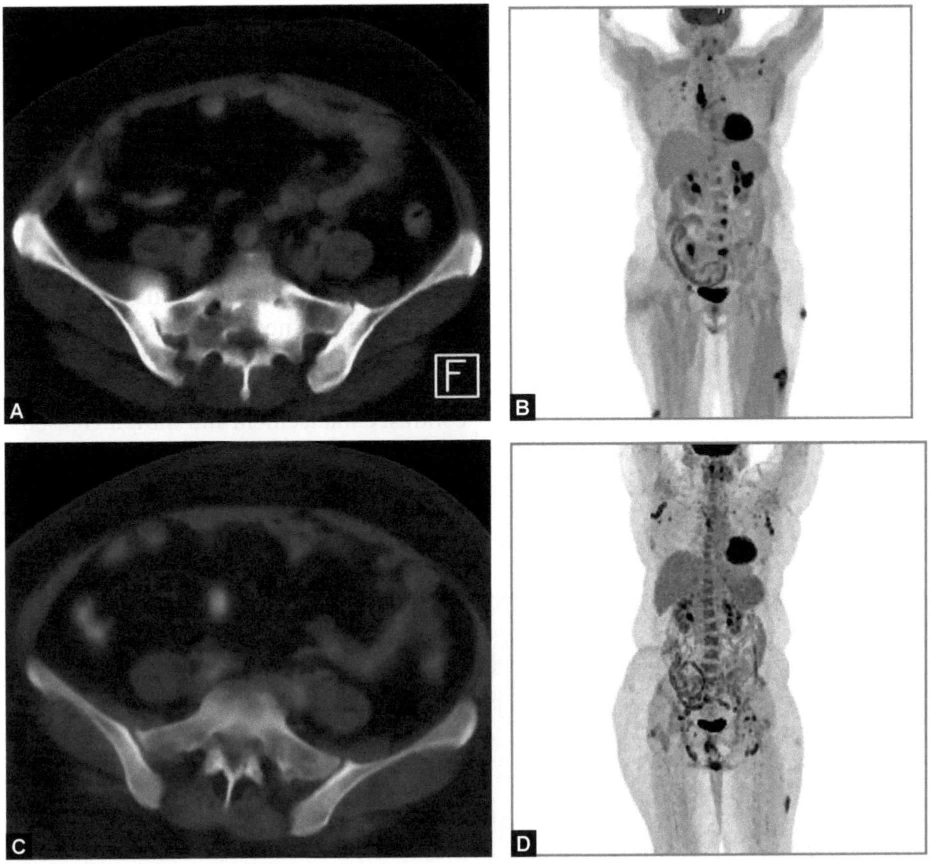

Positron Emission Tomography-Computed Tomography: Does It Have a Role in Tuberculosis?

CT, computed tomography; FDG, fluorodeoxyglucose; PET, positron emission tomography.

FIG. 5: A 23-year-old female presented with miliary disseminated tuberculosis. PET/CT was advised to see the extent of disease which showed lytic lesion with prevertebral soft tissue component and increased FDG uptake, these consistent Pott's spine *(For color version, see Plate 15)*

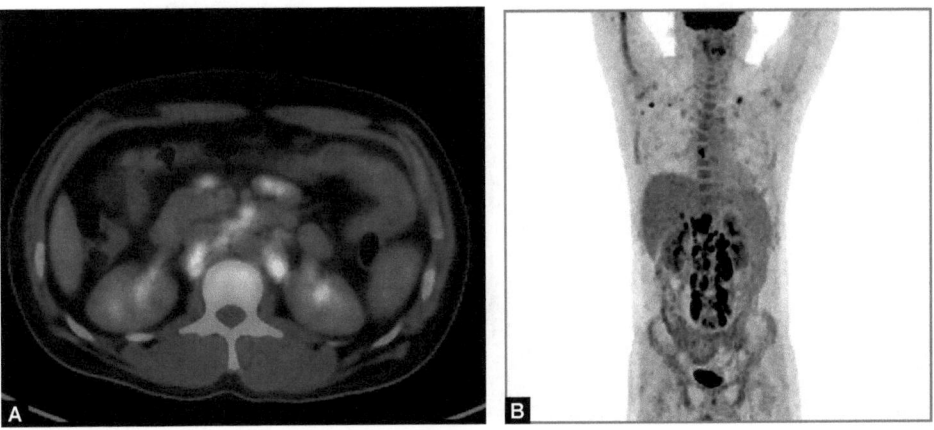

CT, computed tomography; FDG, fluorodeoxyglucose; PET, positron emission tomography.

FIG. 6: A 30-year-old male, presented with abdominal lymphadenopathy, PET/CT scan showing multiple retroperitoneal lymph nodes with increased FDG uptake suggestive of active disease *(For color version, see Plate 15)*

be seen.[46] Perforation may lead to tubercular peritonitis and can be seen as diffuse peritoneal FDG uptake.

Other sites of primary gastrointestinal TB include gastroduodenal TB, isolated colonic TB, and anorectal TB. Gastric TB usually presents as ulcerative gastric lesion with increased FDG uptake and can be confused with gastric carcinoma. Involvement of the duodenum may lead to stricture formation and consequent obstruction.

Isolated colonic TB commonly involves the sigmoid, ascending, and transverse colon and may show multifocal involvement with increased FDG uptake in active lesions.[32,41,45]

Rectal involvement usually leads to stricture formation and active disease shows FDG uptake. Anal TB is rare and frequently leads to formation of fistula-in-ano. These tracts and associated anal lesions show increased FDG uptake in active disease. Nodal involvement is very common with the draining lymph nodes showing enlargement with increased FDG uptake.

Solid Organ Tuberculosis

In patients of miliary TB, the liver and spleen may be studded with small 0.5–2 mm miliary lesions that may not be seen on PET-CT images. Larger lesions are usually 1–3 cm in size and hypodense on CT images with peripheral contrast enhancement and show increased FDG uptake on PET images (Fig. 7). In case of diffuse involvement, diffusely increased FDG uptake may be seen leading to visualization of a "hot" liver on PET images.[47,48]

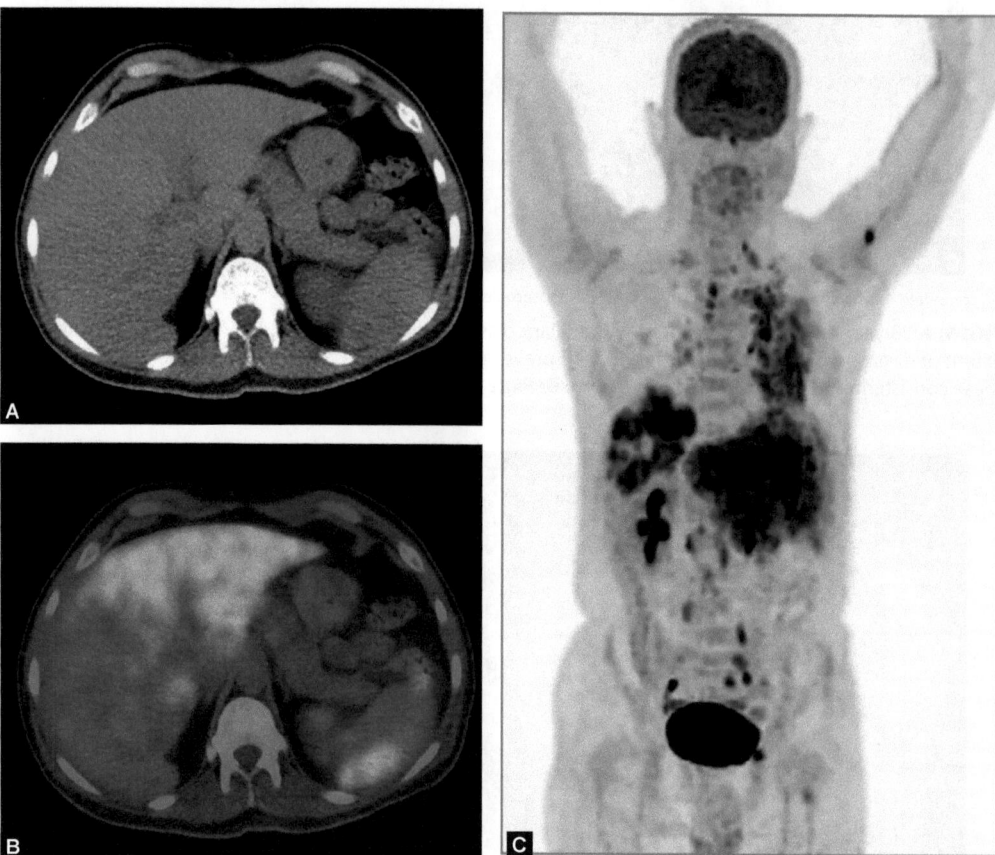

CT, computed tomography; FDG, fluorodeoxyglucose; PET, positron emission tomography.

FIG. 7: A 45-year-old male, known case of Type 2 diabetes, diagnosed as pulmonary tuberculosis, PET/CT scan showing areas of increased FDG uptake in liver and spleen. Projection image show abnormal uptake in lungs and multiple lymph nodes, in addition to liver and spleen *(For color version, see Plate 16)*

Adrenal involvement may lead to asymmetrical enlargement with foci of increased FDG uptake. Later on, atrophy of the gland with calcifications can be seen.[32,46,49,50]

Pancreatic involvement can be visualized as hypodense lesions on CT images showing increased FDG uptake. Peripancreatic lymphadenopathy can also be noted in such patients.[32,46,51]

Genitourinary Tuberculosis

Tuberculosis of the genitourinary system in the male usually involves the kidneys or occasionally the prostate or the seminal vesicles

Due to FDG excretion via the kidneys, lesions of the renal pelvicalyceal system, ureteric or bladder lesions may not be visible. In these cases, a postvoid delayed time point image after injection of a diuretic is very useful in assessing lesions of the genitourinary tract.[52,53]

Infection of the ureter leads to ureter wall thickening with increased FDG uptake. FDG-PET can show increased FDG uptake in ureteric wall in the postdiuretic image. Bladder wall lesions may be visualized on postdiuretic views in FDG-PET as areas of increased FDG uptake.

Male genital tuberculosis

Testicular TB usually occurs due to direct extension from the urinary tract. Testis may have normal physiological uptake. Active lesions show significantly increased FDG uptake.

Female genital tuberculosis

Spread is usually hematogenous and involves the fallopian tubes in the vast majority of the cases, often bilaterally. Tubal involvement may lead to tubal blockage, causing formation of tubo-ovarian abscesses. Diffuse increased FDG uptake may be noted in the tubo-ovarian abscess in active disease. Care must be taken not to confuse physiological ovarian increase in size and uptake with tubal TB.

Uterine TB may lead to increased FDG uptake lesions; however, images must be interpreted taking physiological FDG uptake in the endometrium into account.

Central Nervous System Tuberculosis

Imaging by FDG-PET in central nervous system (CNS) TB has a potential drawback of very high background uptake in the brain parenchyma of FDG. Hence, tracers such as ^{11}C-methionine and ^{11}C-choline may have a potential role in TB of the CNS,[3-5] due to their low background uptake.

On FDG-PET/CT, a tuberculoma appears as a ring enhancing lesion with increased FDG uptake noted in the periphery of the lesion (Fig. 8).

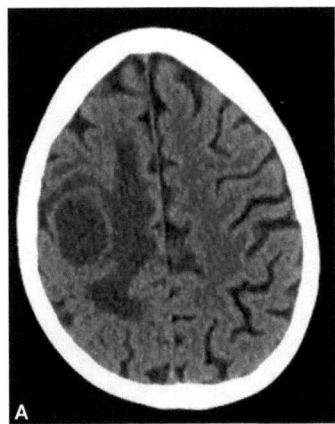 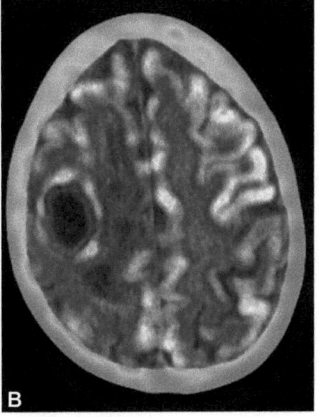

CT, computed tomography; FDG, fluorodeoxyglucose; PET, positron emission tomography.

FIG. 8: A 19-year-old male known case of disseminated multidrug-resistant tuberculosis presented with seizures. PET/CT shows right frontal lesion with perilesional edema and FDG uptake in margins suggestive of active disease *(For color version, see Plate 16)*

Any active disease is seen as areas of increased FDG uptake.

ASSESSMENT OF TREATMENT RESPONSE

The most important clinical application of ^{18}F-FDG PET/CT in TB is the assessment of treatment response of antitubercular therapy especially in patients with extrapulmonary involvement and when drug resistance is prevalent.[21] Some bacillus-negative tuberculomas do not decrease in size and may even increase during treatment, making it difficult for the physician to decide whether or not to modify treatment. In such cases, ^{18}F-FDG PET/CT imaging may help, as the inflammatory activity can be measured by ^{18}F-FDG uptake (Figs 9 and 10). It correlates well with the clinical markers of response.[54] Several studies have confirmed the value of ^{18}F-FDG PET/CT in the follow-up and evaluation of the treatment response. In pulmonary and EPTB, a decrease of approximately one-third in metabolic uptake has been reported after 4 weeks of anti-TB treatment when there is a good response.[55] Metabolic uptake (both early and delayed) of involved lymph nodes and the number of involved lymph node basins are significantly higher in nonresponders than in responders.[15] These findings need further confirmation in larger cohorts of patients. After 4 months of

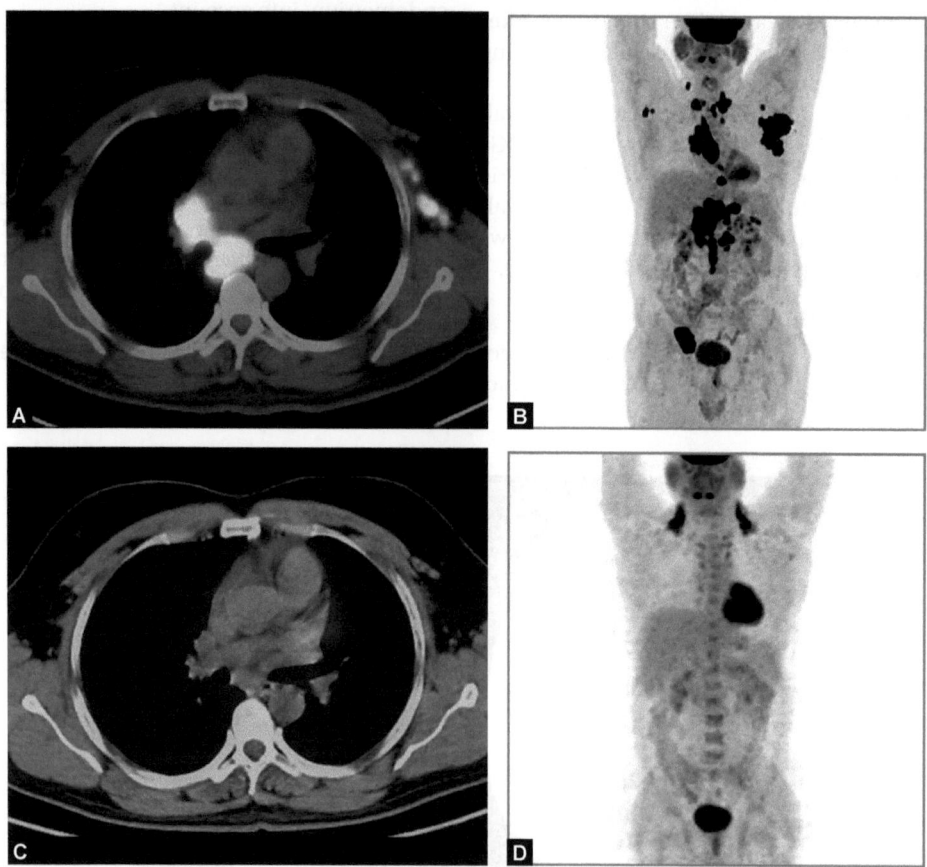

CT, computed tomography; FDG, fluorodeoxyglucose; PET, positron emission tomography.

FIG. 9: A 32-year-old male, disseminated tuberculosis, underwent baseline and 6-months post-treatment PET/CT scan to see therapy response. Baseline PET/CT showed multiple focal areas of increased FDG uptake in multiple lymph nodes (upper row). Post-treatment PET/CT scan showed complete resolution of FDG uptake suggestive of complete response (lower row) *(For color version, see Plate 17)*

Positron Emission Tomography-Computed Tomography: Does It Have a Role in Tuberculosis?

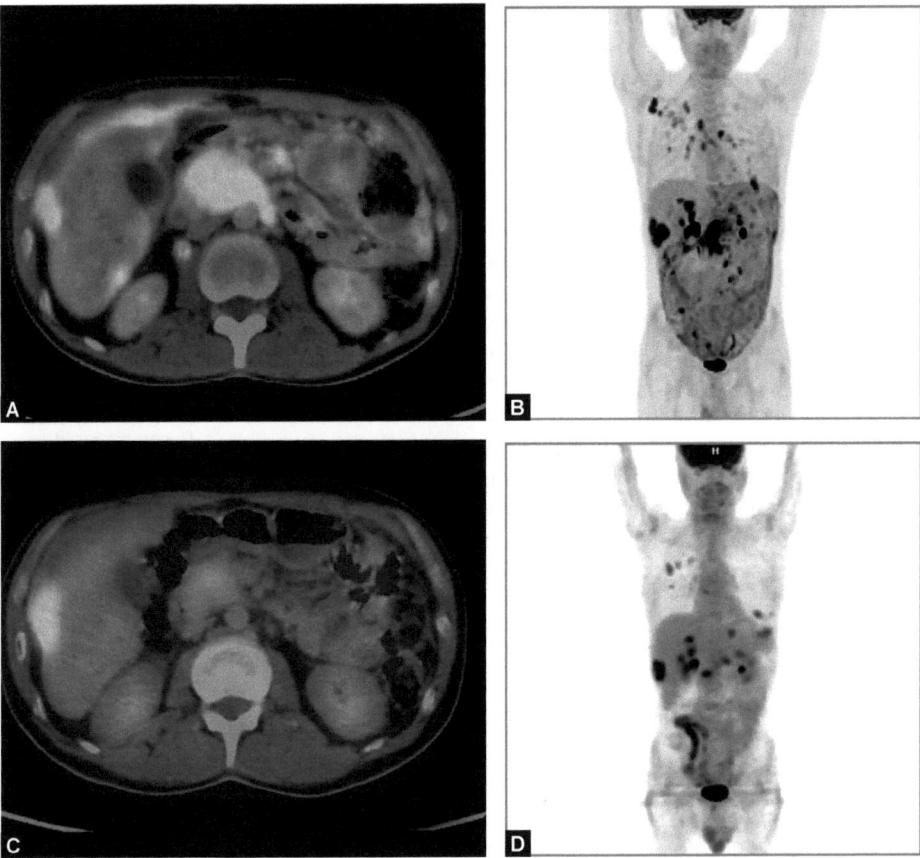

CT, computed tomography; FDG, fluorodeoxyglucose; PET, positron emission tomography.

FIG. 10: A 38-year-old male, disseminated tuberculosis, underwent baseline and 9-month post-treatment PET/CT scan to see therapy response. Baseline PET/CT showed multiple focal areas of increased FDG uptake in multiple lymph nodes and liver (upper row). Post-treatment PET/CT scan showed decrease in FDG uptake suggestive of partial response (lower row) *(For color version, see Plate 18)*

anti-TB treatment, ^{18}F-FDG PET/CT can also evaluate the treatment response in patients with high sensitivity and specificity. ^{18}F-FDG PET/CT also shows encouraging results for the prognosis and detection of residual disease in patients with spinal infection, particularly when magnetic resonance imaging (MRI) is equivocal in distinguishing between degenerative changes and infection.[13]

TREATMENT OUTCOME IN PATIENTS OF MULTIDRUG-RESISTANT TUBERCULOSIS

During drug therapy, TB lesions show substantial decrease in FDG avidity at 2 months after treatment initiation. Definitive clinical trials of new chemotherapies for treating TB require following subjects until at least 6 months after treatment discontinuation to assess for durable cure. PET/CT imaging is useful to predict final treatment outcome in the context of clinical trials of new antitubercular drugs and regimens, early in the course of treatment.[55]

QUANTITATIVE MEASUREMENT OF DRUG EFFICACY

Positron emission tomography/computed tomography imaging may be useful as an early quantitative measure of drug efficacy against TB in human patients. Serial measurements of

PET quantitative parameters such as SUV and total lesion glycolysis may allow quantification and subsequent follow-up of tubercular disease process allowing tailoring of therapy.

CONCLUSION

Fluorodeoxyglucose positron emission tomography/computed tomography is being used to accurately define the full extent of systemic involvement especially in EPTB, and yield material for culture and sensitivity studies (to allow an early diagnosis of drug-resistant TB). PET/CT has a potential utility in assessment of treatment response after antitubercular therapy in selected cases of EPTB and multidrug-resistant TB. PET/CT is able to differentiate active TB focus from old or inactive disease, as active tuberculoma has significantly higher FDG uptake.

REFERENCES

1. Hara T, Kosaka N, Suzuki T, et al. Uptake rates of 18F-fluorodeoxyglucose and 11C-choline in lung cancer and pulmonary tuberculosis: a positron emission tomography study. Chest. 2003;124(3):893-901.
2. Peng ZM, Liu Q, Liu QW, et al. The value of dual time point 11C-choline PET-CT in differentiating malignant from benign lesion of mediastinum. Zhonghua Yi Xue Za Zhi. 2007;87(47):3317-20.
3. Huang Z, Zuo C, Guan Y, et al. Misdiagnoses of 11C-choline combined with 18F-FDG PET imaging in brain tumours. Nucl Med Commun. 2008;29(4):354-8.
4. Hsieh HJ, Lin SH, Lin KH, et al. The feasibility of 11C-methionine-PET in diagnosis of solitary lung nodules/masses when compared with 18F-FDG-PET. Ann Nucl Med. 2008;22(6):533-8.
5. D'Souza MM, Sharma R, Jaimini A, et al. Metabolic assessment of intracranial tuberculomas using 11C-methionine and 18F-FDG PET/CT. Nucl Med Commun. 2012;33(4):408-14.
6. Ahmadihosseini H, Abedi J, Ghodsi Rad MA, et al. Diagnostic utility of 99mTc-EDDA-tricine-HYNIC-Tyr3-octreotate SPECT for differentiation of active from inactive pulmonary tuberculosis. Nucl Med Commun. 2014;35(12):1262-7.
7. Kaim AH, Weber B, Kurrer MO, et al. Autoradiographic quantification of 18F-FDG uptake in experimental soft-tissue abscesses in rats. Radiology. 2002;223(2):446-51.
8. Jones HA, Clark RJ, Rhodes CG, et al. In vivo measurement of neutrophil activity in experimental lung inflammation. Am J Respir Crit Care Med. 1994;149(6):1635-9.
9. Bakheet SM, Powe J, Ezzat A, et al. F-18-FDG uptake in tuberculosis. Clin Nucl Med. 1998;23(11):739-42.
10. Cornelis F, Silk M, Schoder H, Takaki H, et al. Performance of intra-procedural 18-fluorodeoxyglucose PET/CT-guided biopsies for lesions suspected of malignancy but poorly visualized with other modalities. Eur J Nucl Med Mol Imaging. 2014;41(12):2265-72.
11. Fanchon LM, Dogan S, Moreira AL, et al. Feasibility of in situ, high-resolution correlation of tracer uptake with histopathology by quantitative autoradiography of biopsy specimens obtained under 18F-FDG PET/CT guidance. J Nucl Med. 2015;56(4):538-44.
12. Demura Y, Tsuchida T, Uesaka D, et al. Usefulness of 18F-fluorodeoxyglucose positron emission tomography for diagnosing disease activity and monitoring therapeutic response in patients with pulmonary mycobacteriosis. Eur J Nucl Med Mol Imaging. 2009;36(4):632-9.
13. Kim SJ, Kim IJ, Suh KT, et al. Prediction of residual disease of spine infection using F-18 FDG PET/CT. Spine (Phila Pa 1976). 2009;34(22):2424-30.
14. Yang CM, Hsu CH, Lee CM, et al. Intense uptake of [F-18]-fluoro-2 deoxy-D-glucose in active pulmonary tuberculosis. Ann Nucl Med. 2003;17(5):407-10.
15. Sathekge M, Maes A, Kgomo M, et al. Use of 18F-FDG PET to predict response to first-line tuberculostatics in HIV-associated tuberculosis. J Nucl Med. 2011;52(6):880-5.
16. Treglia G, Taralli S, Calcagni ML, et al. Is there a role for fluorine 18 fluorodeoxyglucose-positron emission tomography and positron emission tomography/computed tomography in evaluating patients with mycobacteriosis? A systematic review. J Comput Assist Tomogr. 2011;35(3):387-93.
17. Özmen Ö, Gökçek A, Tatcı E, et al. Integration of PET/CT in Current Diagnostic and Response Evaluation Methods in Patients with Tuberculosis. Nucl Med Mol Imaging. 2014;48(1):75-8.
18. Basu S. 18F-FDG PET/CT as a Sensitive and Early Treatment Monitoring Tool: Will This Become the Major Thrust for Its Clinical Application in Infectious and Inflammatory Disorders? J Nucl Med. 2011;53(1):165.
19. Hofmeyr A, Lau WF, Slavin MA. Mycobacterium tuberculosis infection in patients with cancer, the role of 18-fluorodeoxyglucose positron emission tomography for diagnosis and monitoring treatment response. Tuberculosis (Edinb). 2007;87(5):459-63.
20. Shimizu Y, Hashizume Y. PET/CT for monitoring the therapeutic response in a patient with abdominal lymph node tuberculosis after colon cancer resection. Kekkaku. 2012;87(11):707-12.
21. Tian G, Xiao Y, Chen B, Xia J, et al. FDG PET/CT for therapeutic response monitoring in multi-site non-respiratory tuberculosis. Acta Radiol. 2010;51(9):1002-6.
22. Chen RY, Dodd LE, Lee M, et al. PET/CT imaging correlates with treatment outcome in patients with multidrug-resistant tuberculosis. Sci Transl Med. 2014;6(265):265ra166.
23. Van Dyck P, Vanhoenacker FM, Van den Brande P, et al. Imaging of pulmonary tuberculosis. Eur Radiol. 2003;13(8):1771-85.

24. Soussan M, Brillet PY, Mekinian A, et al. Patterns of pulmonary tuberculosis on FDG-PET/CT. Eur J Radiol. 2012;81(10):2872-6.
25. Yen RF, Chen KC, Lee JM, et al. 18F-FDG PET for the lymph node staging of non-small cell lung cancer in a tuberculosis-endemic country: is dual time point imaging worth the effort? Eur J Nucl Med Mol Imaging. 2008;35(7):1305-15.
26. Razak HR, Geso M, Abdul Rahim N, et al. Imaging characteristics of extrapulmonary tuberculosis lesions on dual time point imaging (DTPI) of FDG PET/CT. J Med Imaging Radiat Oncol. 2011;55(6):556-62.
27. Lee KS, Im JG. CT in adults with tuberculosis of the chest: characteristic findings and role in management. AJR Am J Roentgenol. 1995;164(6):1361-7.
28. Curvo-Semedo L, Teixeira L, Caseiro-Alves F. Tuberculosis of the chest. Eur J Radiol. 2005;55(2):158-72.
29. Rodríguez E, Soler R, Juffé A, Salgado L. CT and MR findings in a calcified myocardial tuberculoma of the left ventricle. J Comput Assist Tomogr. 2001;25(4):577-9.
30. Goo JM, Im JG, Do KH, et al. Pulmonary tuberculoma evaluated by means of FDG PET: findings in 10 cases. Radiology. 2000;216(1):117-21.
31. Heysell SK, Thomas TA, Sifri CD, et al. 18-fluorodeoxyglucose positron emission tomography for tuberculosis diagnosis and management: a case series. BMC Pulm Med. 2013;13(1):14.
32. Burrill J, Williams CJ, Bain G, et al. Tuberculosis: a radiologic review. Radiographics. 2007;27(5):1255-73.
33. Kilborn T, Janse van Rensburg P, Candy S. Pediatric and adult spinal tuberculosis: imaging and pathophysiology. Neuroimaging Clin N Am. 2015;25(2):209-31.
34. Martini M, Ouahes M. Bone and joint tuberculosis: a review of 652 cases. Orthopedics. 1988;11(6):861-6.
35. Rivas-Garcia A, Sarria-Estrada S, Torrents-Odin C, et al. Imaging findings of Pott's disease. Eur Spine J. 2013; 22(Suppl 4):567-78.
36. Skoura E, Zumla A, Bomanji J. Imaging in tuberculosis. Int J Infect Dis. 2015;32:87-93.
37. Schmitz A, Risse JH, Grünwald F, et al. Fluorine-18 fluorodeoxyglucose positron emission tomography findings in spondylodiscitis: preliminary results. Eur Spine J. 2001; 10(6):534-9.
38. Schmitz A, Kälicke T, Willkomm P, et al. Use of fluorine-18 fluoro-2-deoxy-D-glucose positron emission tomography in assessing the process of tuberculous spondylitis. J Spinal Disord. 2000;13(6):541-4.
39. Makis W, Abikhzer G, Stern J. Tuberculous synovitis of the hip joint diagnosed by FDG PET-CT. Clin Nucl Med. 2009;34(7):431-2.
40. Vanhoenacker FM, Sanghvi DA, De Backer AI. Imaging features of extraaxial musculoskeletal tuberculosis. Indian J Radiol Imaging. 2009;19(3):176-86.
41. Ito K, Morooka M, Minamimoto R, Miyata Y, et al. Imaging spectrum and pitfalls of 18F-fluorodeoxyglucose positron emission tomography/computed tomography in patients with tuberculosis. Jpn J Radiol. 2013;31(8):511-20.
42. Xi X, Shuang L, Dan W, Ting H, et al. Diagnostic dilemma of abdominopelvic tuberculosis: a series of 20 cases. J Cancer Res Clin Oncol. 2010;136(12): 1839-44.
43. Tan CH, Kontoyiannis DP, Viswanathan C, et al. Tuberculosis: a benign impostor. AJR Am J Roentgenol. 2010; 194(3):555-61.
44. Takalkar AM, Bruno GL, Reddy M, et al. Intense FDG activity in peritoneal tuberculosis mimics peritoneal carcinomatosis. Clin Nucl Med. 2007;32(3):244-6.
45. Sharma MP, Bhatia V. Abdominal tuberculosis. Indian J Med Res. 2004;120(4):305-15.
46. da Rocha EL, Pedrassa BC, Bormann RL, et al. Abdominal tuberculosis: a radiological review with emphasis on computed tomography and magnetic resonance imaging findings. Radiol Bras. 2015;48(3):181-91.
47. Jeong YJ, Sohn MH, Lim ST, et al. "Hot liver" on 18F-FDG PET/CT imaging in a patient with hepatosplenic tuberculosis. Eur J Nucl Med Mol Imaging. 2010;37(8):1618-9.
48. Wong SS, Yuen HY, Ahuja AT. Hepatic tuberculosis: a rare cause of fluorodeoxyglucose hepatic superscan with background suppression on positron emission tomography. Singapore Med J. 2014;55(7):e101-3.
49. Li YJ, Cai L, Sun HR, Gao S, et al. Increased FDG uptake in bilateral adrenal tuberculosis appearing like malignancy. Clin Nucl Med. 2008;33(3):191-2.
50. Roudaut N, Malecot JM, Dupont E, et al. Adrenal Tuberculosis Revealed by FDG PET. Clin Nucl Med. 2008; 33(11):821-3.
51. Sanabe N, Ikematsu Y, Nishiwaki Y, et al. Pancreatic tuberculosis. J Hepatobiliary Pancreat Surg. 2002;9(4):515-8.
52. Tsai SC, Ou YC, Cheng CL, et al. Reduction of bladder activity on FDG PET/CT scan in patients with urinary bladder carcinoma. A prospective study with a patient-friendly protocol. Nuklearmedizin. 2015;54(1):36-42.
53. Nayak B, Dogra PN, Naswa N, et al. Diuretic 18F-FDG PET/CT imaging for detection and locoregional staging of urinary bladder cancer: prospective evaluation of a novel technique. Eur J Nucl Med Mol Imaging. 2013;40(3):386-93.
54. Dureja S, Sen IB, Acharya S. Potential role of F18 FDG PET-CT as an imaging biomarker for the noninvasive evaluation in uncomplicated skeletal tuberculosis: a prospective clinical observational study. Eur Spine J. 2014;23(11):2449-54.
55. Martinez V, Castilla-Lievre MA, Guillet-Caruba C, et al. (18)F-FDG PET/CT in tuberculosis: an early non-invasive marker of therapeutic response. Int J Tuberc Lung Dis. 2012;16(9):1180-5.

INDEX

Page numbers followed by *f* refer to figure, *fc* refer to flowchart, and *t* refer to table

A

Abdomen 153
 axial contrast-enhanced computed tomography of 134*f*
 central 135*f*
 computed tomography of 194*f*, 195*f*
 contrast-enhanced computed tomography of 133*f*, 134*f*, 136*f*, 137*f*, 141*f*, 207, 216*f*, 219*f*
Abscess 94
 chronic 162
 cold 75
 epidural extension of 78
 paravertebral 76*f*, 77*f*
 pericardial 183, 184*f*
 retropharyngeal 89*f*
 subacute 162
 subligamentous extension of 77*f*
 tubercular 14*t*, 65*f*, 70*f*, 80, 214*f*
Absorption, increased rate of 123
Acetabulum 222*f*
Acid-fast bacilli 9, 25, 30, 73
 analysis 145
 multiple 26*f*
Acid-fast organisms 35
Acinar nodule 107, 210*f*
Acquired immunodeficiency syndrome 2, 47, 121
Adenitis
 bacterial 94
 tuberculous 90, 138*f*
 viral 94
Adenopathy
 abdominal 219, 224*f*
 hilar 223
 mediastinal 223
 necrotic 219*f*
 abdominal 223
Adverse drug reactions 42
Air space nodule 107
Amebic infections 121
Amikacin 22, 41, 46, 49
Aminoglycosides 41, 42
Amoxiclav 44
Amyloidosis 92
Aneurysm
 mycotic 188*f*, 191
 tubercular 186
  mycotic 191
Ankle joints 168, 169*f*
Anorexia 42
Antiretroviral therapy 4, 107
Antitubercular drugs 41, 42
 classification of 41*t*
 currently available 49*t*
Antitubercular therapy 22, 126, 129*f*, 154*f*, 202
 basics of 40
Antitubercular treatment 42, 67, 82, 229*f*
Aorta
 coronal magnetic resonance angiogram of 191*f*
 diffuse wall thickening of 190*f*
 thoracic 190*f*
Aortitis
 active tubercular 190*f*
 acute 191*f*
 variants of 190*f*
Apparent diffusion coefficient 83, 116, 201
Apple core stricture 130
Arachnoiditis 66*f*
 tuberculous 34
Arterial anatomy 73
Artery
 aneurysm, pulmonary 193
 stenosis, abdominal visceral branch 191*f*
Arthritis 161
 advanced 161
 fungal 160
 infective 168
 juvenile idiopathic 160, 168
 monoarticular inflammatory 171
 pyogenic 160, 223*t*
 rheumatoid 160, 168, 171
 tubercular 13, 160, 166, 220, 222*f*, 229
Ascites 133, 224
Asherman syndrome 156
Aspergilloma 109*f*
Atlantoaxial dislocation 68*f*
Atrophy 32*f*, 220
Auramine O stain 18
Autonephrectomy 219
Avascular necrosis 168
Axial computed tomography
 angiography 189*f*
 enterography 131*f*
Axial contrast-enhanced computed tomography 115*f*, 128*f*, 132*f*, 157*f*
Axial transabdominal ultrasound 113*f*
Azithromycin 41

B

Bacilli, tubercular 51, 176
Bacillus calmette-Guérin 2, 7, 155
 vaccination 223
Backache 199*f*
Barium
 enema 122, 130, 130*f*

meal follow through 122, 124f
studies 122, 123, 132
Basal brain parenchyma 53f
Basal meninges 35f
Bedaquiline 41, 49
Bile duct, common 201f
Biliary tract, tuberculosis of 139
Black-blood sequences 179
Bladder 145, 153
Bone scan 78
Bowel
  involvement, length of 126f
  obstruction 124
  perforation 124
Brachial plexopathy 69f
Brain 35f
  abscess, tuberculous 34, 36, 62
  contrast-enhanced computed tomography of 213f, 215f
  parenchyma 52
  parenchymal involvement 165
  tuberculoma 35, 56
Bronchial artery aneurysm 193
Bronchial lesions 27, 28
Bronchiectasis, tubercular 212f
Bronchoalveolar lavage 17
Bronchogenic spread 210f
Bronchopneumonia, tuberculous 27, 211
Bronchopneumonic pattern 223
Brucellosis 84f
Bursitis, tubercular 173

C

Caliectasis 148
  focal 148
Calvarium 165
Capreomycin 22, 41, 44, 46, 49
Carcinoma 121
Cardiac mass 185f
Cardiac tamponade 177
Carotid artery
  internal 192f
  pseudoaneurysm, tubercular 192f
Carpal bones 172f
  multiple 172f
Carpal tunnel syndrome 171
Cartridge-based nucleic acid amplification test 11, 44
Cavernous sinus region 57
Central necrosis 69f, 114f
Central nervous system 7, 11, 34, 44, 51, 211

classification of tuberculosis of 34
Central tubercular lymphadenopathy 116
Centriacinar nodules, extensive 212f
Centrilobular nodules 107
Cerebellar abscess, paramedian 70f
Cerebellum 57f, 59f
Cerebral
  blood volume 62
  hemispheres 54f
  lesions 202
Cerebritis, focal 215f
Cerebrospinal fluid 11, 213
  analysis 52
Cervical
  lymphadenitis 112
  spine 86
Chemotherapy 42
Chest
  computed tomography 178
  contrast-enhanced computed tomography of 211f
  pain 229f
  radiograph 110, 113, 176, 177
    abnormal 223
  wall muscles, anterior 173f
  X-ray 8, 98, 99
Choroid plexitis, tuberculous 54f
Choroidal tubercles 36
Choroiditis 36
Cilastatin 49
Ciprofloxacin 41
Clarithromycin 41, 49
Clofazimine 22, 41, 44, 49
Co-amoxiclav 49
Cocoon formation 124
Collar-stud abscess formation 112
Colony forming unit 20
Color Doppler ultrasonography 122
Common antitubercular drugs, adverse reactions of 42t
Computed tomography 11, 51, 73, 87, 99, 100, 112, 114, 123, 149f-151f, 161, 178, 190f, 197, 204, 207, 217f, 226-236
  angiography 187, 188, 190f
  contrast-enhanced 90f, 98, 99, 114, 123, 142f, 153, 187, 217f, 218, 218f
  enterography 122, 123, 128f

guided aspiration 13
imaging 187, 235
scan 40, 228f
thorax 207
urography 152f
Conglomerate nodal mass 90f
Convulsions 42
Coronal computed tomography enterography 125f
Cranial nerve
  neuropathy 56
  palsies 52
Crohn's disease 121, 126, 127f, 130, 130t, 141
Cycloserine 41, 42, 44, 49
Cystic dilatation 32f

D

Dactylitis, tubercular 165, 222
Delamanid 41, 49
Deoxyribonucleic acid 20, 21
Depression 42
Diabetes 232f, 288f
Diffusion-weighted imaging 55, 63, 83, 115, 153, 162, 197
  role of 162
Directly observed treatment short-course 43, 44, 49
  strategy 2, 40
Discitis, tuberculous 78f
Dizziness 42
Doppler study 177
Dorso-lumbar spine, fat suppression of 67f
Drug sensitivity testing methods 22
Drug susceptibility 22
  testing 22, 44
Dynamic cine magnetic resonance imaging 181
Dysplasia, fibrous 163

E

Echocardiography 177, 184
  transesophageal 178
Edema
  perifocal 59f
  perilesional 60f, 233f
Ehionamide 42t
Elbow 171
  joint 171f
Electrolyte imbalance 42
Empyema 103, 211f
Encephalopathy, tuberculous 34

Index

Endocarditis, tuberculous 186
Enteroliths 128*f*
Enzyme-linked
   immunosorbent assay 21
   immunospot assay 21
Epididymis 145, 155
   acute infection of 155
Epidural disease 86
Epigastric discomfort 42
Epithelioid cells 26*f*, 74
Epithelioid histiocytes, slipper-shaped 27*f*
Esophagus
   middle third of 132
   tubercular involvement of 132
Ethambutol 41, 42, 44, 49
Ethionamide 22, 41*t*, 44, 49
Ethylenediamine 41*t*

F

Fever 140*f*, 142*f*, 203*f*, 204*f*
Fibroatelectasis 103
Fibrobronchiectasis 108*f*
Fibrosis 156, 161
   mediastinal 104
Fibrotic stricture 128*f*
Fine-needle aspiration cytology 40, 173*f*
   ultrasonography-guided 155*f*
Fleischner's sign 123
Flexible bronchoscopy 9*f*
Fluorescent staining 18
Fluorodeoxyglucose 197, 204*f*, 230-235
   positron emission tomography 100, 156, 161, 226, 227, 236
   scan 82
   study 204*f*
Fluoroquinolones 41, 42
Foot joints 168
Fractures, multiple 163
Fungal infections 121

G

Gadolinium, role of 162
Gallium scan 78
Gastric
   aspirate 17
   lavage 17
Gatifloxacin 49
Gen-probe amplified mycobacterium tuberculosis direct test 20
Ghon's complex 27*f*
Ghon's focus 100, 208
Glenoid fossa 170*f*
Granular calcification, amorphous 147*f*
Granuloma
   eosinophilic 163
   epithelioid 29*f*, 33*f*, 34*f*
   necrotizing 31*f*
Granulomatosis 92, 95
Granulomatous infection, chronic 84*f*
Granulomatous infiltrate, thin layer of 35*f*

H

Hallucination 42
Hard granulomas 25
Headache 203*f*, 204*f*
Healing 161
   early 82
   late 82
Heart, globular enlargement of 177*f*
Hematoma, intramural 190*f*
Hemophilia 168
Hemoptysis 228*f*
Hepatitis 42
   granulomatous 30
Hip joint 166
Hounsfield unit 118, 133, 153, 216
Human immunodeficiency virus 1, 2, 4, 7, 9*f*, 14, 40, 44, 46, 47, 52, 89, 111, 157, 186, 197
Hybridization protection assay 21
Hydrocephalus 52, 116*f*
Hydronephrosis 148, 151*f*
Hypersensitivity reaction 42
Hypertrophic granulation 36
Hyperuricemia 42
Hypodense mass lesion 143*f*
Hypokalemia 42
Hypothyroidism 42
Hysterosalpingography 156

I

Ileocecal valve 125*f*
Imipenem 49
Immunocompromised host 156
Immunodeficiency diseases, primary 222
Infarction, hemorrhagic 54*f*
Infection, tubercular 80
Inferior vena cava 180, 195*f*
Infertility 157*f*
Inflammation
   chronic 156
   granulomatous 32*f*, 33*f*
   necrotizing granulomatous 34*f*
   tuberculous granulomatous 33*f*
Interferon-gamma release assays 21
Interstitial disease, diffuse infiltrating 183
Intestinal obstruction 218*f*
Isoniazid 22, 41, 42, 47, 49
   high-dose 44
Ivory vertebra 80

J

Joint
   ankylosis, partial 166*f*
   infection, tubercular 160

K

Kanamycin 22, 41, 44, 46, 49
Kaposi's sarcoma 9*f*
Kerr's kink 148
Kidney 145, 153
Kissing sequestra 160
Knee joint 168
Kuttner tumors 92

L

Lacrimal gland 94
Langhans giant cell 26, 26*f*, 29, 32*f*-34*f*, 35*f*
   multinucleated 27*f*
Laryngeal swab 17
Laryngitis, tuberculous 91
Late gadolinium enhancement 179, 184*f*
Legg-Calve-Perthes disease 168
Levofloxacin 22, 41, 44, 49
Light-emitting diode
   fluorescent microscopy 19
   technology 19
Linezolid 41, 44, 49
Lipoarabinomannan 23
Loop-mediated isothermal amplification test 21
Lowenstein-Jensen media 44
Lumbar spine 76*f*, 77*f*, 84*f*
   computed tomography of 84*f*
Lumbosacral spine 77*f*
Lung 98
   disease, interstitial 117*f*
Lymph nodal disease 209*f*

Lymph nodes 3, 11, 29f, 89, 98, 111, 113f, 115f, 131f, 197
  calcified 91
  enlarged 92f, 125f
    mesenteric 30f
    popliteal 168f
  enlargement 101f
  hilar 117f
  hypodense 194f
  involvement 208
  lower para-aortic 126
  mesenteric 113f
  multiple 232f, 234f, 235f
    enlarged necrotic 138f
    necrotic 143f, 195f
    retroperitoneal 231f
    small mesenteric 218f
Lymphadenitis, tubercular 3, 10, 11, 29, 29f, 112, 114f, 118
Lymphadenopathy 102, 113, 117, 208, 219f
  abdominal 231f
  hypodense mediastinal 105f
  left hilar 208f
  mesenteric 30f
  peripheral tubercular 116
  tuberculous 118
Lymphatic drainage routes 118
Lymphoid tissue, abundant 123
Lymphoma 94, 95, 117f, 118, 121, 137, 184

M

Macrolides 41
Magnetic resonance 151, 189
  angiography 55, 189
    three-dimensional 57f
  cardiovascular 188
  cholangiopancreatography 140, 201f
  enterography 122, 128f
  imaging 11, 12, 40, 51, 65, 67, 73, 78, 81, 82, 82f, 87, 99, 112, 115, 116, 123, 151, 153, 161-163, 169f, 171, 172, 172f, 178, 181f, 183, 184f, 188, 197, 207, 220, 235
  cardiac 179, 185
  contrast-enhanced 153
  studies 188
  whole body 162, 198
  spectroscopy 60, 215
  urogram 152f
  urography 151
Mantoux test 7, 8, 15, 40

Mediastinitis, fibrosing 104
Melanoma 95
Meninges 35f
  calcification of 70
Meningitis 58f, 203f, 213f
  classical basal 116f
  spinal 34
  tubercular 3, 12, 34, 35f, 52, 53f, 55f, 213, 213f
Menstrual disturbances 42
Meropenem 49
Mesorectal fascia 132f
Metastasis 121
Midtarsal bones 169f
Molecular diagnostic tests 12
Mono-ostotic involvement 166
Moth-eaten appearance 148
Moxifloxacin 22, 41, 44, 49
Multidetector computed tomography 77, 148, 149
Multidrug-resistant tuberculosis, burden of 46
Multilocular cystic mass lesions, bilateral 157f
Multiplanar reconstruction 131f
Multiple hypodense parenchymal cavities 150f
Mycobacteria
  culture positive 19
  growth indicator tube 19, 44, 47, 48
  nontuberculous 20
Mycobacterial infection, nontubercular 174, 107
Mycobacterium
  abscessus 20
  biochemical identification of 19
  bovis 157
  chelonae 20
  fortuitum 20
  identification of 20
Myeloma 163
Myelomalacia 220
Myeloradiculopathy 34
Myosarcoma 184
Myositis, tuberculous 96f
Myxoma 184

N

N-acetyl-l-cysteine 18
National Tuberculosis Program 43
Nausea 42
Necrosis 113f

Nephrotoxicity 42
Nephrotuberculosis 31
Neurocysticercosis 215t
Neuropathy 42
  cranial 56f
Neurotuberculosis 11
  parenchymal 12
Nitroimidazole 41
Nodular disease, caseating 183
Nodules, multiple 223
Nuclear imaging 191
Nuclear medicine 161
Nucleic acid
  amplification test 21
  hybridization tests 20

O

Ofloxacin 22, 41, 49
Omentum, thickening of 133f
Orbit 93
Orbital cellulitis, pyogenic 94
Orchitis, tuberculous 33f
Osteitis
  tuberculosa multiplex cystica 162
  tuberculous 222
Osteoarticular disease 73
Osteoid osteoma 168
Osteomyelitis 34f, 222
  chronic 222f
  chronic recurrent multifocal 163
  extraspinal tubercular 160
  multifocal tubercular 160
  tubercular 95f, 159, 160, 162, 163f
Osteopenia, diffuse 169f, 172f
Ototoxicity 42

P

Pachymeningitis 55
  diffuse 55
  focal 55
Pain
  abdominal 140f, 142f
  neck 89f
  recurrent abdominal 138f
Para-aminosalicylic acid 41, 42, 44, 49
Paradiscal disease 74
Paraspinal disease 86
Paraspinal lines, displacement of 76f
Parenchymal involvement 100, 208

Index

Parrot's beak 83
Pauciarticular type 160
Pelvic bones 164
Pelvicalyceal system 147
Pelvis
  radiograph of 166f, 167f
  soft tissue window, axial contrast-enhanced computed tomography of 164f
Penumbra sign 162
Pericardiac fat 178f
Pericardial calcification 180f
  amorphous 180f
Pericardial effusion 176, 177, 183
Pericarditis
  acute 176
  constrictive 176, 177, 179, 179f, 183f
  effusive-constrictive 183
  magnetic resonance findings of 180
  tuberculous 3, 37f, 176
Pericardium 178f
  thickened 37f, 179f, 180, 181f
Periosteal reaction 169f
Peripheral hypointense rim 60
Periportal hypodensities 224
Peritoneal cocoon formation 135f
Peritoneum, parietal 136f
Peritonitis
  sclerosing encapsulating 133
  tuberculous 3
Petroff's method 18
Peyer's patches 29, 30
Phantom calyx 148
Photosensitivity 42
Phototoxicity 42
Pipe-stem ureter 219
Pneumonia
  fibrocavitary 207
  lobular 27
Polyangiitis 92, 95
Polymerase chain reaction 20, 21
Porta hepatis 114f, 194f
Positive tuberculin skin test 9
Positron emission tomography 100, 161, 197, 226, 228-235
  whole body 204
Pott's disease 229
Pott's paraplegia 34
Pott's puffy tumor 165
Pott's spine 34, 230f, 231f
Pretomanid 41

Progressive primary disease 8, 208, 210f
Prostate, magnetic resonance imaging of 156
Prothionamide 41, 42, 49
Pseudoaneurysm
  large 194f
  tubercular 189f
  pulmonary 194f
Pulse sequences 161
Pyelography spot, intravenous 147f
Pyogenic infections 137
Pyrazinamide 22, 41, 42, 44, 49

Q
Quantiferon-TB gold in-tube 10

R
Radiotracers 226
Radius, distal end of 172f
Ranke's complex 113, 208
Rash 42
Real-time elastography 114
Rectum 132f
Renal cortex, thinning of 32f
Renal pelvis 150f
Renal toxicity 42
Restriction enzyme analysis 20
Retroperitoneum 143f
Revised National Tuberculosis Control Programme 40, 43, 44, 211
Rhabdomyosarcoma 184
Ribosomal ribonucleic acid 20
Ribs 163
Rifabutin 41
Rifampicin 41, 42, 49
Rifampin 22
Rifamycins 41
Rifapentine 41

S
Sacroiliac joint 172, 172f
Sacroiliitis, tubercular 33f, 172
Sarcoidosis 92, 117f, 121
Scapula 164
  glenoid part of 82f
  superior aspect of 164f
  tubercular
    involvement of 164
    osteomyelitis of 223f
Scarred calculi 148
Sclerosis 77f

Seizures 233f
Short-course chemotherapy 42
Shoulder 170
Sinonasal cavities 94
Sinus tract formation 112
Skin rash 42
Small bowel
  loops, clumping of 134f
  obstruction 122f, 128f
Snow-storm appearance 103
Sodium hydroxide
  method 18
  solution 18
Soft granuloma 25, 26f
Soft tissue 168f
Solitary saccular aneurysm 57f
Sonography 146, 153
Spina ventosa 166
Spinal tumor syndrome 81
Spine, thoracic 66f
Spondylitis 159
  chronic healed tuberculous 77
  early tuberculous 67f
  tuberculous 66, 68f, 69f, 81f, 82, 83, 220
Spondylodiskitis, tuberculous 221f
Sputum
  collection 17
  specimens, storage of 18
Squamous cell carcinoma 90, 95
Stenotic lesion 190f
Sterile pyuria 147f
Sternum 165
Stierlin's sign 123
Stomach 130
Streptomycin 41, 49
Suicidal tendency 42
Surgery, role of 49
Sutezolid 41
Swelling 89f
Sylvian fissure cistern 213f
Synovitis 161

T
Takayasu arteritis 186
Technetium -99m-methylene diphosphonate scan 161
Tendinopathy 42
Tenosynovitis 173
  tubercular 160, 162, 173f
Terizidone 49
Testis 145
Thalidomide 41
Thimble bladder 151

Thioacetazone 41t, 49t
Thoracic aorta, descending 186, 188f
Thoracic aortic wall, descending 191f
Thoracoabdominal aorta 191f
Thromboembolism, venous 193
Thrombus 184
Thumb, distal phalanx of 163f
Thyroid carcinoma 103
Tibia, tubercular osteomyelitis of 162f
Tibiotalar joint 170f
Tracheobronchial tree 104
Transbronchial biopsy 17
Transtracheal biopsy 17
Transurethral resection, histopathological examination of 155
Tree-in-bud
  appearance 210f
  sign 228f
Tremor 42
Tubercles
  bacilli 74, 186
  formation of 160
  granulomatous 112
Tubercular lymphadenopathy, region specific 116
Tubercular meningeal enhancement, complications of 214
Tuberculoma 26, 35f, 54f, 57, 58f, 59, 61f, 62, 66f, 94, 103, 183, 213f-215f, 215t
  cardiac 184, 185f
  central nervous system 34
  cerebellar 203f
  heterogeneous 64f
  intracranial 56, 57, 214
  intramedullary 66f
  magnetic resonance imaging
    appearance of 214
    features of 215t
  Meckel's cave 57
  miliary 27, 57f
  multiple 54f, 60f
    miliary 63f
  nonosseous spinal 34
  parenchymal 70
  right cerebellar 59f
  variegated 62f
Tuberculosis 1, 4, 7, 14, 17, 25, 40, 44, 46, 51, 86, 91, 93, 95, 98, 99, 101f, 104, 107, 121, 128f, 130, 138, 141, 145, 183, 159, 176, 193, 194f, 197, 207, 222, 226-228
  abdominal 12, 29, 117, 121, 137f, 141f, 193, 195f, 216, 218f, 219f, 230
  active 105f, 106, 229
  adrenal 154, 154f
  ankle 169f, 170f
  anorectal 126
  aortic 187fc
  articular, stages of 161t
  bladder 31
  bones 14, 14t, 159
  bowel 230
  cardiac 176
  cardiovascular 37, 176, 195
  cavitary 2
  central nervous system 11, 11t, 51, 208, 213, 213f, 233
  central type of 81f
  cervical spine 86, 221f
  chest 98, 99, 104, 106, 106t
  classification of 2
  clinical features 7
  colonic 126, 130f, 131f
  complications of 109f
  congenital 223, 224f
  conjunctival lesions of 36
  cranial 52
  direct test, mycobacterium 20
  disseminated 14, 14t, 25, 116f, 212f, 234f, 235f
    multidrug-resistant 233f
  drug resistant 4, 40, 43, 47
  duodenal 132, 132f
  elbow 171f
  endobronchial 8
  endophthalmitis 36
  epidemiology of 1
  eradication of 5
  esophageal 132
  extensively drug-resistant 46
  extranodal mediastinal 104
  extrapulmonary 2, 3, 25, 98, 111, 145, 207, 211, 226, 229
  extraspinal
    musculoskeletal 159, 159fc
    osteoarticular 174
    skeletal 34
  female genital 31, 33, 156, 157f, 233
  fibrocaseous 27, 28f
  flat bones 163
  foot 169f
  gastric 130
  gastrointestinal 13t, 217
  genitourinary 13, 13t, 151, 158, 219, 220f, 233
  granuloma of 27f
  head and neck 36, 86
  healed 106, 108f
  hepatic 3, 139f, 140f
  hepatobiliary 30
  hepatosplenic 138
  hip 166f, 167f
  histopathology of 25
  ileal 30f, 126f
  ileocecal 12, 123, 124f, 125f, 129f
  iliac bone 164f
  immunological diagnosis of 21
  inactive 229
  infection 207
    latent 9, 10, 21
  intestinal 31f, 218f
  intracranial 34, 213
  intraspinal 64
  joint 14, 14t, 159
  kidney 31
  knee 168f
  laryngeal 3
  localized 14
  long bones 163
  lung 27, 28
  lymph node 11t, 29, 111
  male genital 31, 32, 154, 155f, 233
  march 8t
  metatarsal 166f
  midtarsal 169f
  miliary 3, 8, 28, 28f, 62, 103, 183, 211, 212f
    brain 62
    disseminated 231f
  molecular
    diagnosis of 17
    pathology of 35
  multidrug-resistant 4, 22, 43, 46-48, 48t, 235
  multifocal 82f, 163f
    skeletal 162
  muscles 173, 173f
  musculoskeletal 219
  mycobacterium 1-4, 7, 9, 14, 17, 19-22, 25, 31, 40, 46, 51, 112, 157, 159, 197, 207
  myelitis 65
  myocardial 183
  nasopharynx 37

Index

neural arch 80
new technology for detection of 23
nodal 90f
nodular 27
nonosseous spinal cord 36
ocular 36
orbital 94
osteal 3
osteoarticular 34, 160
pancreas 140
pancreatic 143f
paranasal sinuses 37
pathology of 25
pediatric 224
pelvis 31
pericarditis 104
peritoneal 12, 132, 133f, 134f, 216, 216f, 217f
  carcinomatosis mimicking abdominal 137f
pleural 10t
pleurisy 2
pneumonia, primary 2
postprimary 25, 100, 227
  pulmonary 27
primary 25, 209f, 227
  pulmonary 26, 208
progressive primary 25
pulmonary 2, 8, 10t, 25, 26, 98, 191, 207, 208, 209fc, 227, 228f, 229f, 232f
rectal 132f
renal 3, 31, 32f, 151
ribs 164f
sacroiliac joint 172f
scapular 164f

short bones 165, 222
shoulder 170f
skeletal 13, 68f, 229
small bowel 123
small intestinal 12
solid organ 138, 232
spinal 34, 36, 64, 73, 74, 229
splenic 141f, 142f
sputum-negative pulmonary 226
sternal 165f
thoracic 116
thyroid 92f
tracheobronchial 104
treatment of 41, 44
ureter 31
urethra 31
urinary tract 31, 145, 146f, 147f, 149f-152f, 157, 219
urogenital 31, 145, 156
vascular 186
visceral 219, 219f
whole body imaging in 197
wrist 172f
Tubo-ovarian mass lesions 156
Tumors
  pedunculated 36
  vascular 184
Typical water bottle appearance 177f

U

Ulceration 36
Ulcerative lesions 30
Ulcerohypertrophic type 30
Ultrasonography 98, 122, 154, 161

Ultrasound 77, 112, 113
  contrast-enhanced 114
Ultraviolet light 18
Ureter 145, 153
Ureteric strictures, multiple 152f
Ureteric wall thickening 152f
Urethra 145
Urinary lipoarabinomannan antigen detection 23
Urography, intravenous 147, 147f, 153, 219

V

Valvular involvement 186
Vascular endothelial growth factor 35
Vasculitis 51, 53, 54f, 55f
Vasculopathy, tuberculous 34
Vertebral body, concentric collapse of 80
Vertigo 42
Vesicoureteric junction 219
Vesphene 18
Villonodular synovitis, pigmented 168
Visual disturbance 42
Vomiting 42

W

Watermelon skin sign 156
Weight loss 142f
Whipple's disease 118, 137
Winking owl sign 83
Wrist joint 222f

Z

Ziehl-Neelsen staining 18, 26f, 40

Printed by Libri Plureos GmbH in Hamburg, Germany